Managing
Low Back Pain

Managing Low Back Pain

Edited by

W. H. KIRKALDY-WILLIS
M.A., M.D., F.R.C.S.(Edin.)(C)

Emeritus Professor
Department of Orthopaedic Surgery
University Hospital
University of Saskatchewan
Saskatoon, Saskatchewan, Canada

Churchill Livingstone
New York, Edinburgh, London, and Melbourne   1983

Acquisitions editor: Lewis Reines
Copy editor: Ann Ruzycka
Production editor: Charlie Lebeda
Production supervisor: Larry Meyer
Compositor: The Kingsport Press
Printer/Binder: The Murray Printing Co.

© Churchill Livingstone Inc. 1983

All rights reserved. No part of this publication may be reproduced, stored in a retrieval system, or transmitted in any form or by any means, electronic, mechanical, photocopying, recording, or otherwise, without prior permission of the publishers (Churchill Livingstone Inc., 1560 Broadway, New York, N.Y. 10036).

Distributed in the United Kingdom by Churchill Livingstone, Robert Stevenson House, 1–3 Baxter's Place, Leith Walk, Edinburgh EH1 3AF and by associated companies, branches, and representatives throughout the world.

First published 1983

Printed in USA
ISBN 0-443-08189-1
  7   6   5

Library of Congress Cataloging in Publication Data

Main entry under title:

Managing low back pain.

  Bibliography: p.
  Includes index.
  1. Backache. I. Kirkaldy—Willis, W. H.
[DNLM: 1. Backache—Diagnosis. 2. Backache—Therapy. WE 755 M2665]
RD768.M37   1983   617'.56   83-14286
ISBN 0-443-08189-1

Manufactured in the United States of America

Contributors

R. C. Bowen, M.D., F.R.C.P.(C)
Associate Professor, Department of Psychiatry, University Hospital, University of Saskatchewan, Saskatoon, Saskatchewan, Canada

C. V. Burton, M.D., F.A.C.S.
Medical Director, Institute for Low Back Care and the Low Back Clinic of the Sister Kenny Institute, Minneapolis, Minnesota

A. J. R. Cameron, Ph.D.
Associate Professor, Department of Psychology, University Hospital, University of Saskatchewan, Saskatoon, Saskatchewan, Canada

H. F. Farfan, M.Sc., M.D., C.M., F.R.C.S.(C)
Adjunct Professor of Electrical Engineering, Concordia University; Orthopaedics Department, St. Mary's Hospital, Montreal, Quebec, Canada

W. H. Kirkaldy-Willis, M.A., M.D., F.R.C.S.(Edin.)(C)
Emeritus Professor, Department of Orthopaedic Surgery, University Hospital, University of Saskatchewan, Saskatoon, Saskatchewan, Canada

L. F. Shepel, Ph.D.
Head, Department of Psychology, University Hospital, University of Saskatchewan, Saskatoon, Saskatchewan, Canada

S. Tchang, M.D., F.R.C.P.(C)
Professor, Department of Diagnostic Radiology, University Hospital, University of Saskatchewan, Saskatoon, Saskatchewan, Canada

J. H. Wedge, M.D., F.R.C.S.(C)
Professor and Head, Department of Orthopaedic Surgery, University Hospital, University of Saskatchewan, Saskatoon, Saskatchewan, Canada

K. Yong-Hing, M.B., Ch.B., F.R.C.S.(Glasg.)(C)
Assistant Professor, Department of Orthopaedic Surgery, University Hospital, University of Saskatchewan, Saskatoon, Saskatchewan, Canada

Preface

Though written mainly by orthopaedic surgeons, the aim of this book is to help all those involved in the treatment of patients suffering from low back and leg pain. We believe it will also be of help to postgraduate and undergraduate students.

Richard Foster wrote, "Books are best written in Community." For the thoughts that led to the writing of this book the writer is indebted to a number of different communities; to an outstanding teacher and to students in a biology class at high school in England; to surgeons in London and Edinburgh who were stimulating teachers; and to the staff and patients of a mission hospital in a primitive part of East Africa and of the central hospital in Nairobi: the problems presented by bone and joint tuberculosis and by poliomyelitis were new to the writer and no previous surgeon had tackled them. During the past 18 years he has been working in an entirely different environment in North America. The variety and diversity of these situations has again and again compelled the writer to think hard about each series of problems, often with reluctance, starting from essential principles.

The subject addressed is the degenerative lesion of the lumbar spine produced by repeated minor trauma, as this is the most common. Some space is devoted to the role of developmental lesions. Other lesions, congenital, inflammatory, neoplastic, rheumatoid, and metabolic, are mentioned only for purposes of exclusion. These have been dealt with elsewhere in a thoroughly adequate way.

Throughout this book, more attention has been given to the importance of making an accurate assessment of the patient's problem and, on this foundation, to the formulation of a logical regimen of treatment than to any other aspect of the problem. In the writer's opinion, a logical rather than an empirical approach is most important.

The natural history of spinal degeneration is considered first. Understanding this makes it possible for the physician and therapist to estimate the prognosis in each case and therefore to help the patient grasp the nature of his or her problem and the extent to which treatment may be expected to be of help. For the patient it is important to understand the limitations as well as the benefits of treatment.

Considerable space has been allocated to a consideration of biomechanics, pathology, and pathogenesis. Study of these subjects has helped us to comprehend the nature of the problem and we believe that the physician and therapist need the same fundamental knowledge.

Turning our attention to the clinical picture and to diagnosis, emphasis is placed on the fact that there are at least three aspects to be considered: the framework in which the lesion is found—the personality of the patient; the actual syndrome or lesion present in each patient; and the presence or absence of abnormal movement of the affected segment.

Any decision as to the most rational and suitable form of treatment for each individual is based on the three aspects of the problem mentioned immediately above and the stage, (a) dysfunction phase (decreased movement), (b) unstable phase (increased abnormal movement, or (c) stability phase (stabilization), to which the lesion has progressed.

Details of types of treatment, such as the Spine Education Program, physiotherapy, occupational therapy, manipulation, mobilization, immobilization, and the description of operative techniques, are considered in the third section of the book.

A wise man, Ecclesiastes, writing more than 2,500 years ago, said, "Much learning is a weariness of the flesh." Certainly a great deal has already been written about the problem of low back pain. May it be of some comfort to the present reader to know that while knowledge is undoubtedly required, even more important is the ability to discern the needs of the individual patient and in what way can these be met most effectively.

W. H. Kirkaldy-Willis

Acknowledgments

It is impossible to acknowledge all the help I have received over many years that has led to the writing of this book. I would, however, like to record my thanks to the following.

The staff and residents of the Department of
   Orthopaedic Surgery, Pathology and Human Diagnostic
Imaging at the University Hospital in Saskatoon
The contributing authors
Mrs. Shirley Stacey, for the illustrations
Mrs. Deanne Woodrow, for typing the manuscript
Mr. John Junor, Mr. David Mandeville, and
   Mr. R. Van den Buecken, for the photography
Dr. David Cassidy, for a great deal of help with
   pathology and manipulative therapy
My wife, for so much help and encouragement

W. H. Kirkaldy-Willis

Contents

Essential Principles

    1. The Natural History of Spinal Degeneration   3
        J. H. Wedge, M.D., F.R.C.S.(C)

    2. Biomechanics of the Lumbar Spine   9
        H. F. Farfan, M.Sc., M.D., C.M., F.R.C.S.(C)

    3. The Pathology and Pathogenesis of Low Back Pain   23
        W. H. Kirkaldy-Willis, M.A., M.D., F.R.C.S.(Edin.)(C)

    4. The Perception of Pain   45
        W. H. Kirkaldy-Willis, M.A., M.D., F.R.C.S.(Edin.)(C)

The Clinical Picture

    5. Introduction   53
        W. H. Kirkaldy-Willis, M.A., M.D., F.R.C.S.(Edin.)(C)

    6. Psychological Assessment   63
        A. J. R. Cameron, Ph.D. and L. F. Shepel, Ph.D.

    7. The Three Phases of the Spectrum of Degenerative Disease   75
        W. H. Kirkaldy-Willis, M.A., M.D., F.R.C.S.(Edin.)(C)

    8. The Site and Nature of the Lesion   91
        W. H. Kirkaldy-Willis, M.A., M.D., F.R.C.S.(Edin.)(C)

    9. Diagnosis   109
        W. H. Kirkaldy-Willis, M.A., M.D., F.R.C.S.(Edin.)(C)
        and S. Tchang, M.D., F.R.C.P.(C)

   10. Differential Diagnosis of Low Back Pain   129
        J. H. Wedge, M.D., F.R.C.S.(C) and S. Tchang, M.D., F.R.C.P.(C)

Treatment

   11. A Comprehensive Outline of Treatment   147
        W. H. Kirkaldy-Willis, M.A., M.D., F.R.C.S.(Edin.)(C)

   12. Spine Education Program—Intensive Therapy—The Pain Clinic   161
        W. H. Kirkaldy-Willis, M.A., M.D., F.R.C.S.(Edin.)(C)

   13. Manipulation   175
        W. H. Kirkaldy-Willis, M.A., M.D., F.R.C.S.(Edin.)(C)

14. Supports and Braces 185
    W. H. Kirkaldy-Willis, M.A., M.D., F.R.C.S.(Edin.)(C)

15. Gravity Lumbar Reduction 191
    C. V. Burton, M.D., F.A.C.S.

16. Surgical Techniques 199
    K. Yong-Hing, M.B., Ch.B., F.R.C.S.(Glasg.)(C)

17. Psychological Treatment of Back Pain and Associated Problems 229
    A. J. R. Cameron, Ph.D., L. F. Shepel, Ph.D., and R. C. Bowen, M.D., F.R.C.P.(C)

18. Neuroaugmentive Surgery 241
    C. V. Burton, M.D., F.A.C.S.

19. Back Pain and Work 251
    W. H. Kirkaldy-Willis, M.A., M.D., F.R.C.S.(Edin.)(C)

Index 255

Managing Low Back Pain

Part I Essential Principles

1 The Natural History of Spinal Degeneration

J. H. Wedge

INTRODUCTION

The ubiquitous nature of pain originating in the low back is accepted by those involved in treating this complaint regardless of their individual disciplines. Beyond this statement, however, there is little agreement on the nature and size of the problem. The lack of diagnostic precision, the variation in the perspective of those studying the problem, the poor correlation of symptoms, radiological findings, and pathological changes, and the application of uniform treatment programs to a heterogeneous group of disorders all lead to confusion.

Chronic backache in the setting of a family medicine unit, sciatica with neurological deficit in the context of a specialist practice, and back pain following trivial industrial accidents seen in occupational medicinal practice are widely varying problems and are associated with so many complicating psychosocial factors that useful studies of the natural history of degenerative disease of the spine have been virtually impossible. Statements such as "10% of all patients attending a family practice clinic over a 3-year period present with back pain," "50 to 80% of workmen will have experienced back pain in the previous year," or "spinal disorders are the second leading cause of time lost from work in industry" are probably true and serve to emphasize the magnitude of the problem but give us no clues as to what pathological lesions produce clinical symptoms.

An attempt to understand and correlate the pathomechanics of the spine with the clinical presentation is essential if we are to develop rational and effective treatment. This chapter will not belabor what is *not* known about the lumbar spine but rather will attempt to tie together the small amount of available information about the natural history of spinal degeneration.

An understanding of the biomechanics (chapter 2) and of the pathology (chapter 3) is essential to the process of following the natural history through the stages of spinal degeneration. The spectrum of degenerative change in an intervertebral joint is divided into three phases: Phase I—Dysfunction—is the earliest. Minor pathology results in abnormal function of the posterior joints and disk. Phase II—Instability (the unstable phase)—is intermediate. Progressive degeneration due to repeated trauma produces laxity of both the posterior joint capsule and the annulus. Phase III—Stabilization—is the final stage in the process. Fibrosis of the posterior joints and capsule, loss of disk material, and formation of osteophytes render the segment stable because move-

FACET JOINTS | | **I.V. DISC**

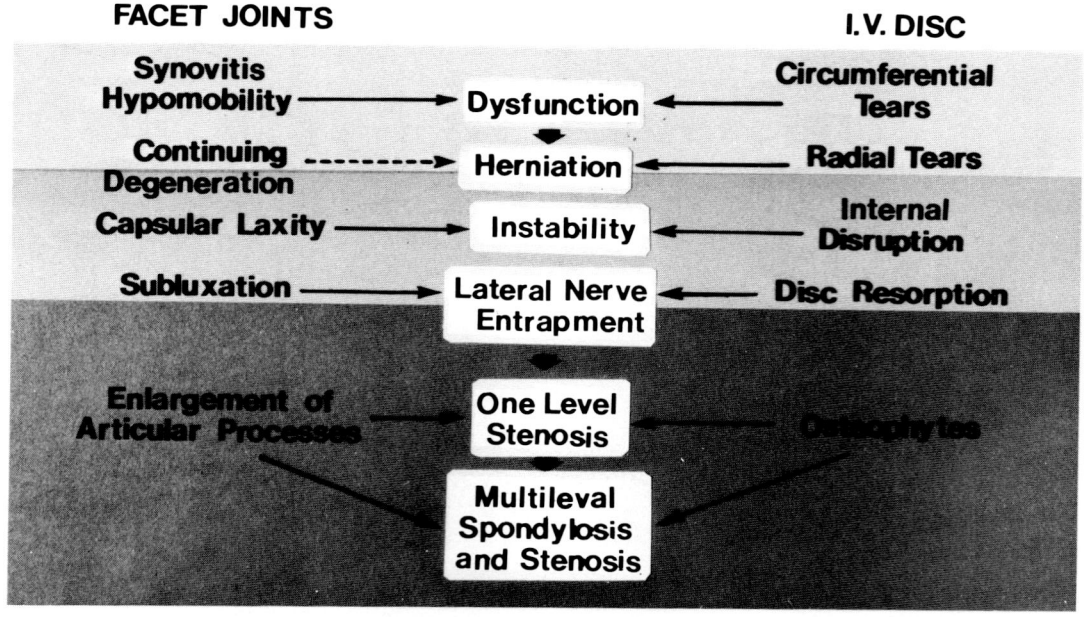

- Synovitis / Hypomobility → Dysfunction ← Circumferential Tears
- Continuing Degeneration ⇢ Herniation ← Radial Tears
- Capsular Laxity → Instability ← Internal Disruption
- Subluxation → Lateral Nerve Entrapment ← Disc Resorption
- Enlargement of Articular Processes → One Level Stenosis ← Osteophytes
- → Multilevel Spondylosis and Stenosis ←

Fig. 1-1. The spectrum of pathological changes in facet joints and disk and the interaction of these changes. The upper light horizontal bar represents dysfunction, the middle darker bar instability, and the lower dark bar stabilization.

ment is reduced. In Figure 1-1 the natural history is superimposed on the scheme of pathogenesis. The symptoms, clinical course, and treatment are correlated with the stages in the pathogenesis. This correlation makes it possible to predict the degree to which the natural history can be modified by different treatment methods.

PATHOLOGY

Radiological and postmortem studies suggest that the degenerative changes described in chapter 3 are progressive and almost universal. The morbidity associated with these changes, however, is episodic and many people never experience symptoms at all. Figure 1-2 is a graphic illustration of the pathogenesis. While the degenerative changes are progressive, the rate of progression is not linear and those factors that alter the rate are poorly understood. Sex, body weight, body habitus, posture, and occupation all probably play a role.

SYMPTOMS

Attempts to correlate symptoms with degenerative changes have met with little success. The peak incidence of disabling symptoms occurs between the ages of 35 and 55. This does not parallel the progression of degeneration. The lack of correlation would suggest that the later stages in the degenerative process have a protective effect and are nature's mechanism for compensating for damage. This teleological explanation has led to the concept of the phases of degeneration, the central theme of this book.

In Figure 1-3 the symptoms of low back pain are plotted against age through the phases of spinal degeneration. The repair reaction can result in return to a symptom-free state in all three phases but is less likely to do so as one moves from one phase to another.

In the phase of dysfunction, return of the facet joint to the normal position or repair of a capsular tear prevents further damage. A fracture in the lamina may unite without deformity. Each of these examples may represent a single episode

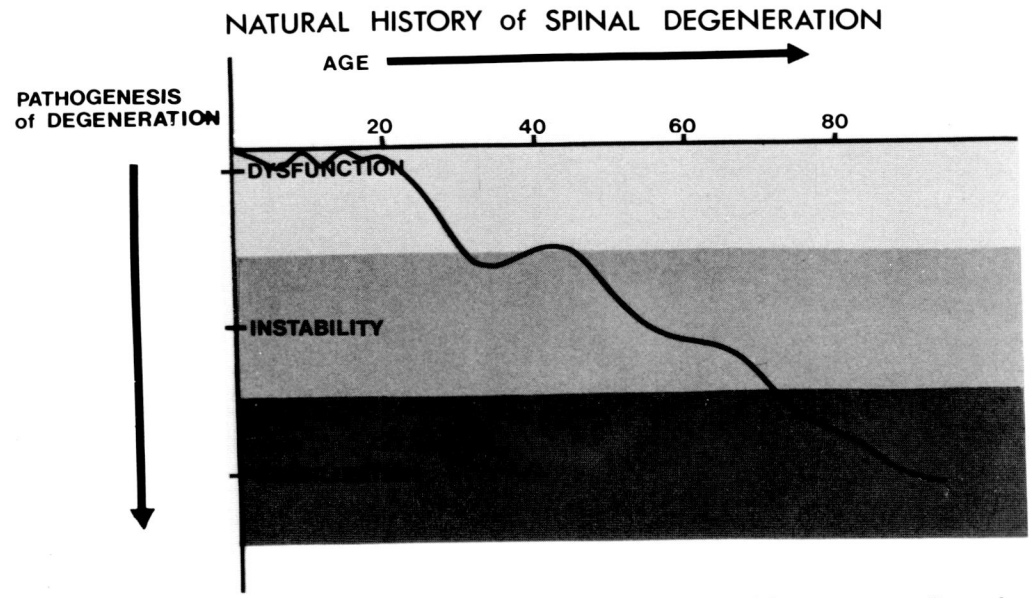

Fig. 1-2. The degenerative process throughout life can be represented diagrammatically as shown. The minor initial lesions may heal, but with time healing is no longer complete.

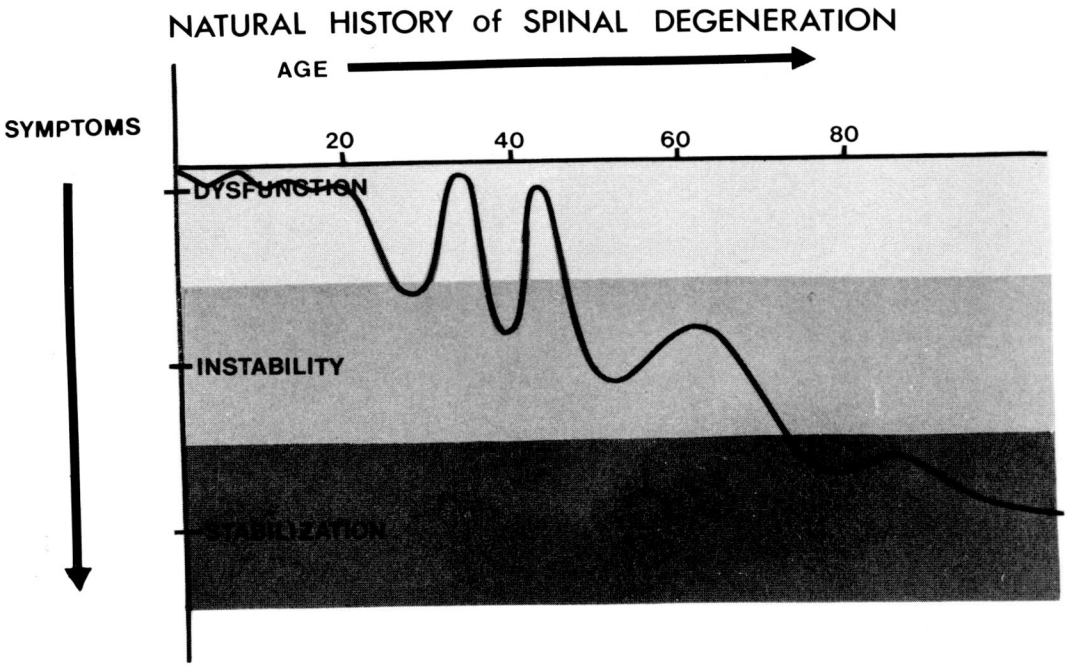

Fig. 1-3. Symptoms through the phases of pathogenesis do not correlate well with the pathological changes. Relief from pain can occur despite the presence of permanent damage. In the later phases, however, symptomatic recovery may not occur.

of symptoms in a lifetime in the fortunate individual. Injury may occur at more than one level, giving a possible explanation for why several or many acute attacks may not lead to chronicity.

However, if the damage exceeds the capacity of the repair reaction, the condition may pass on to the unstable phase. More severe damage to the three-joint complex can lead to a lengthier period of symptoms and eventually to chronic difficulty. Disk herniation, dynamic lateral entrapment, or other sequelae may occur. Thus a return to a symptom-free state may not occur, but instead a background state of mild chronic symptoms may exist with superimposed acute attacks from time to time. The picture of the natural history may be complicated by the simultaneous or sequential occurrence of the same process at one or more levels in the lumbar spine.

In the final phase a proliferative repair response may result in stabilizing the segment. This may explain the decreased incidence of disabling symptoms later in life. However, symptoms may diminish simply because activity is reduced and aggravating factors are avoided.

It is unlikely that the damaged segment can be stabilized in all individuals. This could explain the small group of patients who have continuing severe difficulty late into old age. In addition, the proliferative repair response may lead to compromise of the neural elements, which results in spinal stenosis, the culmination of the degenerative process for an unfortunate few.

TREATMENT

In Figure 1-4 the various forms of treatment are superimposed on the three phases of spinal degeneration. The indications for different treatment will be dealt with in depth in later chapters. An understanding of which forms of treatment are more likely to meet with success throughout the natural history is obviously important if we are to develop a rational plan of management for the individual patient. In general, relatively simple nonsurgical management is likely to meet with success early in the natural history whereas operative procedures may be necessary later. The nature of the surgery obviously depends on the pathology encountered in the later two phases of spinal degeneration.

RESULTS OF TREATMENT

Unfortunately, in the past both nonoperative and operative treatment have been based on the training, discipline, and bias of the individual physician rather than on an understanding of the pathology and the natural history of the disease. Patients have too often been led to believe that a form of treatment is an "all or nothing" phenomenon and that therapeutic methods from different disciplines are mutually exclusive. Counseling the patient should include a realistic explanation of what he or she can expect from a particular form of treatment at that stage in the pathology of spinal degeneration. For example, removing an extruded disk may dramatically relieve suffering but may not significantly alter the progression of pathological changes or the longterm clinical picture.

Figure 1-5 is a graph superimposed on the three phases. Treatment is more likely to result in a return to a symptom-free state and to have more longterm benefit in the earlier stages of the degenerative process. The expectations for a particular method of treatment are less optimistic as we move along the course of the natural history. Ideally, intervention should take place as soon as it becomes obvious that spontaneous recovery is unlikely or that it will be unacceptably prolonged. In the later stages the patient must understand that expectations are for significant general improvement or relief of a particular part of the problem rather than for a "cure."

CONCLUSION

An attempt has been made to correlate pathological changes, symptoms, diagnosis, and treatment throughout the whole spectrum of degenerative change in the lumbar spine that forms what we call the natural history of the disease. In doing this we find that often there is little correlation between the patient's disability and the degree of damage to the tissues. Factors such as the per-

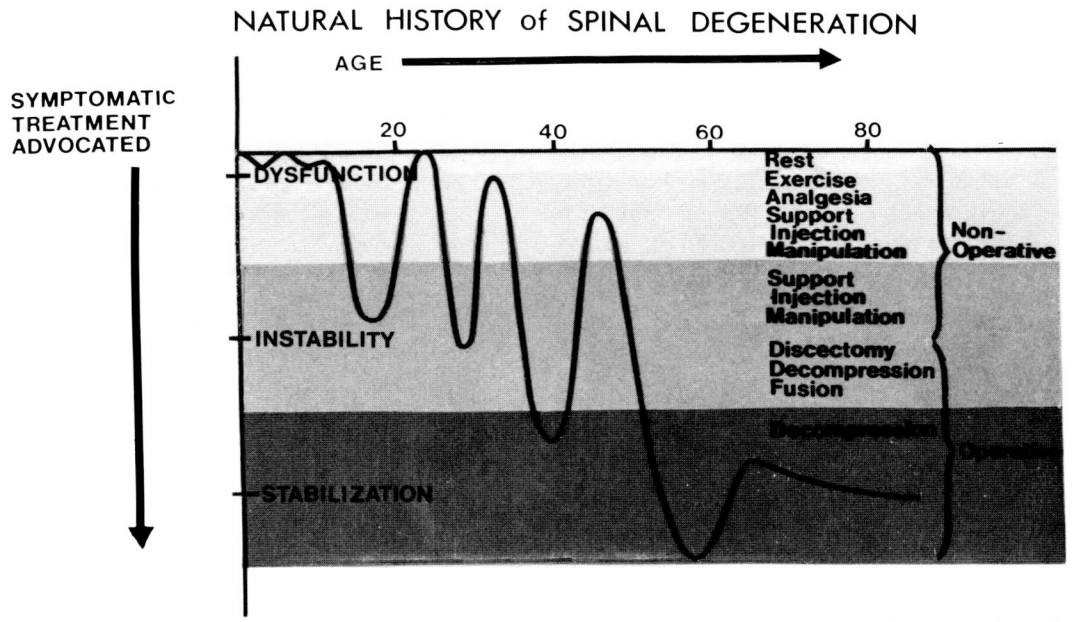

Fig. 1-4. Diagrammatic demonstration of the types of treatment that are likely to meet with success in the different stages of pathogenesis. The curve on the graph represents symptoms.

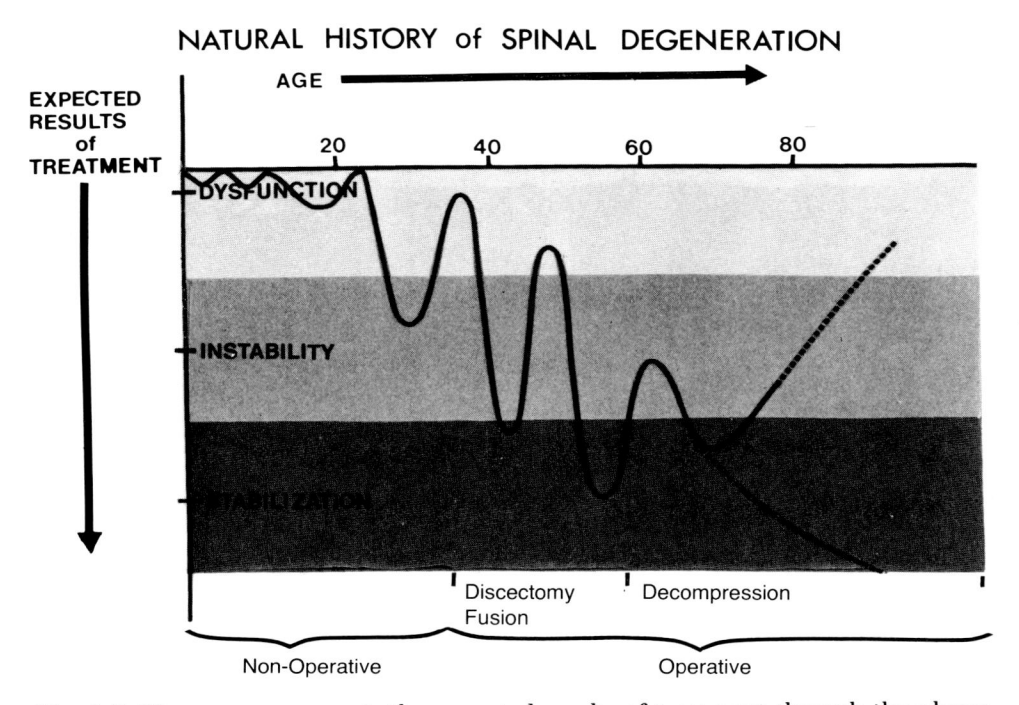

Fig. 1-5. The curve represents the expected results of treatment through the phases of degeneration. Initially nonsurgical measures are almost universally successful in relieving symptoms. In the late stages even surgery is unlikely to result in complete relief of symptoms.

sonality of the patient, secondary gain, and expectations for the future make the picture more complex.

Study of the natural history of this disease enables the physician to gain insight into the disease process, to make a more complete and accurate diagnosis, to formulate a more rational regime of treatment, and to inform the patient in simple terms what may be expected from conservative or operative treatment and even more important what the future holds.

In the final analysis, with cooperation between physician and patient it is possible occasionally to effect a cure, often to arrest the progress for a long time, and nearly always to alleviate the suffering of the patient.

2 Biomechanics of the Lumbar Spine

H. F. Farfan

INTRODUCTION

Some understanding of biomechanics, difficult as this is for many clinicians, enables us to define the etiology of the lesion in the lumbar spine. It is of special value in deciding if the cause of injury is compression, with fracture of a cartilage disk plate followed by a slow degenerative process in disk and posterior joints, or torsion, involving more rapid failure of posterior joints and disk.

To date there is no consensus on the normal mechanism of the spine. This lack creates a very real problem. How can we understand the abnormal when the normal is not known? In the absence of a method to measure internal stresses directly, a possible approach to understanding the normal mechanism is by mathematical simulation. The more closely the simulation approximates in vivo observations, the more confidence we have that the simulation is a true representation. In scientific endeavor the descriptive hypothesis remains just that until it can be formulated in terms that can be treated rigidly in mathematical terms and subjected to rigid experimental proof. In this presentation a mathematical formulation of the normal lumbar spinal mechanism is presented in descriptive terms.

In the body all motion is initiated through the agency of active muscle contraction, which in turn is controlled and coordinated by the central nervous system (CNS). While ligament and capsule may be called on to support a load, these tissues remain passive and unable to initiate a motion. Almost without exception, it is these passive elements that are injured. It therefore falls to the muscular system and its control mechanism to protect the organism from injury.

Mechanical structures fail because they are unable to support the stresses induced by the loads applied to them. Two systems are involved: the passive structural members that provide local support and the appropriate muscle groups that act to minimize the risk of failure.

Because the lumbar tissues are undoubtedly injured more often than those of the extremities in performing an upper extremity task, the spinal mechanism becomes a pertinent example of the interaction between muscle on the one hand and ligament, bone, and joint on the other.

THE SPINAL MECHANISM

Among special adaptations in humans are the modifications that permit them to maintain an upright posture—a capability shared with other anthropoids, notably the chimpanzee and the gibbon. Humans, however, are unique in their ability to lift and carry heavy objects and to perform, in bipedal stance, the accelerated trunk movement necessary for throwing objects.

Hip Extensor Muscle

The main muscle power for maintaining the trunk upright resides in the hip and thighs. The muscles of the hips and lower extremities have been studied extensively in relation to bipedal motion, but surprisingly little attention has been paid to their function in supporting the trunk, upper extremities, and head.[1]

In humans, the relatively long anteverted femoral neck puts the gluteal attachments well behind the center of rotation of the hip, giving them extension power regardless of the degree of hip flexion. The extensive attachment of the gluteus maximus to the iliotibial band further increases the leverage of this muscle. By far the most significant modification is the greatly increased anterior–posterior (A–P) diameter of the pelvis, which permits the posterior migration of the glutei, increasing both their leverage and their bulk.

The effectiveness of the hip extensors is somewhat diminished when the hip is fully flexed, as in the squatting position. Thus, flexion at the knees to below the 90° position is not a good method of lifting.

We may estimate, using a conservative force density of muscle contraction (50 lb/in²), that the glutei and hamstrings together can generate a moment greater than 15,000 in-lb, which is enough for men in the 50th percentile by weight to manage their own weight above the pelvis (one-half body weight) plus an external load of three times body weight. This estimation is supported by results of weight-lifting championships, where the 150-lb athlete lifts 450 lb, developing a maximum external moment of the order of 10,000 in-lb. No other sport imposes such high moments on the spinal mechanism. In rowing for example, the maximum moment is only equivalent to a 200-lb lift.

If we examine the weight lift in greater detail, we see that maximum moment occurs early in the lift when the barbell clears the knees. The attitude of the trunk as measured by a line drawn through hip and shoulder is approximately 70° to the vertical. As the upright position is obtained,

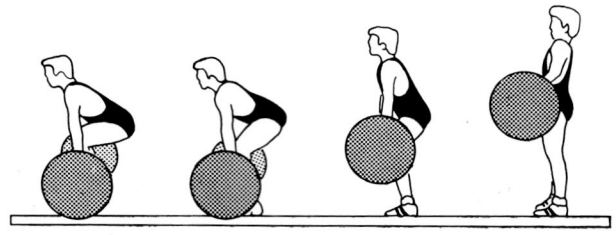

Fig. 2-1. Dead lift. The maximum moment occurs when the barbell clears the knees. Raising the weight above the head does not involve large moments.

the moment decreases to zero. To raise the weight above the head does not require the balancing of large moments but rather an enormous coordination to maintain the moments near zero (Fig. 2-1).

Trunk Musculature

Surprisingly, the trunk musculature is much weaker than the hip extensor system. The spinal musculature has a cross-sectional area of approximately 10 in², firing at a density of 50 to 100 lb/in² at approximately 2–2.5 in. behind the center of the disk. It can generate a moment of only 2000 to 3000 in-lb, which is only 20% of that required for a 450-lb lift. Though the extensor muscle system in humans is proportionally more developed than that in other anthropoids, it is still grossly inadequate to handle the large moments that are required.

The paraspinal muscles, such as the sacrospinalis, run at a slight angle to the long axis and therefore in contracting generate a small component of shear in the plane of the disk. This component is too small to balance the shear of 525 lb induced by the combination of body weight and barbell.

The Ligamentous Systems

The missing moment is supplied by the ligamentous system, which may conveniently be considered as two separate but interdependent systems. The first consists of the midline ligaments, the supra- and interspinous ligaments, the facet joint capsules, the ligamentum flavum, and the posterior longitudinal ligament, and the second consists of the lumbodorsal fascia (LDF).

No tension is present in these ligaments unless they are stretched. Stretching occurs through forward rotation of the intervertebral joints. With the hands gripping the barbells, the hip extensors rotate the pelvis backward while the spine rotates forward. As pointed out above, ample hip extensor power to rotate the pelvis and stretch the ligaments to the required tension is present.

It is essential that the hip be free to extend. Should hip extension be limited by arthritis or flexion contracture, the important posterior ligament tension is no longer available. In these instances, the individual must resort to using the spine extensors, with the reduced capacity to lift thus further increasing the stress on the intervertebral joints. Hence the common problem of a back disorder complicating the diseased hip (Fig. 2-2).

The supraspinous–interspinous ligament system has an angulated attachment to the spinous process. Below the level of L3, the continuation of these ligaments is placed behind the spinous process of L4, L5, and first-to-third sacral segments. This arrangement also is unique to humans among the primates. It ensures that when these ligaments

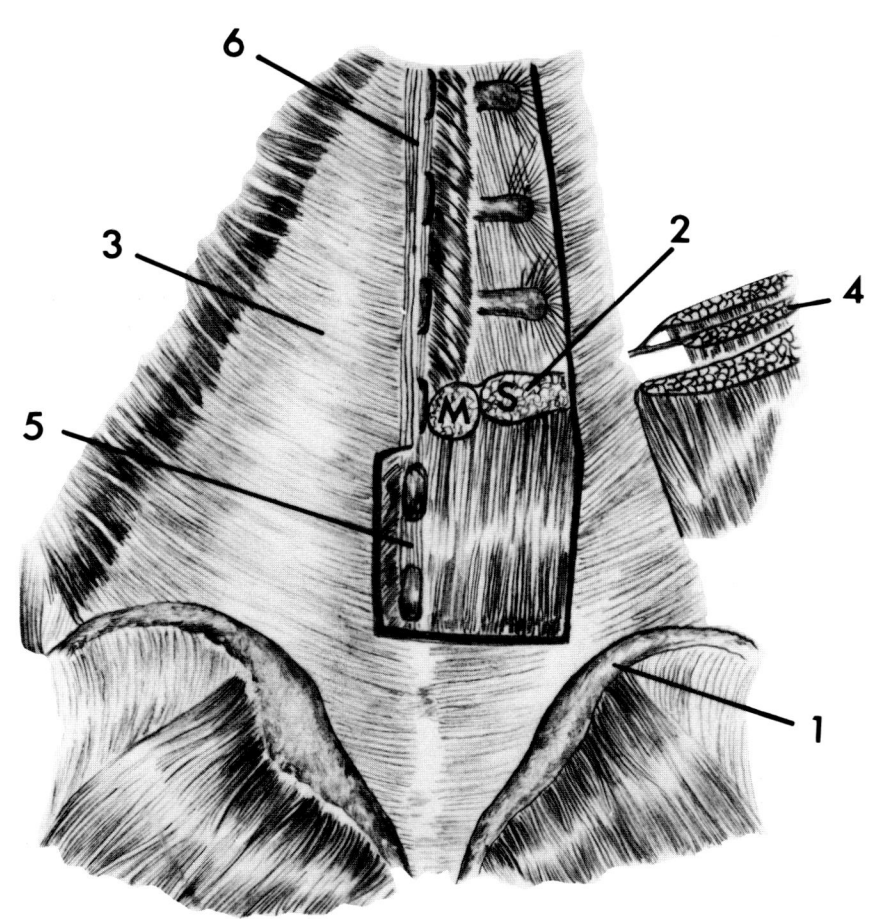

Fig. 2-2. The ligamentous system. 1. Iliac Crest. 2. Sacrospinalis and multifidus. 3. Lumbo-dorsal fascia. 4. Internal oblique and transversus abdominis attached to lumbo-dorsal fascia. 5. Interspinous ligament. 6. Supraspinous ligament.

are stretched, they exert a component of shear force backward on each vertebra, more than sufficient to counteract the shear caused by body weight and barbell.

The Posterior Lamella of the Lumbodorsal Fascia

At the posterior midline the LDF blends with the midline longitudinal ligaments. Below the level of the posterior iliac spine, the lateral margin of the sheet is firmly attached to the ilium. Above L2, it is attached to both the tips of the transverse processes and the ribs. However, between the levels of L2 and iliac crest, its lateral edge forms the posterior attachment of the internal oblique and transversus abdominis muscles.

With flexion, this ligamentous sheet is stretched and—precisely because it is stretched—should also become narrowed. However, bony restraints at the upper and lower ends prevent narrowing while contraction of internal oblique and transversus abdominis muscles contribute the restraint for the mid-portion.[3]

Preventing the lumbodorsal fascia from narrowing as it is stretched causes its longitudinal tension to increase. Thus with the powerful internal oblique muscle attached to its margin, the probability exists that tension can be generated in the lumbodorsal fascia by abdominal muscle contraction, even without flexion of the spine. This means that in the first arc of rotation, when the midline ligament is still slack, useful tension may be present in the fascia. The efficiency of this system is low in normal upright lordosis and high when the spine is flexed. The efficiency of the internal oblique muscle in this regard will be greatest if its pull is in the tangential plane of the lumbodorsal fascia. This obtains when the abdominal cavity is rounded by a small internal pressure.

This ligamentous sheet, because it follows the contour of the spine, does not create shearing forces; the internal oblique and transversus abdominis muscles, because they lie almost transversely to the spine, do not produce compression. Thus these muscles produce extensor moment without adding appreciably to the compression or shear felt by the intervertebral joint.

The Balance between Muscle and Ligament

Both the ligamentous systems described above are placed behind the musculature. The muscle acting at the center of cross-sectional area has a much shorter lever arm. Therefore, muscle contraction produces a greater compressive force on the disk than an equivalent tension in the ligament. It is important to realise that the penalty of using the paraspinal muscle instead of the ligament is increased stress at the intervertebral joint.

Consider a simple diagram of the spinal mechanism (Fig. 2-3). Both muscle (M) and ligament (L) forces are used to balance the body weight (BW) and the barbell (W). It is clearly more efficient to manage the load with ligament tension alone, because compression stress is less than when muscle is used.

Mathematically there may be an infinite number of ways to combine ligament and muscle tensions or strategies to balance a given weight. However, physiologically there are constraints. To lift a very heavy load, a technique that depends almost entirely on using the ligament is preferred because stress levels are lowest. For maximal external loads, we *must* rely on a ligament strategy. Therefore, there is a unique method of lifting the maximal weight, and no variation can be tolerated. Evidence that the proper use of ligament strategy is an acquired skill exists.

Relying solely on the ligament has its drawbacks. The first is that in many body positions the ligament is largely inoperative because it is slack for the first 45° of forward flexion. For smaller

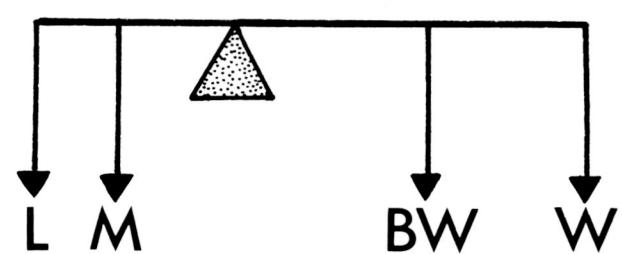

Fig. 2-3. Moments due to external loads are balanced by moments generated internally. External loads: BW, body weight above disk acting through center of gravity of upper body; W, weight held in hands. Internal loads: L, tension developed in ligamentous system; M, tension developed in trunk musculature.

external loads (BW + 50 lb) a ligament strategy can be used, but the spine must be in a flexed position. Secondly, the ligament is a passive structure, whereas muscle contraction implies some measure of active control and hence a mechanism that may act to prevent injury. Even with heavier lifts the trunk muscles remain active, remaining available to provide fine control in case of accident. Using a muscle strategy permits greater variation in trunk attitude. However, for this increased freedom the body tends to pay the price of increased spinal stress because the muscle is used.

Does this mean that the stresses in the spine vary with the choice of strategy? Not necessarily, if a system exists whereby stresses caused by intermediate strategies can be minimized. We believe that this is the role of the abdominal muscle mechanism. As mentioned above, the abdominal musculature produces longitudinal posterior tensions with reduced compression and shear. Calculations show that when the abdominal mechanism functions properly, it tends to reduce stress when the midline ligaments are unavailable.

STABILITY OF THE LUMBAR SPINE

It has been determined that the unsupported upright spinal column can support only 5 lb before it buckles or collapses. With the body in an upright relaxed stance, the center of gravity of the upper half of the body is some 14 inches above the lumbosacral joint. This is equivalent to balancing a weight of approximately 75 lb at the end of a 14-inch flexible rod. Clearly this feat cannot be accomplished without some mechanism of stabilization. There is no problem with the thoracic segments that are stabilized at the back, front, and sides by the ribs. The only available support system for neck or lumbar regions is the musculature. No means of maintaining the trunk and upper extremities in a given position could exist without the stabilizing effects of the peripheral trunk musculature, especially if the ligamentous system is slack.

In the absence of muscle and ligament support, we can expect the spine to buckle under body weight. Buckling in the saggital plane would be motion in the normal mode and therefore not dangerous (Fig. 2-4).

Buckling in the lateral or vertical modes, however, could endanger the intervertebral joints. In both instances, the tendency to buckling is increased as the imposed load is increased, and the intervertebral joint is rotated laterally (sidebend). With lateral rotation, the facet joints induce a dangerous torsion at the joint.

The paravertebral muscles are poorly placed to counteract the dangerous types of buckling. The abdominal muscles, particularly the lower digitations of the external oblique, seem well placed to control buckling by lateral bend and the psoas to protect against vertical collapse. The obliques are ideally placed to counteract torque. The amount of torque contributed by the abdominals is very small (approximately 300–400 in–lb). This small contribution is sufficient to afford some valuable protection for the intervertebral joint.

The generation of torque, by pitching a ball, for example, is produced from motion imparted to the pelvis by the lower extremities and transmitted to the upper extremities through the trunk, which must become rigid at the crucial moment. The torque at the upper extremities, therefore, derives principally from the angular momentum imparted to the trunk by the lower extremities. However, this torque must be transmitted to the upper extremities via a rigid torso.

The stability of the spine depends greatly on the conditions obtaining at the joint itself (the point "P" in Fig. 2-5). Redraw Figure 2-5 so that P is free to move between stops S and S1, representing an increased abnormal motion at the joint, as caused by injury, for example. Any tendency to lateral bend would immediately cause P to move towards the appropriate stop, and this motion cannot be controlled satisfactorily by muscle acting at a distance to P. The point "P" is mechanically unstable. This instability results not so much because the joint permits movement—slight degrees of motion (called deformation) are normal—but rather in the fact that when 1 mm of deformation is called for, the joint yields more than this (Fig. 2-5).

We see, therefore, that the integrity of the spinal mechanism depends on the controlled interac-

14 *Managing Low Back Pain • 2*

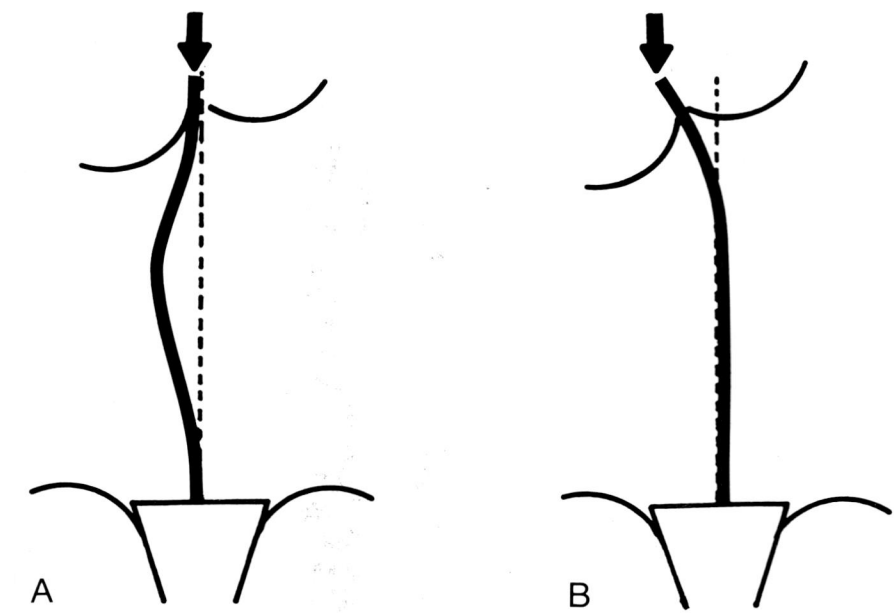

Fig. 2-4. Two forms of buckling under increased axial load. (↓) (A) Axial buckling prevented by the psoas muscles. (B) Lateral bend controlled by laterally placed musculature. Both forms of buckling induce a torsion at the intervertebral joints because lateral bend is accompanied by axial rotation.

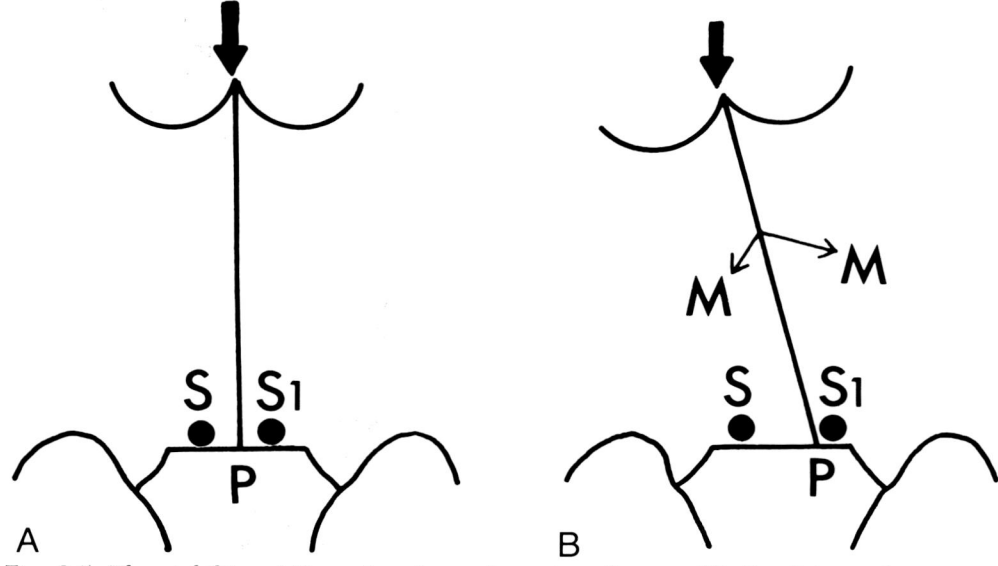

Fig. 2-5. The stability of the spine depends on two factors. (A) Conditions obtaining at the joint (P). P can move between the stops S and S1. (B) Any tendency to lateral bend causes P to move toward the appropriate stop, and this motion cannot be controlled by muscle acting at a distance to P. The point P is mechanically unstable.

tion between the musculature: on the hip extensors for the power for heavy exertion, on the paraspinal musculature for lighter tasks, and on the abdominal musculature for the balance between ligament and spinal motion and for adjusting the whole system to the task to be performed. A loss of efficiency in any of these components leads to a loss of control that may precipitate an injury at the intervertebral joint.

THE INTERVERTEBRAL JOINT

The disk, facet joints, and their complementary ligament and muscle systems all appear to respond to stress at the intervertebral joint. The stress at that joint can be represented in general terms as:

$$\text{Stress} = \sqrt{C^2 + S^2}$$

where C is compression force and
S is shear force.

The amount of stress at the joint can be manipulated by changing the spinal geometry through muscle action. Calculations show that in life normal spinal function can be achieved by choosing the combination of ligament tension and muscle force that produces the minimum stress at the intervertebral joint. This simulated system is not very sensitive to compression. This is to be expected, because the column must withstand very high compressive loads, often more than 1 ton. On the other hand, the system is very sensitive to shear. Correspondingly, in the laboratory, we find that the intervertebral joint is relatively much weaker in shear. Basically, then, the organism seems to respond to imposed loads by attempting to reduce shear to a minimum and to equalize stress at all joints.

AXIAL COMPRESSION LOADING: THE DISK

The main support for a compression load is the vertebral body annulus column. The upper lumbar facet joints are unable to support a compression force in the axial direction. At the two lower intervertebral joints, the facets may support up to 20% of the axial compression.

The compression strength of the vertebral body resides virtually in its thin cortical shell, which per unit cross-sectional area is as strong as the femur. The cancellous core of the vertebral body may increase the strength of the unit by a hydraulic mechanism. Under a slowly increasing compression load, the fluid content of the vertebral body may be squeezed out into extracellular space through the veins or through small canals through the cortex. When the rate of deformation is increased, these channels are not large enough to permit the greater rate of outflow. Therefore, the internal pressure in the vertebral body rises, making the whole structure more rigid. This hydraulic system depends on the rate of loading and makes the vertebral body the shock-absorbing system for the disk, which is stiffer and stronger than that body. Shock absorption is a role sometimes erroneously ascribed to the disk.

The endplate of the vertebral body is the weak point of the disk. It is the site of failure when compression loads become excessive. The endplate may be overstressed by two different mechanisms. First, when compression is applied peripherally to an oval-shaped plate, stresses develop in the plate in the line of its long axis. Fissure fractures in the endplate can be created experimentally by this method of compressing the annulus in the absence of the nucleus. Second, in the presence of a hydrostatic nucleus or when the disk cavity contains sufficient firm material, compression may cause the nuclear material to act as a punch as the endplates are forced closer together. The result is a depressed fracture. The endplate itself is reinforced around its periphery at the point where the annulus is attached.

Compression Loading

After a compression load is applied, the nucleus of the disk takes approximately 1 sec to attain its highest pressure. The annulus therefore takes on the initial load, and as it deforms under the load, the nucleus pressure develops to redistribute the load to the best advantage. This mechanism explains why the disk may function quite successfully without a nucleus.

The concentric arrangement of the collagenous

layers of the annulus ensures that when the disk is placed in tension, shear, or rotation, the individual fibers are always in tension. When compressed in the presence of a functioning nucleus, the annular fibers are again stressed in tension. This arrangement ensures that should the annulus fail, the failure would be at the annulus–endplate interface where, as with other ligamentous attachments, healing is most likely to occur.

Motion at the Disk

Motion is a function of the properties of the annulus and does not depend on the nucleus. The functioning annulus can be depicted diagrammatically as in Figure 2-6. There is a point in the disk at which, when compression is applied, the disk is compressed but no forward, backward, or sideways rotation occurs. We may call this the neutral point. When the load is applied eccentrically away from this point, the joint rotates (flexes) in the direction of the eccentric load. In the symmetric disk, applying the load in the sagittal plane results in forward or backward rotation, with no tendency for lateral bending. In this situation, all the applied force goes to provide the desired motion, and we may call this the preferred line of the axis of motion. In the symmetric vertebra, this preferred line lies in the saggital plane. In either scoliotic or asymmetric joints, the preferred line apparently does not coincide with the sagittal plane.

The eccentricity of the applied load in the normal disk cannot be further forward than the midpoint of the annulus. A load applied in front of the annulus will put the posterior annulus in tension. This can occur accidentally as in a sudden fall on the backside. The combination of rising nucleus pressure and tension in the posterior annulus may cause the disk to rupture and its contents to explode into the neural canal.

The fact that the point of load application remains within the confines of the annulus implies that the disk itself has no need to support a moment. Indeed in the laboratory, the maximum moment supportable by the annulus is of the order of 200 to 300 in-lb.

Compression Failure

It can be seen from the above discussion that with axial loading the disk is always compressed with a force approximately equal to the weight of the body supported by the joint and that additional compression due to ligament or muscle tension results whenever the spine moves from the neutral upright position. Thus, at L5–S1 the average force in men is BW/2, or 75 lb, and the disk area approximately 2.5 to 3.0 in^2. This is equivalent to a pressure of 25 to 30 lb/in^2. Pressure is increased with forward flexion because of the tension in muscle and ligament needed to support the body in this position. When failure occurs, it is not the annulus but the endplate that fails. It is extremely difficult to cause annular failure by compression.

The spinal mechanism seems well equipped to support and to react to compression load. An accidental axial overload can be imposed by an uncoordinated lift when the spinal musculature takes on too much load. Asymmetries in the disk and/or the facet joints may act to concentrate the stresses, thereby increasing the risk. Less frequently, increased axial load may occur accidentally as in a fall onto the backside. Details of traumatic injuries depend on an analysis of forces obtaining at the time of trauma and are outside the scope of this discussion.

SHEARING FORCES AND TORSION: THE FACET JOINTS

As stated above, the midline posterior ligamentous system develops posterior shearing forces at the disk to counteract the forward shearing forces due to body weight that arise when the body bends forward. Muscles such as the sacrospinalis, multifidus, and psoas may also create shear forces that combine to produce a smaller posterior shear force.

The neural arch and its appendages are so arranged as to add considerable resistance to forward shear. The disk, with its large central cavity, does not appear to be an ideal structure for supporting shear force. In fact, its shear strength is probably less than 200 lb. Under normal circum-

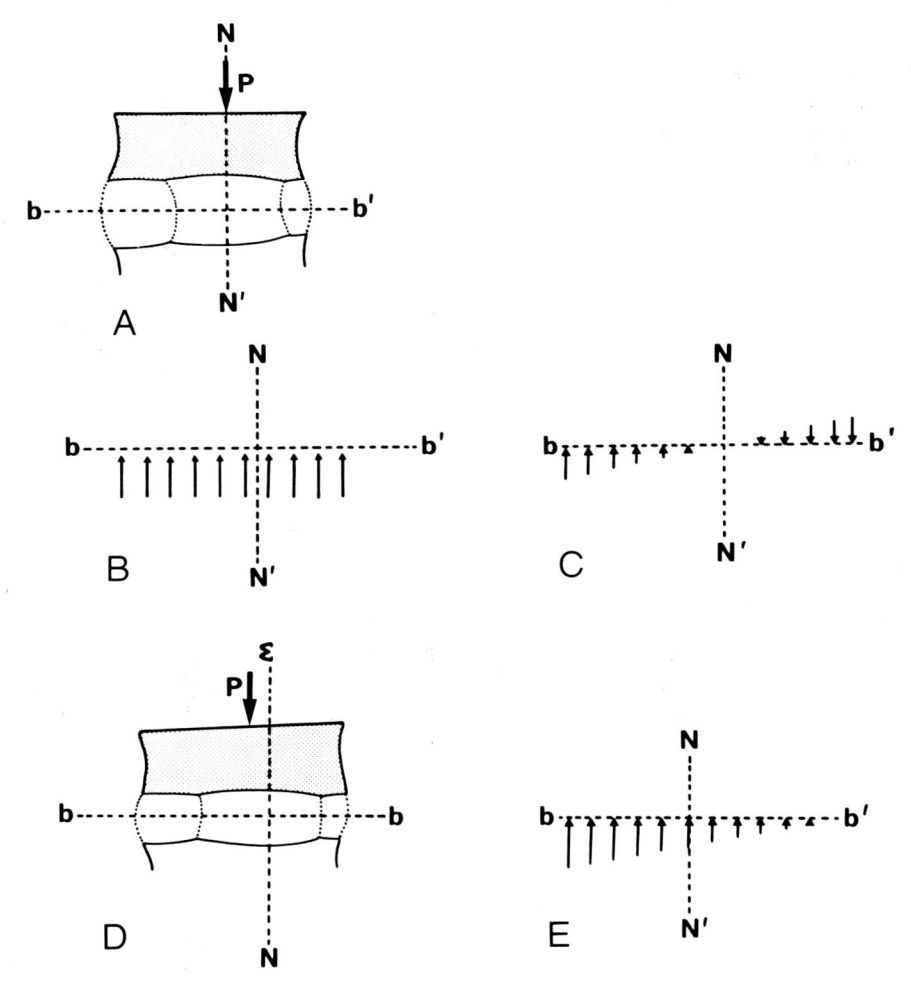

Fig. 2-6. (A) NN¹, the neutral axis of the IV joint; bb¹, the bisector of the disk. When force P is applied in the neutral axis, the joint has no tendency to rotate, flex, or extend. (B) The load P is supported over the cross-sectional area of the disk, as shown diagrammatically. (C) If a pure rotation (or a moment)—flexion, for example—could be applied to the disk, the distribution of stress would appear as shown here. (D) When the disk is flexed, stress is distributed by applying the force P at some eccentricity (ϵ) from the neutral axis. Thus both compression and moment act on the disk, and the posterior annulus does not go into tension. (E) As shown in diagram E, this is obtained by adding algebraically the arrows in B and C.

stances, it is doubtful that any shear is felt by the disk, because of the protection afforded by ligament, muscle, and facet joints.

Axial torsion is not a normal motion of the lumbar spine. In fact much of its design appears to be anti-torsional. The center of axial rotation is within the nucleus of the disk. The greatest bulk of the annulus and the two facet joints are disposed around this center, well located to counteract torsion.

The Facet Joints

The facet joints are carried on articular processes that themselves arise from the neural arch. The *superior articular process* is squat and strong. Because of this, it shows little deflection when loaded at 90° to its articular surface. Its facet joint projects above the endplate just far enough to allow the joint's center to lie in the transverse plane of the disk.

The *inferior articular process* is much longer and extends over the back of the vertebral body in such a way that the center of its articular surface lies in the transverse plane of the disk. Because of its length, this process is more easily deflected by load and may deflect as much as 8 to 9° before fracture occurs. The articular process, pedicle, and neural arch all exhibit proportionally the same strength as femoral bone. However, it is always difficult to visualize the fact that some deflection of bone normally occurs.

The *synovial joint* has a very low coefficient of friction. Its design is such that it can support a load at 90° to the plane or curved surface in which motion takes place. The facets may therefore support a load in the plane of the disk. They are clearly capable of supporting shear forces when the spinal column is in the flexed position. They are also oriented 90° to the direction of motion imposed by axial torsion, because the center of this motion is within the disk. Thus, like all synovial joints, the facet joints are weight-bearing. By virtue of this function, these joints are capable of absorbing some 700 to 800 lb of shear force whereas the disk probably supports less than 200 lb. The maximum shear that the intervertebral joints may be called on to support is probably less than 500 lb. The facet resistance to torsion nearly doubles the torque strength of the whole intervertebral joint. Thus loss of function by the facet joints may have a serious impact on the strength of the whole joint, and it is not difficult to understand why the intervertebral joint deteriorates when a facet joint is damaged.

Stable and Unstable Injuries to the Intervertebral Joint

In the case of injury resulting in endplate failure, a "back-up" system—namely, the posterior midline ligaments, the facets, and the disk annulus—is present to protect against a repetition of damaging forces. Should injury occur, this system survives and is available at the site of injury to maintain a certain degree of spine stability (as in Fig. 2-5A).

In the case of accidental torsional injury, simultaneous damage to the disk annulus and facet joints removes the local back-up mechanism of stabilization. Except for the anti-torsional activity by abdominal muscles, the joint has no protection against torsion. The muscles, however, are too far removed from the site of injury to control the local effects at the intervertebral joint (see Fig. 2-5A).

The proper function of the facet joints depends on the integrity of their articular processes, which in turn rely on the integrity of the neural arches that support them. Therefore, it is important to understand the forces that affect the neural arch as a whole.

The normal force impinging on the neural arch is shown in Figure 2-7. The shear force pushing back on the inferior articular process and the downward pull of the midline structures create a stress concentration at the pars interarticularis. The stress is magnified when torsional forces are added to the facet joints in the direction of axial

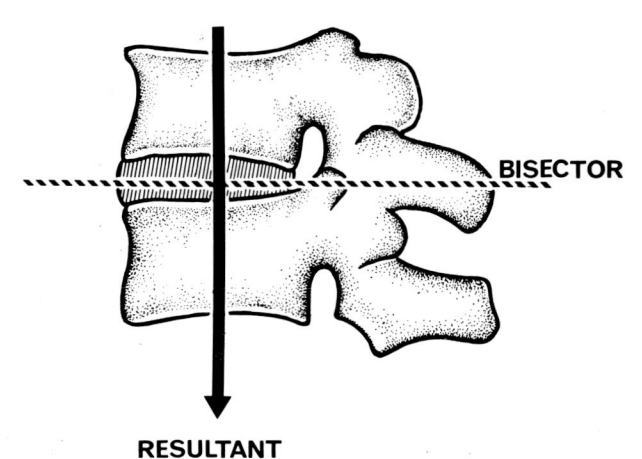

Fig. 2-7. The muscles and ligaments apply tension to the spine while the facet joints support the shear force in the plane of the disk. The forces combine to apply a twisting force to the neural arch so that stress is concentrated at the pars inter articularis.

rotation of the intervertebral joint. It is predictable, therefore, that a torsional injury is the most likely cause of spondylolysis. The second most likely cause is overload with the spine in the flexed or almost fully flexed position, particularly if the erector spinae muscles contract strongly at the same time.

THE THREE-JOINT COMPLEX

Because the facet joints form two of the three articulations of an intervertebral joint, motion at one site must reflect motion at the other two. The instantaneous center of motion for the whole intervertebral joint—for flexion, extension, and torsion—has been found to be near the center of the disk. This must also be the center of motion for the facet joints. The facet joints do not interfere with flexion or extension but are squarely opposed to axial rotation, allowing only approximately 2 to 3° of rotation. When rotation is forced, the facets impose a flexion or forward rotation at the disk and a lateral bend towards the side of the impacted facet joint (coupled motion).

TORSIONAL FAILURE

The force required to induce 3° of axial rotation is generally large enough to deform the neural arch appreciably or even to produce crush injuries to the facet joint.

The forward rotation imposed by the facet joints is not normal in the sense that the annulus is forced into tension or, rather, into reduced compression. The tensile stress added to the torsional stress imposed by the axial rotation together render the annulus more vulnerable. This vulnerability is reduced if the compression load is simultaneously increased to compensate. The difference can make a 20% difference to the torque strength. Hence the inadvisability of doing torsional exercises without either muscle control or some external load.

Forced rotation of 2 to 3° may also damage the annulus. In torsion only half of the annulus is loaded in tension because of the alternating arrangement of its fibers. The highest stresses are attained first in the outermost fibers and predictably, they fail at the ligament–bone interface. As predictably, they fail at the posterolateral angles, which act as "stress risers." The distortion and tearing of the outer annular fibers are greatest at these points and are sufficiently large to interfere with the neural canal content.

AGING AND DEGENERATION

A very high percentage of in vitro experimentation has been on intervertebral joints obtained at autopsy. The average age of the specimens is 60 to 65 yr. It thus happens that, theoretically at least, we should know more about the damaged intervertebral joint than the normal. However, it is precisely because we are not sure of the normal that we have problems interpreting the laboratory results and separating "aging changes" from "degeneration."

In my opinion, considerable evidence exists to support the point of view that aging and degenerative changes are not synonymous and that degenerative changes do not appear unless the joint has been damaged by trauma. Many elderly joints prove to be just as strong in torsion or compression as the younger ones. Furthermore, degenerated joints appear to be stiffer than normal but fail before the healthier ones. This is a typical mechanical characteristic of scar tissue and scar implies injury.

THE RESULT OF COMPRESSION AND TORSIONAL INJURY

Compression Overload

As shown above, the failure in compression overload is a fractured endplate. Little or no damage to the annulus or the facet joints occurs. Should the fracture seal off and no damage to the nucleus ensue, we may conclude that joint function is restored to normal. However, this is usually not the case, because the scar in the endplate remains a weakness and the character of the nucleus undergoes a change that renders it less efficient. The net result is loss of stiffness of the annulus and therefore of the whole joint. In mechanical terms, greater deformation results for any given load. Under such conditions the facet joints become abnormal because of the abnormal call for weight bearing on their surfaces, which are not optimized for this function. This would be especially true of spines submitted to repeated axial loadings, such as is the case with truck drivers and farmers.

The joint with a fractured endplate also shows a reduced resistance to torsion and in the appropriate circumstances tends to be prone to torsional strains.

Creep

Because the intervertebral joint loses stiffness following injury, the "creep" characteristics of the joint are changed. "Creep" is the gradual deformation of the intervertebral joint under a constant load. Creep deformation is greater and occurs more rapidly in the injured joint, which tends to creep in the direction of the injury. Thus, with a fractured endplate, the disk creeps to a reduced thickness. With torsional failure, the joint tends to creep into the rotated position of injury. This phenomenon accounts for the appearance of symptoms as the day passes by.

Loss of Stiffness

The loss of joint stiffness affects the entire function of the joint. For instance, the center of motion may be markedly shifted from its normal position. This affects the system of forces acting in the joint, upsetting the normal muscle–ligament balance and the resultant joint motion.

Loss of Annular Substance

The gradual loss of annular substance and of facet articular cartilage leads to a permanent loss of vertical height of the disk. The vascular portions of disk and facet joint act to proliferate scar and at the capsule or peripheral annulus—where ligament is inserted into bone—osteophyte formation is induced. The mechanical importance of these changes is that mechanical deformation at the joint is reduced and joint strength is improved.

Torsion

The second and major mode of injury is torsion. Abnormal motions may occur because asymmetries are present in the intervertebral joint, disk, or facet joint; minor torque forces may develop when the intervertebral joint is compressed; or else, in the presence of a minor asymmetry a torque may be induced at the intervertebral joint in the performance of a task. In torsional injury, damage occurs simultaneously to the peripheral annulus and the facets. The neural arch may be deformed. Torque resistance at the joint is reduced by this injury. The surviving structures of the intervertebral joint are not able to compensate for the injury and abnormal deformations may occur at the joint.

Severe Injury

When the intervertebral joint is badly damaged, the degree of axial rotational deformation is uncontrollable and therefore the joint is mechanically unstable. Because all local torque-resistant structures are damaged simultaneously, the organism has no replacement mechanism to tide it over until healing is complete. The only surviving anti-torque mechanism is that provided by the abdominal muscles, which cannot react fast enough to protect from the unexpected overload.

At first the remaining intact deeper layers of annulus offer a resistance to further torsion as do the deformed facet joints. However, the reduced diameter of the remaining undamaged annulus and the acquired deformation of neural arch do not offer the original resistance to torque. Also, a greater degree of rotation can occur before the undamaged annular fibers and deformed neural arch offer any resistance. The damaged annular layers heal with scar formation, but the deformed neural arch does not correct. The intervertebral joint is left with a reduced resistance to torque at the annulus and an abnormal amount of motion permitted by the neural arch.

The deformed neural arch permits the intervertebral joint to settle in a new position, and should the annulus heal, we have a stabilized deformity that at best is weak, in which the neural arch has returned to its relatively normal appearance but with the vertebral bodies displaced relative to each other.

CONCLUSIONS

Mechanical failures are predictable when the functions of the individual structural members are understood within the confines of the whole system. A knowledge of the mechanical behavior of each member allows the site of failure to be predicted.

When the precise location of failure has been determined, a knowledge of pathology makes it possible to predict local reactions to the injury and therefore the pathogenesis of the symptomatology.

At this stage of our understanding we can say that injury occurs in one of two modes: first by direct force or axial overload with initial damage to the disk alone, either through compression that causes the endplate to fracture or tension, tensile rupture of posterior annulus with explosive rupture of the disk; or, second, by indirect force or torsional overload with the initial damage occurring simultaneously to facet and annulus.

We may also add that bending overload equals torsional overload because of coupled motion; that the direct and indirect force overload may be combined but the features of torsional overload predominate; and that because the site of failure depends on stress distribution and on local geometric features, we must distinguish injuries at the L4–5 from those at the L5-S1 joints.

These diagnoses are precise *etiological* diagnoses and not to be confused with syndromes such as low back pain, combined low back pain and sciatica, or sciatica. The clinical syndrome can never be a scientific basis for a disease classification. For this we must have the etiological diagnosis.

The clinician must relate the symptomatology to the etiologic diagnosis. Various modes of treatment can then be related to etiology in a rational way rather than to symptomatology, as is all too common at present.

REFERENCES

1. Farfan HF: Biomechanical advantage of lordosis and hip extension for upright activity in man compared with other anthropoids. Spine 3: 336, 1978
2. Farfan HF, Gracovetsky S, Lamy C: Mechanism of the lumbar spine. Spine 6: 249, 1981
3. Farfan HF, Gracovetsky S: The abdominal mechanism. Spine (Accepted for publication)

3 The Pathology and Pathogenesis of Low Back Pain

W. H. Kirkaldy-Willis

INTRODUCTION

It is important to study the etiology, pathology, and pathogenesis of low back pain for several reasons. Such study helps the physician and therapist to understand the nature of the process and to correlate it with the clinical picture. The knowledge gained makes possible an accurate and complete diagnosis and facilitates formulating a logical plan for treatment.

The necessary knowledge is acquired by studying autopsy specimens, clinical symptoms and signs, stress radiograms, and CT scan images, sometimes supplemented by myelograms.

In this chapter we are concerned with a description of changes seen in autopsy specimens and at operation.

PATHOPHYSIOLOGY

The initial cause of lumbar spine dysfunction must be found in pathophysiology, i.e., abnormal function of the lower lumbar intervertebral joints. We know less about this than about the pathological changes that are seen sequentially as the degenerative process unfolds and progresses. Abnormalities of function occur first and lead later on to structural abnormalities.

Two aspects of abnormal function can be identified. Clinical examination of the patient with early dysfunction reveals the presence of a contracted segment of posterior lumbar spinal muscle. Stress radiographs sometimes demonstrate abnormal intervertebral joints; fixation with or without rotation of one joint complex may be present; lateral bending to one side may be reduced.

From these findings we can extrapolate that either the muscles activating an intervertebral joint or the joint itself may be responsible for the patient's symptoms. Often both are involved. We do not know whether a strain to the joint comes first and is followed by contraction of muscle to protect the joint or whether the initiating factor is abnormal muscle function, which then leads to a joint strain.

Early Changes in the Joint Structures

The changes seen in the posterior joints and the disk are discussed and illustrated below in this chapter. In the very earliest stages of Dysfunction (Phase I, see chapter 1) the changes are less pronounced than those shown below. In fact it may not be possible to demonstrate any changes. It is possible to postulate that such changes include (1) synovitis of a posterior joint, (2) stretching of ligaments and annulus, (3) minor tears of ligaments and annulus that heal without a trace of previous injury, (4) minor subluxations that can be easily reduced. The reader will appreciate that the stage of abnormal function merges imperceptibly into that of abnormal structure.

The Role of Muscle

Little attention has been given to this aspect of the problem, probably because investigation of muscle function and structure, other than by electromyographic studies, has proved difficult. We can postulate two ways in which abnormalities of muscle function operate to cause low back pain.

First, when posture is poor, the posterior extensor muscles work harder than the anterior flexor muscles. The result is that the spine is hyperextended. The posterior joints are jammed together. A small synovial fold may be nipped, resulting in synovitis. Muscle changes occur first; abnormal function of the joint follows. Reflex contraction (spasm) of muscle results.

Second, at each level, slips of multifidus muscle pass from the base of the spinous process obliquely downward and outward to the capsule of the posterior joint at the level concerned and also to the capsule one level lower. The multifidus is not under voluntary control. Uncoordinated contraction of the muscle may well initiate strains and minor subluxations of posterior joints.

Three factors may predispose to uncoordinated action of these muscles: stress and anxiety, heat, and cold. Thus a patient under stress or tension is more prone to develop low back pain: Muscle contraction and spasm can follow exposure to the sun on a hot summer day—this is especially likely in the tropics; and exposure to cold because of inadequate protective clothing can also lead to contraction and spasm.

Much of pathophysiology is speculative at present. When, in a later chapter, we come to consider the role of the Spine Education Program we shall see that dealing with abnormalities of function is most important in both treating and preventing lumbar spine dysfunction.

THE MECHANISM OF INJURY

Two different mechanisms are involved: rotational strains and compressive forces. Rotational strains affect mainly the L4–5 joint because of the alignment of the posterior facets and because the L5–S1 joint is often protected by the bony architecture and strong ligaments, thus causing rotational stresses to fall on the L4–5 joint. Compressive forces such as falls onto the buttocks most commonly affect the L5–S1 joint, because it is often protected and because the disk is wedge-shaped. Rotational stresses lead to changes in both posterior joints and disk. Compressive forces affect the disk first and changes are not seen in the posterior joints until a later stage.

THE LEVEL AT RISK

The earliest changes are seen in the L4–5 joint in approximately two-thirds of patients and in the L5–S1 joint in the remaining third. The L5–S1 joint is often protected because it is seated deep in the pelvis and because the L5 transverse processes are large, with short, strong ligaments connecting them to the ilium.

THE THREE-JOINT COMPLEX

At any one level the intervertebral joint is made up of three parts, formed by two posterior facet joints and a disk. Changes affecting the posterior joints also affect the disk and vice versa. The rotational stresses mentioned above most often result in injury to all three parts. They will be described below. Compressive forces usually result in fractures of the cartilage plates of the disk; these are followed by slow degeneration of the disk and resultant stress on the posterior joints at a later date. They may also cause the annulus to rupture explosively at its insertion into the vertebral body bone.

THREE PHASES IN THE DEGENERATIVE PROCESS

The spectrum of degenerative change in an intervertebral joint can be divided into three phases: Dysfunction, Instability (the Unstable Phase), and Stabilization (Fig. 3-1). In Phase I, normal function of the three-part complex is inter-

Fig. 3-1. The three phases of the degenerative process. Dysfunction, pale grey; Unstable Phase, darker shade; Stabilization, darkest shade.

rupted as the result of injury. Examination of the patient reveals that on one or other side of the spine at either L4–5 or L5–S1 the segmental posterior muscles are in a state of hypertonic contraction. Normal movement is restricted in one or other direction. In Phase II, examination of the patient demonstrates the presence of abnormal increased movement. Laxity of the posterior joint capsule and of the annulus fibrosus is seen in autopsy specimens. As degenerative changes become advanced (Phase III) the unstable segment regains its stability because fibrosis is present and osteophytes form around the posterior joints and within and around the disk.

CHANGES IN THE POSTERIOR FACET JOINTS

The changes that occur in the posterior facet joints (Figs. 3-2, 3-3) are the same as those seen in any diarthrodial joint. The earliest change is *synovitis,* which may persist with the formation of a *synovial fold* that projects into the joint between the cartilage surfaces. Later on minimal *degeneration of articular cartilages* occurs and this gradually but increasingly becomes more marked. Sometimes an *intra-articular adhesion* is seen passing from one articular surface to the other. Still later *the capsule becomes lax.* Increasing laxity allows *subluxation* of the joint surfaces to occur. Continuing degeneration (due to repeated rotational strains) results in the formation of subperiosteal osteophytes. These produce *enlargement of both the inferior and the superior facets.* The end result is that the joints become grossly degenerated with almost complete loss of articular cartilage, the formation of bulbous facets (due to subperiosteal new bone formation), and marked periarticular fibrosis. This, together with similar changes in the disk, produces a stable segment with much reduced movement.

The progressive changes are shown in Figure 3-2. It will be appreciated that the early changes occur during Phase I, intermediate changes during Phase II and late changes during Phase III. For simplicity the three phases are shown in horizontal blocks of different shades of gray. In fact there is a gradual transition from Phase I to II and from II to III. These changes are illustrated in Figures 3-3A to H.

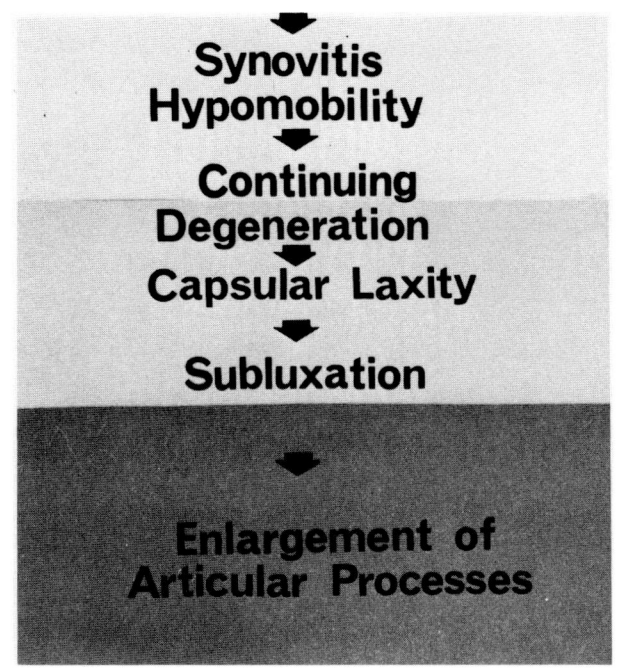

Fig. 3-2. Progressive degenerative changes in the facet joints. The three phases are colored as in Fig. 3-1.

26 *Managing Low Back Pain • 3*

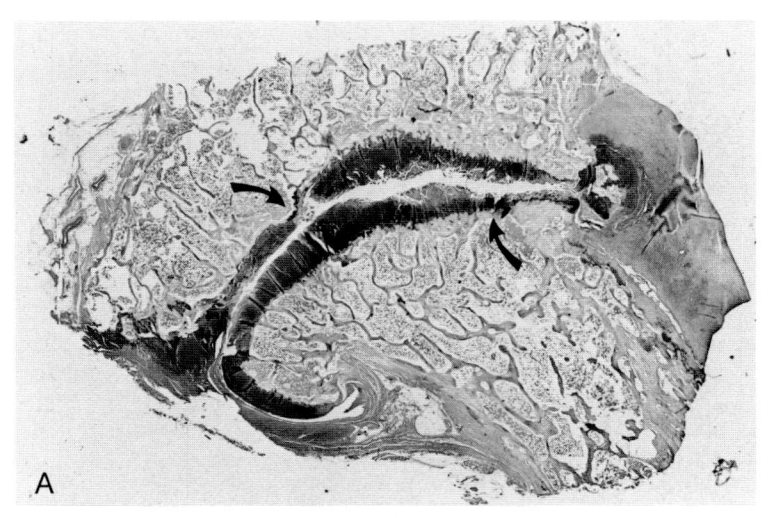

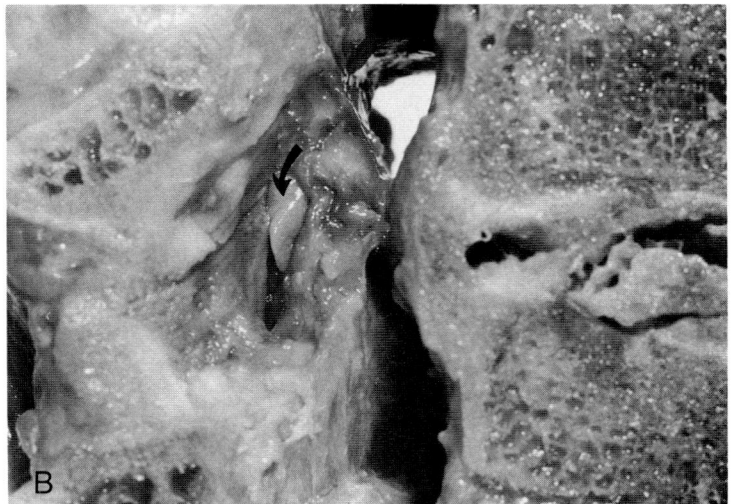

Fig. 3-3. Pathological changes in the facet joints. (A) Histological section. The inferior facet (below) shows thinning of cartilage and crevice formation (arrow); the superior facet (above) shows thinning of cartilage at each end of the section and erosion in the center (arrow). (B) Macroscopic parasagittal section. A large synovial tag is present in the upper part of the posterior facet (arrow). (C) Histological section. Marked subluxation of the dark staining cartilage surfaces and a large intraarticular synovial fold (arrow) are present. (Figure continues).

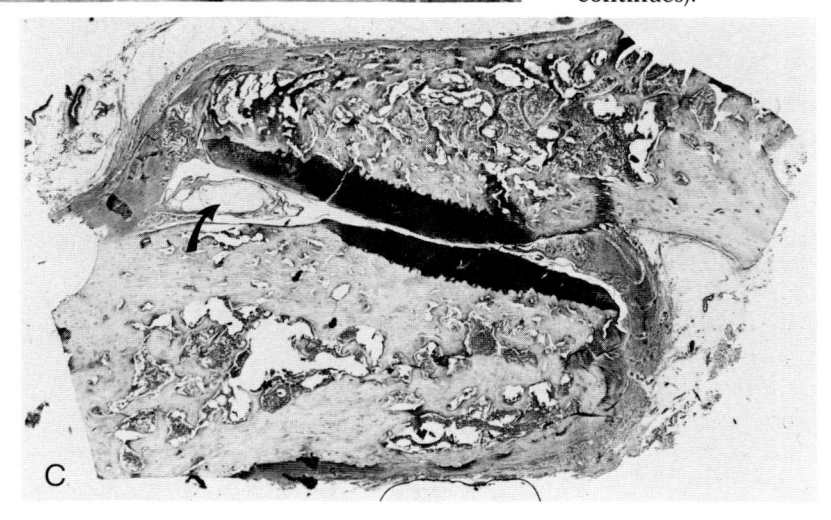

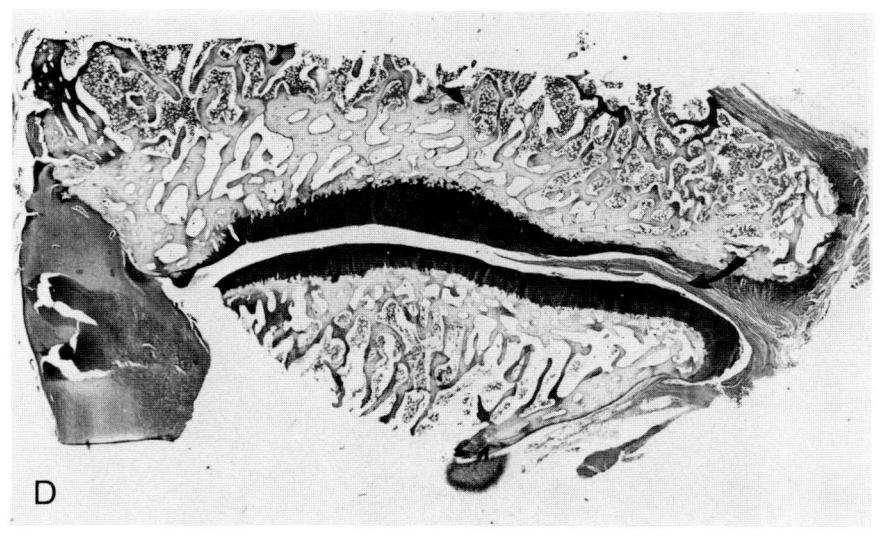

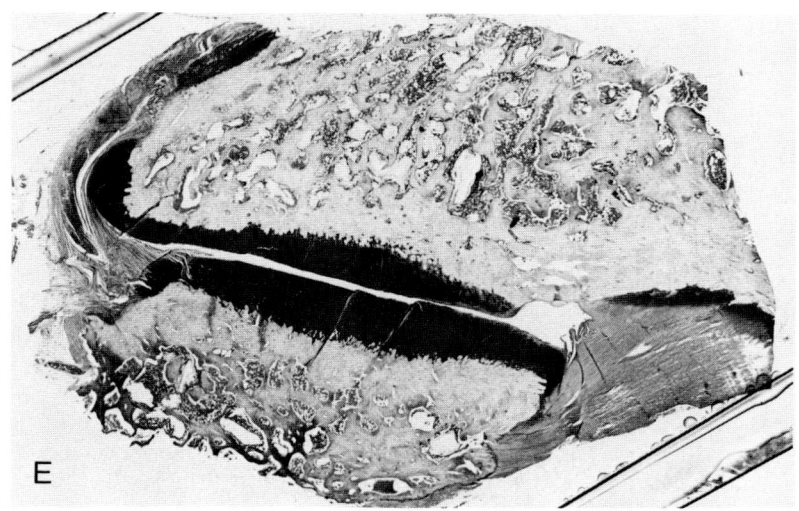

Fig. 3-3 (*Continued*). (D) Histological section. Note the long fibrous fold between the cartilage surfaces (arrow). (E) Histological section. The dark staining cartilage surfaces are markedly subluxated. (F) Histological section demonstrating capsular laxity and instability. A large space that extends deep to the lax capsule is present on the left (arrow). ((F) from Cassidy JD, Potter GE: Motion examination of the lumbar spine. Manipulative Physiol Therapeut, 2:151, 1979) (Figure continues).

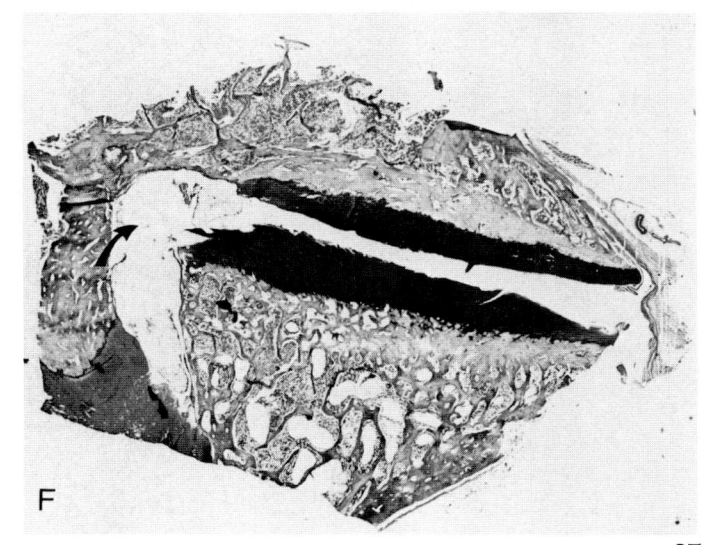

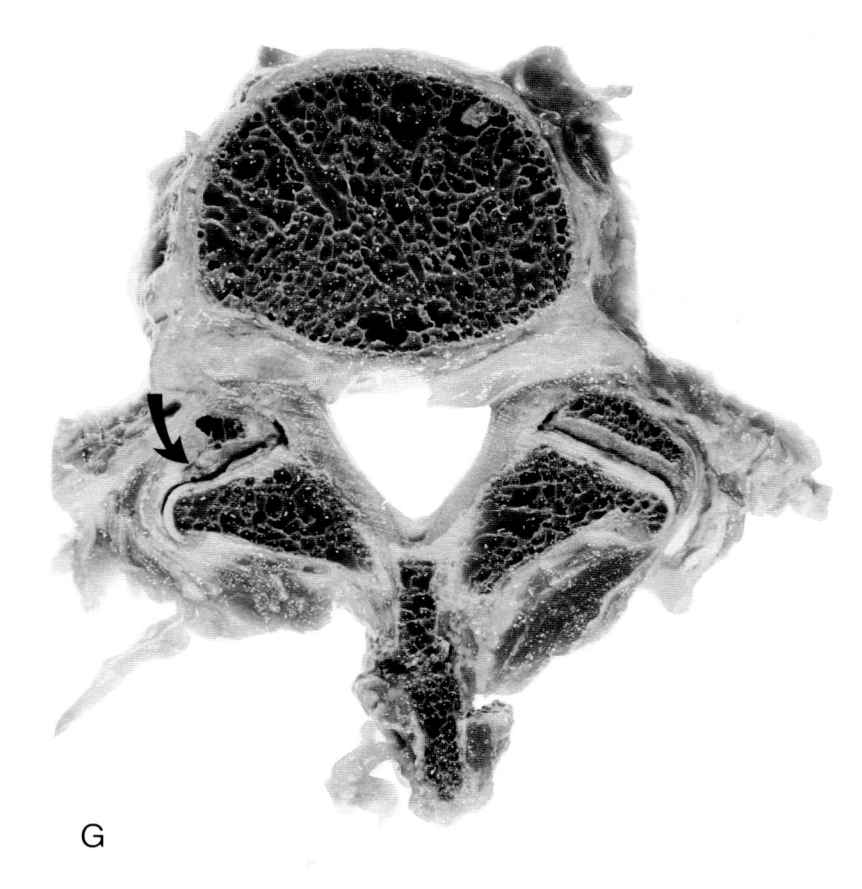

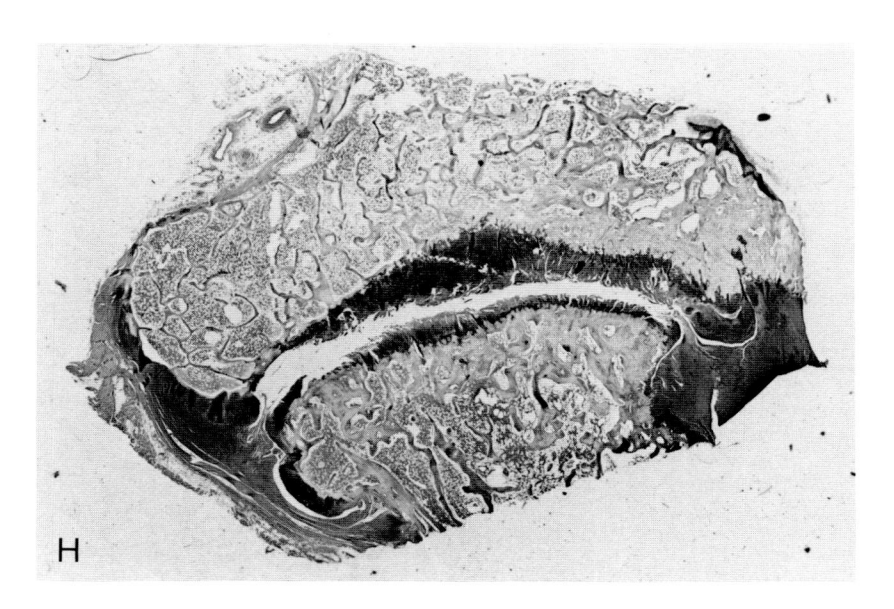

Fig. 3-3 (Continued). (G) Macroscopic transverse section at L5–S1. Marked degeneration of the facet joint is present on the left; the articular cartilage is thin and irregular (arrow); the facet joint on the right is normal. (H) Histological section. The superior articular facet (upper picture) is enlarged; marked degeneration is present on both cartilage surfaces.

Circumferential Tears
⬇
Radial Tears
⬇
Internal Disruption
⬇
Disc Resorption
⬇
Osteophytes

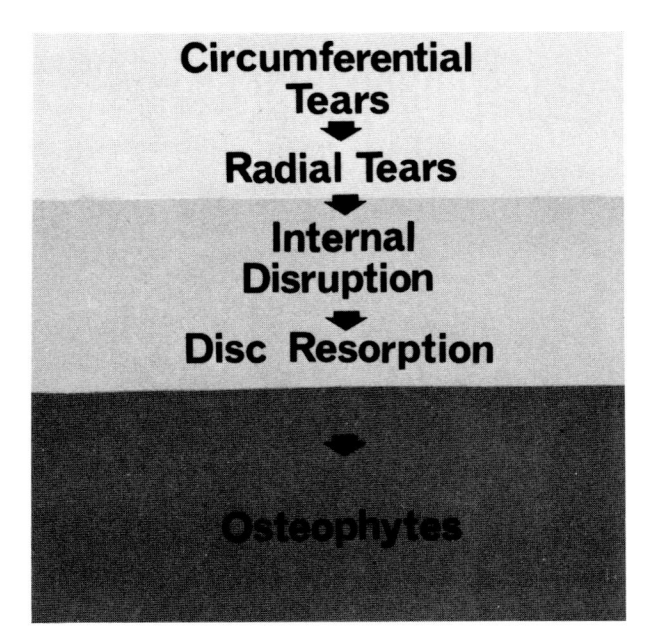

Fig. 3-4. Progressive degenerative changes in the disk. The three phases are colored as above.

CHANGES IN THE INTERVERTEBRAL DISK

Figure 3-4 schematizes the sequence of changes seen in the disk and demonstrates the phases during which they occur. Here again there is no hard and fast delineation between Phases I and II or Phases II and III.

Recurrent rotational strains produce first a number of small *circumferential tears* in the annulus fibrosus. Later on these become larger and coalesce to form *radial tears* that pass from the annulus into the nucleus pulposus. At a still later stage these tears increase further in size until the disk is completely disrupted internally. The large tear now passes from front to back and side to side of the disk. The normal disk height is greatly reduced because of loss of proteoglycans and water from the nucleus. The annulus becomes lax and bulges right around the circumference of the disk. This generalized bulge must be distinguished from a disk herniation, which is a local protrusion. With further degeneration and loss of disk contents the disk space is represented by a thin slit between the vertebral bodies filled with fibrous tissue. Vertebral body bone on either side of the disk is dense and sclerotic. This condition is called *disk resorption*. Finally, the disk is anchored by peripheral osteophytes that pass around its circumference. Occasionally the end result is bony ankylosis. The changes described above are shown in Figures 3-5A to F.

THE INTERACTION OF CHANGES IN FACET JOINTS AND DISK

In some patients the changes seen during the course of the progressive degenerative process affect mainly the facet joints. In others they affect mainly the disk. More commonly the whole three-joint complex at L4–5 or at L5–S1 is affected; posterior joint changes produce a reaction on the disk and vice versa.

The process of change is illustrated in Figure 3-6. The light gray upper horizontal bar represents Dysfunction, the darker middle bar the Unstable phase, and the darkest lower bar Stabilization. The vertical column on the left shows changes in the facet joints, the right column changes in the disk, and the center column the interaction of changes in the component parts of the complex.

The earliest changes—synovitis and minor strains in the facet joints (with hypomobility) together with minor rotational strains of the annulus leading to the formation of circumferential tears—produce a state of dysfunction. As this dysfunction becomes more severe, leading to the formation of radial tears in the annulus, a localized bulging or protrusion of the annulus that is called a disk herniation may occur, often caused by relatively minor further trauma. The disk contents protrude into the spinal canal. The tear in the annulus may be complete, with the disk contents extruded into the canal. As seen in Figure 3-6, disk herniation occurs most commonly at the end of Phase I or at the beginning of Phase II, but it may occur during Phase III as well. Continuing degeneration that produces capsular laxity of the posterior joints and causes internal disruption of the disk results in segmental instability (Phase II). This phase is characterized by *abnormal increased movement* of the spinal segment, as opposed to the *abnormal decreased movement* found during Dysfunction (Phase I).

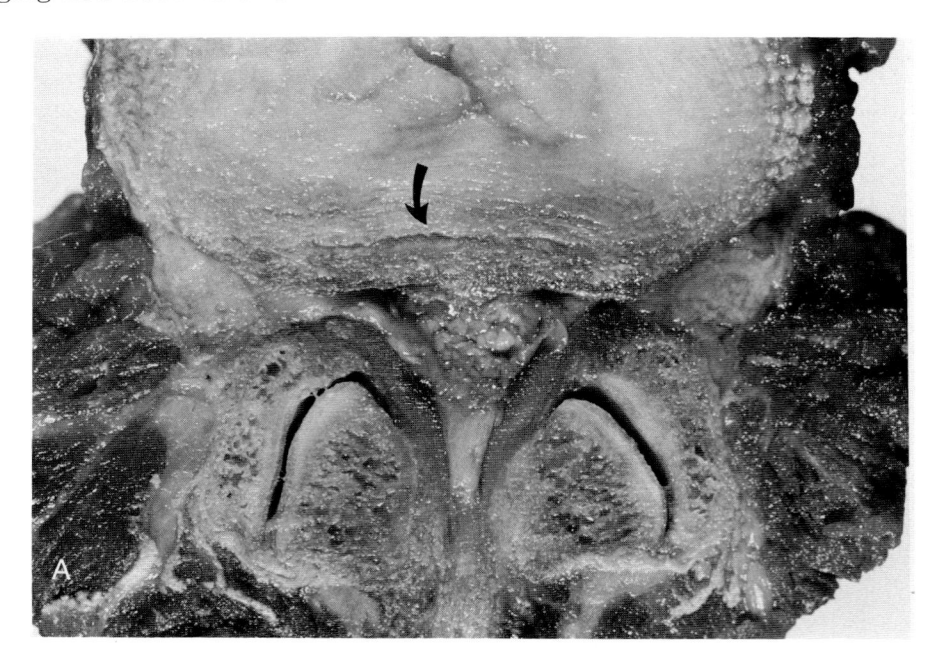

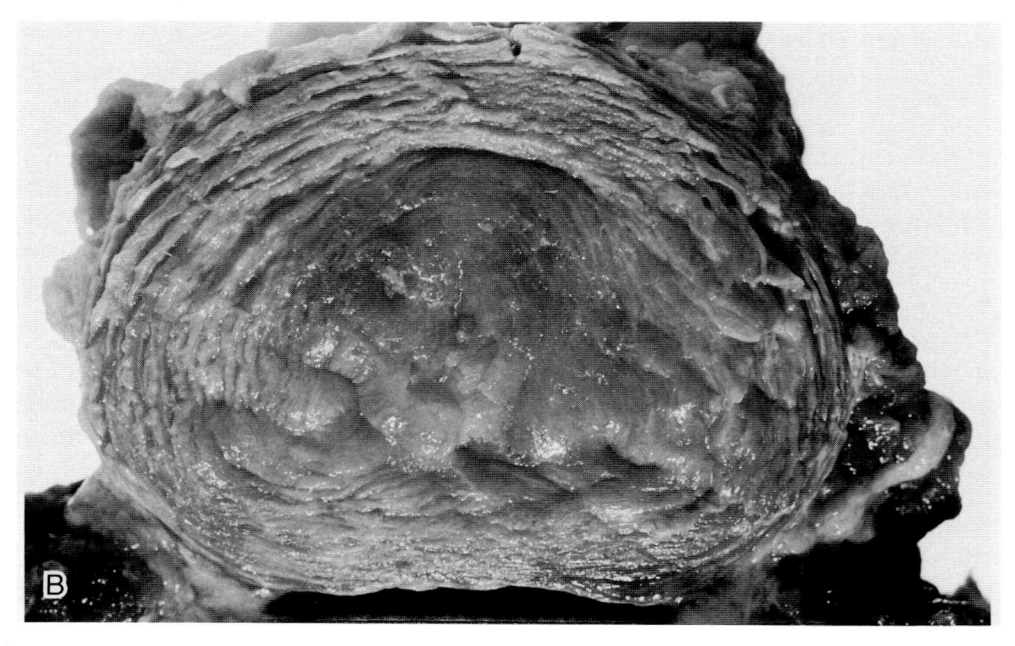

Fig. 3-5. Pathological changes in the disk. (A) Macroscopic transverse section at L4–5. Part of the disk is shown above and the facet joints are shown below. A transverse circumferential tear is seen in the annulus fibrosus (arrow). (B) Macroscopic transverse section at L4–5 to show the whole disk. Numerous circumferential tears are visible, especially in the upper part of the picture. (Figure continues).

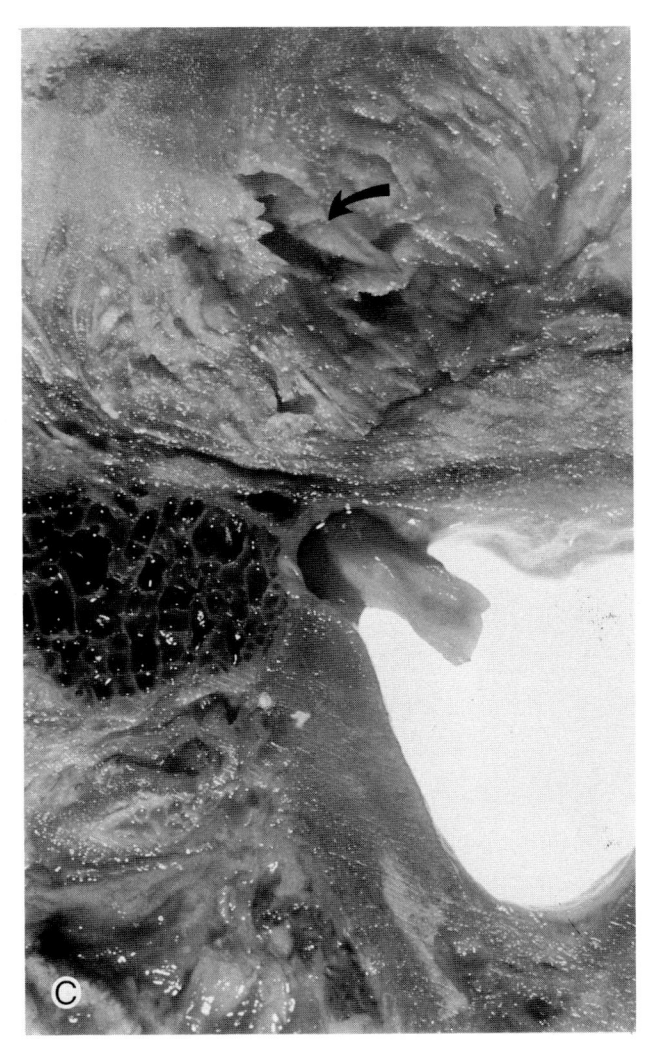

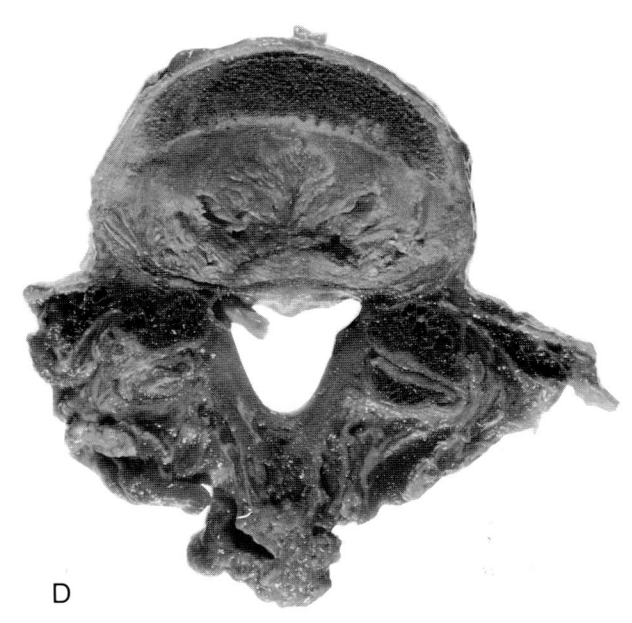

Fig. 3-5 (Continued). (C) Macroscopic transverse section at L4–5 showing part of the disk (above). The arrow points to one large radial tear. (D) Macroscopic transverse section at L4–5. Several radial tears are coalescing; early signs of internal disruption are present. (Figure continues).

Lateral Spinal Nerve Entrapment

Lateral spinal nerve entrapment, a relatively common lesion, is seen either late in Phase II or early in Phase III; that is, sometimes we encounter this type of nerve entrapment when the spine is unstable and on other occasions when it is again stabilized (see Fig. 3-6).

The nerve canal is shown in diagrammatic form in Figure 3-7D. It extends from the dura to the foramen. The lateral part of this canal, in which lateral nerve entrapment takes place, runs from the medial edge of the superior facet to the foramen.

Lateral Entrapment with Instability. As described above and shown in Figure 3-8, the capsule of the posterior facets is lax and permits subluxation of these joints to occur. In the disk internal disruption results in loss both of height and stability, with annular bulging. The sequelae of loss of disk height are fourfold: subluxation of the facet joints; upward and forward displacement of the superior on the inferior facets; diminution in size of the intervertebral foramen; and, even

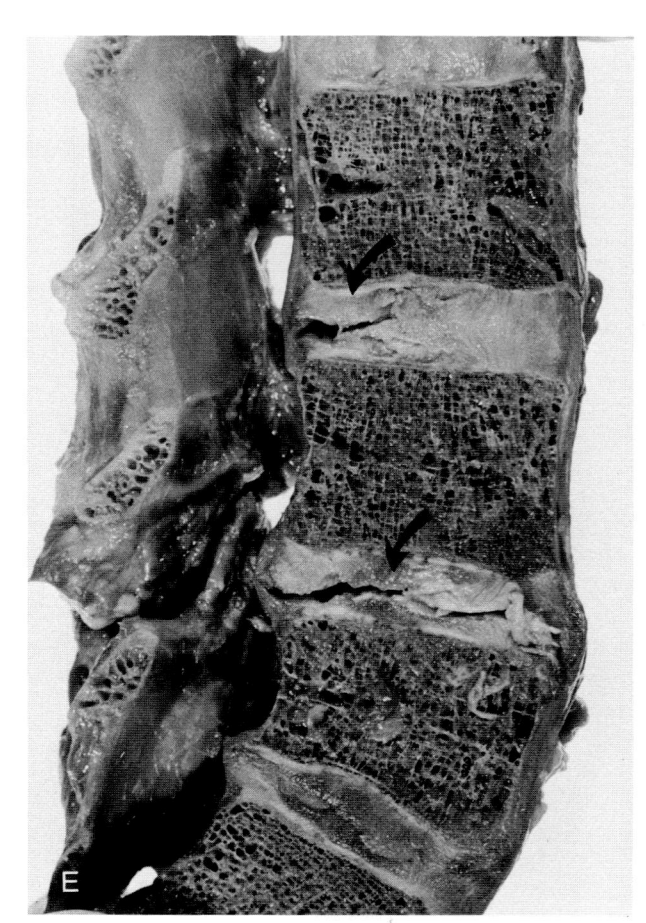

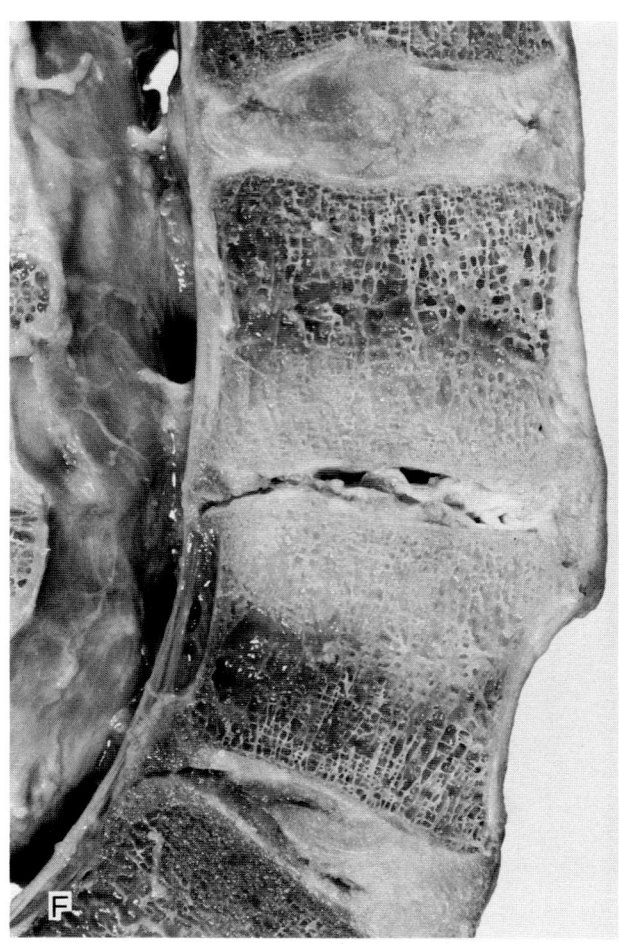

Fig. 3-5 (Continued). (E) Macroscopic sagittal section of the lumbar spine. The upper arrow points to a disk showing early internal disruption; the lower arrow points to a disk characterized by severe internal disruption. (F) Macroscopic sagittal section of the lumbar spine. The central disk demonstrates marked resorption; the disk itself is a narrow slit; vertebral body bone on either side is sclerotic. ((F) from Kirkaldy-Willis WH, Wedge JH, Yong-Hing K, Reilly J: Pathology and pathogenesis of lumbar spondylosis and stenosis. Spine 3:323, 1978)

more important, narrowing of the lateral canal medial to the foramen.

The way in which the foramen is diminished in size is shown in Figure 3-7E. The two vertebrae in the upper picture are positioned to demonstrate normal alignment of the facet, a normal disk height, and a normal foramen. In the lower picture the vertebrae have been approximated to simulate loss of disk height, subluxation of facets, and narrowing of the intervertebral foramen. In the presence of instability the lax facet capsule allows the superior facet to move backward and forward with rotation. This is illustrated in Figures 3-8A and B. In Figure 3-8A, a sagittal section of an autopsy specimen, the posterior joint at L4–5 is markedly eroded and the capsule appears to be very lax. Note the distance between the anterior aspect of the superior facet and the posterior surface of the annulus. This is the lateral canal. In Figure 3-8B, from the same specimen, the spinous process of L5 has been rotated; the superior facet has moved anteriorly; the joint space has opened; the anterior aspect of the superior facet is now almost touching the annulus; and the lateral canal is markedly narrowed. The same phenomena are shown in cross-section in Figures 3-8C

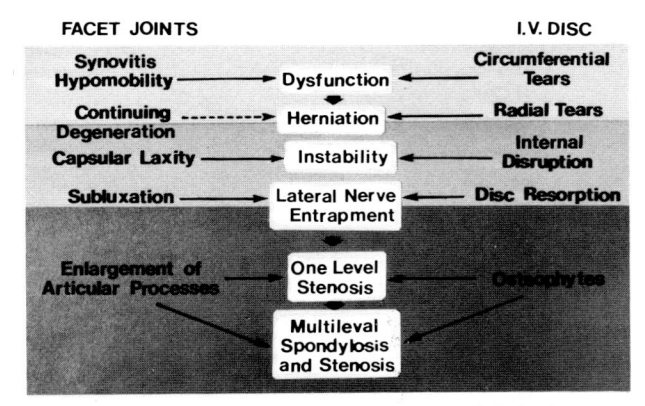

Fig. 3-6. The interaction of facet joint and disk changes. Changes in the facet joints appear on the left and changes in the disk on the right. Lesions that occur as a result of the interaction of these changes are seen in the center.

and D. In this kind of entrapment, each time that rotation occurs between L4 and L5 the superior facet impinges on the spinal nerve in the lateral canal. We can thus call this lesion a recurrent dynamic entrapment. Abnormal flexion–extension movement can produce the same effect. As will be seen in chapter 9 this type of lesion can be demonstrated by the CT scan.

Lateral Entrapment with a Fixed Deformity. Fixed-deformity lateral entrapment occurs in a similar way to that described above. It is encountered during Phase III at a point when the degenerative changes are sufficiently advanced to stabilize the affected segment (Fig. 3-9A). Little or no movement takes place at the affected level. Thus the narrowing of the lateral canal is fixed because of a permanent deformity. Two factors are involved in producing the entrapment: subluxation of posterior facets, which allows the superior facet to move upward and forward (Fig. 3-7E), and enlargement of this facet by osteophytes, which further narrows the lateral canal (Figs. 3-9A,B). The importance of lateral entrapment will be seen when we consider diagnosis and treatment.

Central Stenosis

At One Level. Stenosis is encountered mainly at the L4–5 level but also occurs at the L3–4, L5–S1, and other levels. The pathogenesis of this lesion is similar to that of lateral entrapment (lateral stenosis). Narrowing of the central spinal canal is produced mainly by osteophytic enlargement of the two inferior facets, but the superior facets may also contribute. Central stenosis and lateral stenosis may occur as separate entities. They may also be combined. Central stenosis may be seen during Phase II in an unstable spine. It occurs more commonly during Phase III, when the spine is again stabilized as shown in Figure 3-6. The cauda equina and its blood vessels are often compromised to a greater extent than individual spinal nerves.

Spread of Changes to Affect Several Levels. In the early stages the lesion is confined to one level, as stated above, but later on the degenerative process spreads to involve several levels. The way in which this takes place is not well understood. It is thought that either increased or decreased movement at one level predisposes to strains at levels above and below this. Some experimental work supports this view. In Figure 3-9F, a longitudinal sagittal section of an autopsy specimen obtained many years after a successful posterior fusion from L3 to the sacrum, the disks below the site of fusion are normal. At L2–3, just above the top of the fusion, the posterior joints are markedly degenerate and the disk is disrupted internally. The stiffness produced by the fusion from L3 to the sacrum protects this area and subsequent strains affect the L2–3 level, with resultant spondylosis and stenosis at this level. Involvement of a second and then of subsequent levels first produces the changes seen in Phase I, progresses to Phase II, and in the end reaches Phase III. In some cases the whole lumbar spine becomes spondylotic, and stenosis—both central and lateral—may be present at several levels. Frequently some degree of scoliosis with a rotational element is present.

Developmental Stenosis. Abnormal development of the spine during the growth years frequently results in a central canal that is smaller than normal. This may involve one segment, one part, or all of the lumbar spinal canal. The coronal or saggital diameter or both may be affected. A severe form of this abnormality is seen in achondroplasia. More commonly the cause of the narrowing is unknown. Figures 3-9C and D demonstrate one type of developmental stenosis. Of itself

34   *Managing Low Back Pain • 3*

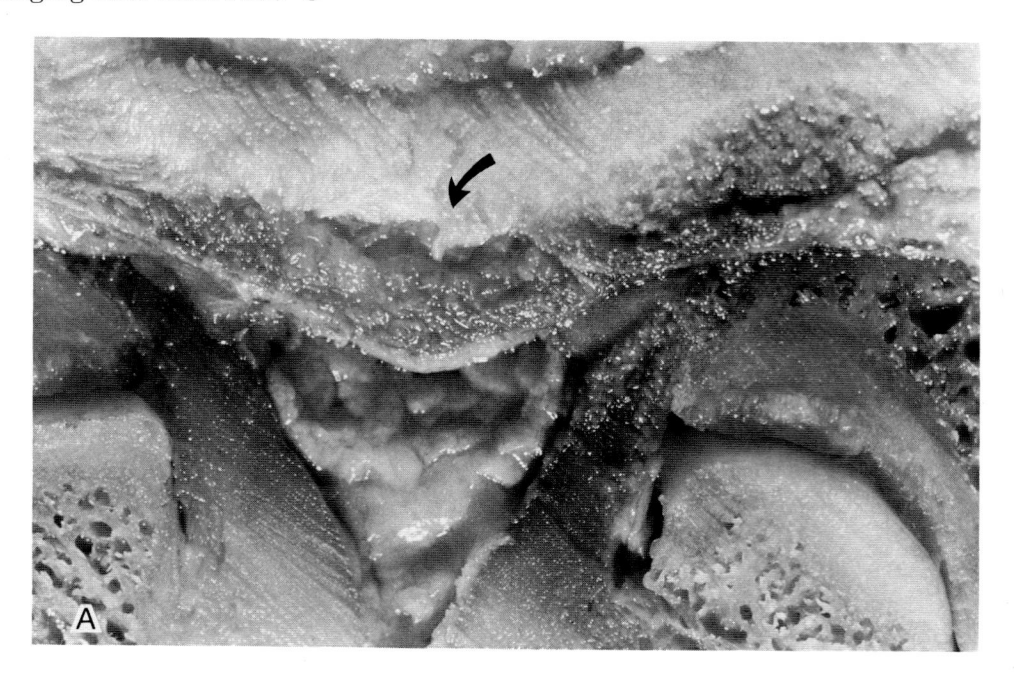

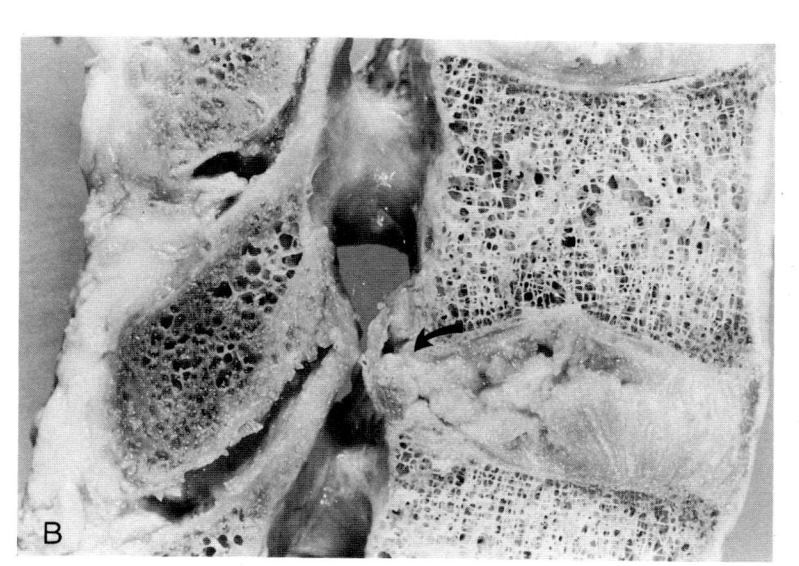

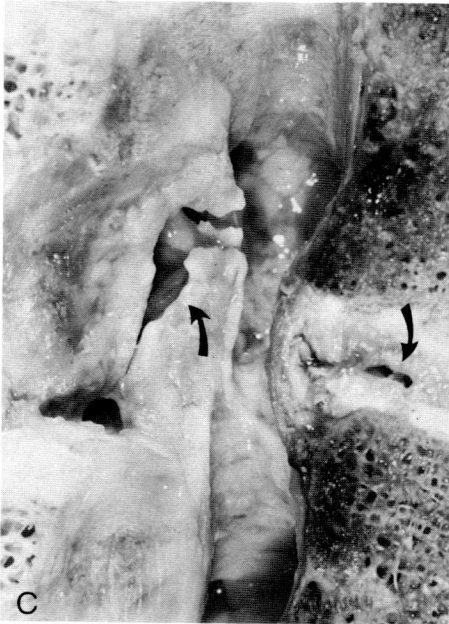

Fig. 3-7. Lesions occurring as a result of the interaction of changes in facets and disk. (A) Macroscopic transverse section at L5–S1. The arrow points to a large central disk herniation. (B) Macroscopic sagittal section at the L4–5 level demonstrates the presence of a large disk herniation (the arrow), which has ruptured into the spinal canal. (C) Macroscopic sagittal section of facet joint and posterior disc at L4–5 demonstrates the presence of instability, the result of marked degeneration of the facet joint (left arrow) and of internal disruption of the disk (right arrow). ((C) from Kirkaldy-Willis, Wedge JH, Yong-Hing K, Reilly J: Pathology and pathogenesis of lumbar spondylosis and stenosis. Spine 3:319, 1978) (Figure continues).

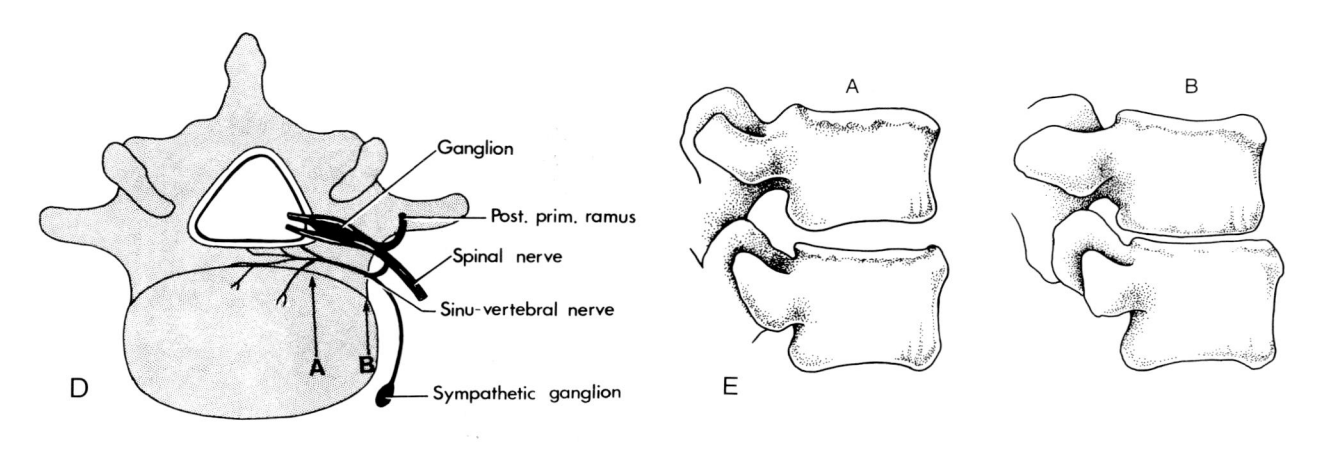

Fig. 3-7 (Continued). (D) Diagram of transverse section of the lumbar spine. The lateral part of the nerve canal—the site of lateral nerve entrapment—is between the two arrows. (E) Drawings of two vertebrae. A shows a normal disk. Note the size of the foramen. B shows marked reduction of disk height, retrospondylolisthesis of the upper on the lower vertebra, subluxation of posterior facets and reduction in size of the foramen. (F) Macroscopic sagittal section of the lumbar spine showing degenerative changes at several levels. The L1–2 disk is normal. The L2–3 disk shows marked internal disruption. The L3–4 disk shows early disruption. The L4–5 joint demonstrates very marked disruption. The L5–S1 disk shows resorption. There is marked encroachment on the central canal at the lowest three levels.

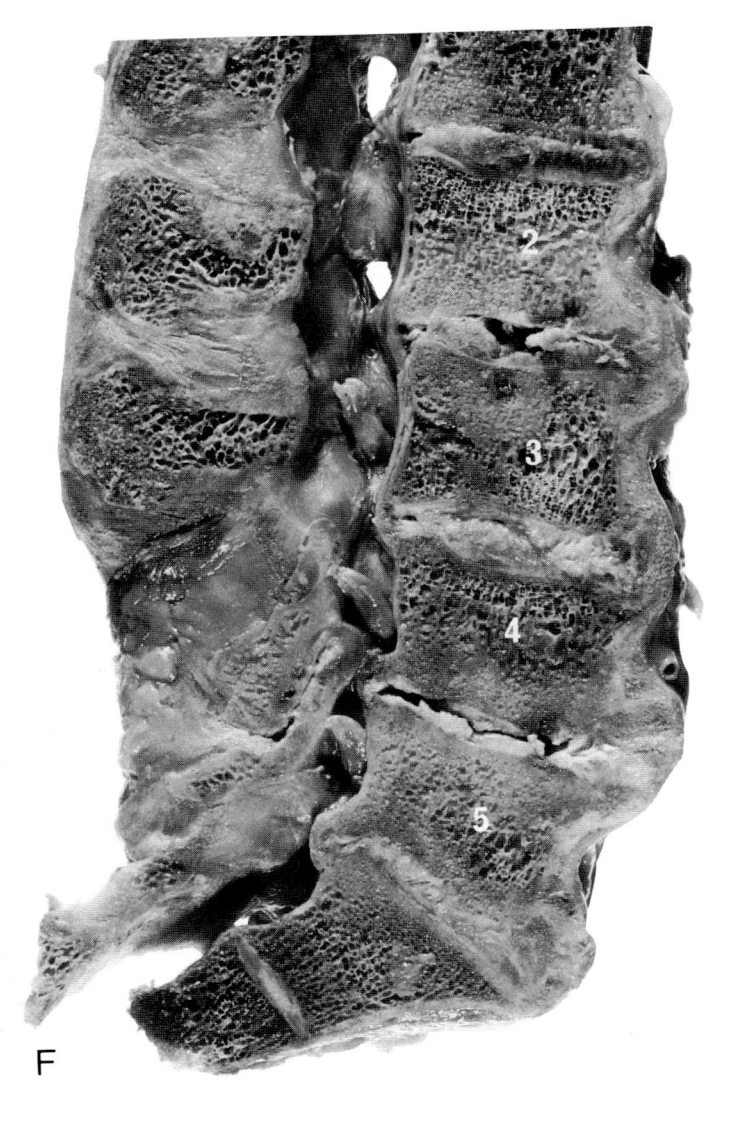

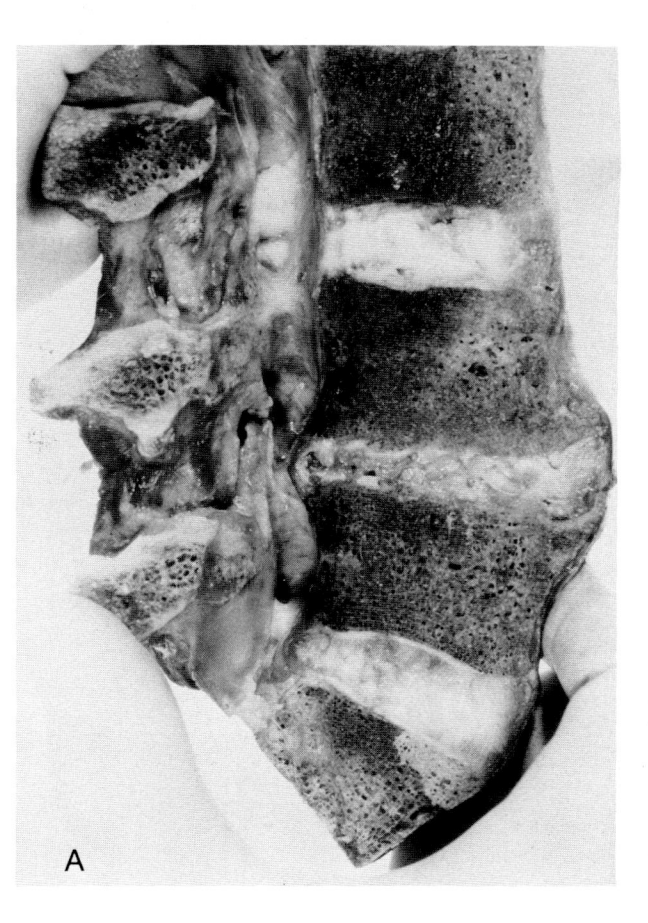

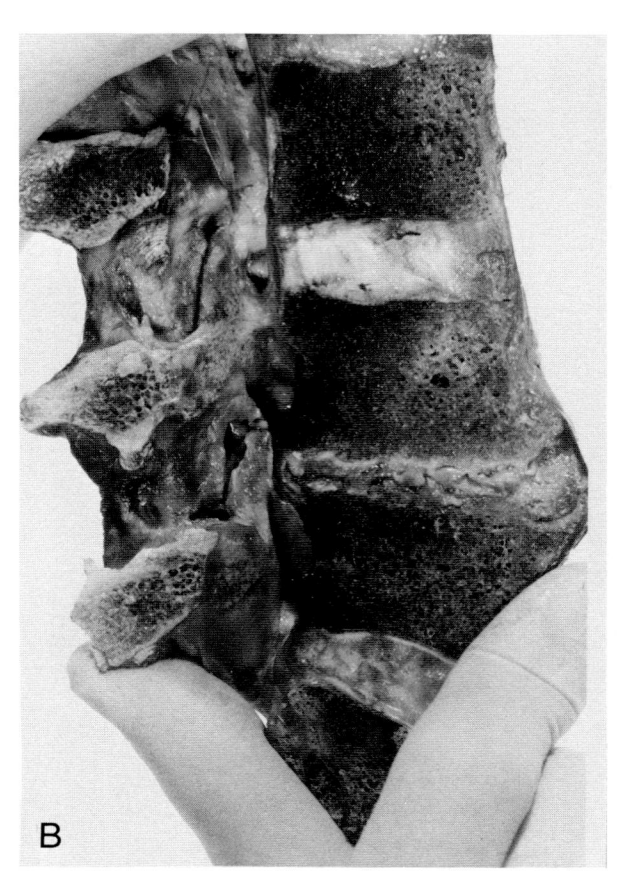

Fig. 3-8. Dynamic lateral stenosis with instability. (A) Macroscopic sagittal section of the lumbar spine. At the L4–5 level there is erosion of the facet joint and internal disruption of the disk. This joint complex is unstable. Note the size of the lateral canal between the anterior surface of the superior facet and the posterior aspect of the disk. (B) The same specimen. The spinous process of L5 has been rotated toward the observer. The facet joint has opened, the superior facet has rotated toward the back of the disk, and the lateral canal has become narrow. (From Reilly J, Yong-Hing K, MacKay RW, Kirkaldy-Willis WH: Pathological anatomy of the lumbar spine. Disorders of the Lumbar Spine. Edited by Helfet AJ, Gruebel-Lee DM. Philadelphia, JB Lipincott, 1978) (Figure continues).

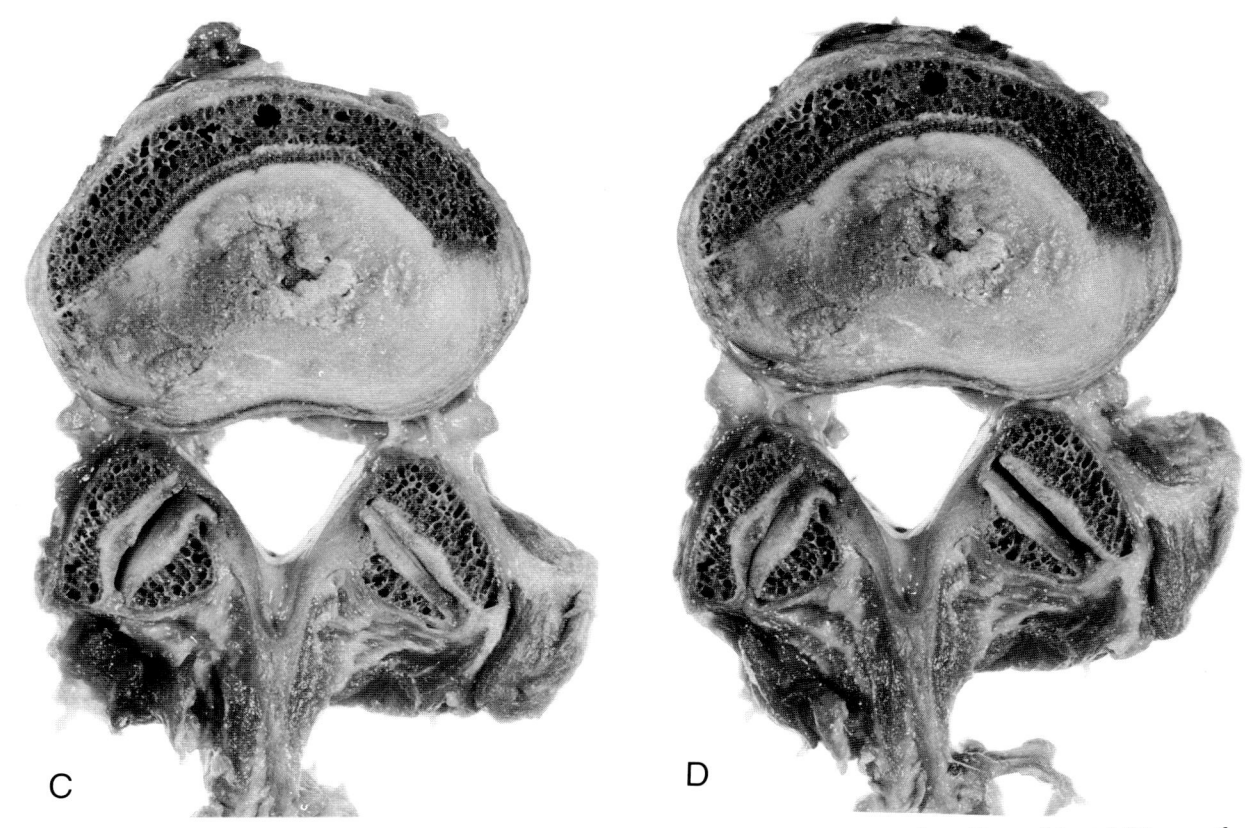

Fig. 3-8 (Continued). (C) Macroscopic transverse section at L4–5 demonstrates the effect of instability on the lateral canals. Rotation has opened the left facet joint; the left superior facet has shifted toward the back of the disk, the left lateral canal is narrow. (D) The same specimen. Rotation in the opposite direction has opened the right posterior joint; the right superior facet has moved toward the back of the disk; the right lateral canal is narrow.

this change does not produce symptoms. Together with a small disk herniation or minor degenerative stenosis severe symptoms may result. Thus developmental stenosis is regarded as an enhancing factor.

LESIONS THAT ACT DIRECTLY TO PRODUCE STENOSIS

Certain lesions can produce stenosis in a direct way without degenerative or developmental narrowing of the central or lateral spinal canals. Stenosis may be produced by a *vertebral body fracture*. Late changes following fracture may result in narrowing the canal (Fig. 3-9E). In *degenerative spondylolisthesis*, commonly seen at the L4–5 level, the L5 spinal nerve may be entrapped between the inferior articular facet of L4 (which has slipped forward) and the back of the body of L5. (Fig. 3-10A). In *isthmic spondylolisthesis* at the L5–S1 level the L5 nerve may be entrapped by the pars interarticularis just cranial to the fracture (Fig. 3-10B). *Following laminectomy* fibrous tissue scarring may compress the dura and cauda equina or involve spinal nerves. *Fusion operations* may result in stenosis. Most frequently stenosis is caused by continuing degenerative changes at the cranial end of the fusion, but hypertrophic

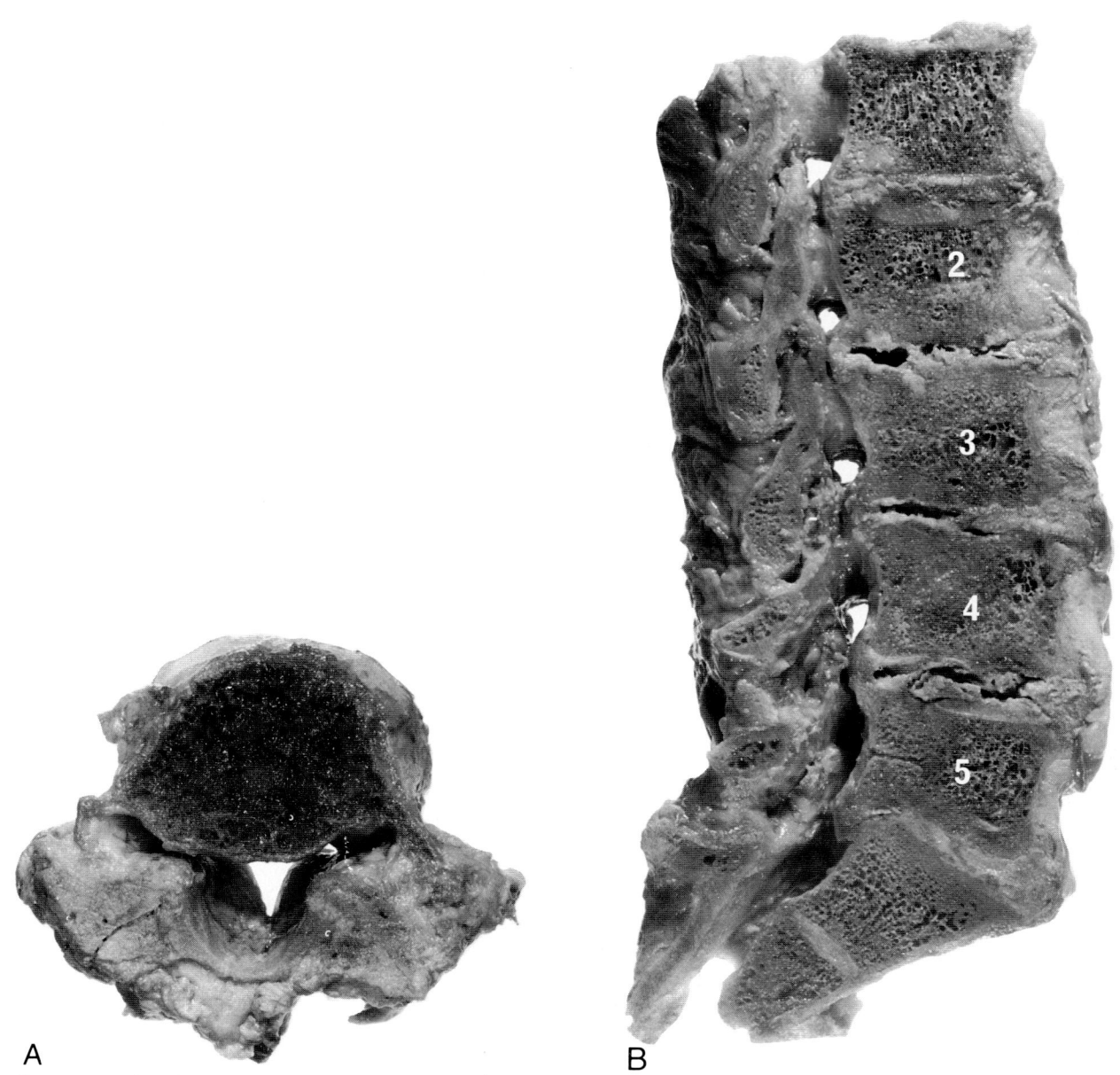

Fig. 3-9. Other lesions in the lumbar spine. (A) Fixed central and lateral stenosis. Macroscopic transverse section at L5–S1 demonstrates fixed central and lateral stenosis seen in Phase III (Stabilization). The central canal is markedly narrowed by enlarged inferior facets; the right lateral canal is narrow because of facet subluxation; the left lateral canal is very narrow from both subluxation and osteophyte formation. (B) Multilevel stenosis. Macroscopic sagittal section of lumbar spine shows internally disrupted disks at the L2–3, L3–4, and L4–5 levels and resorption at the L5–S1 level, with retrospondylolisthesis of L5 on S1. The lateral canals are narrow at every level. (Figure continues).

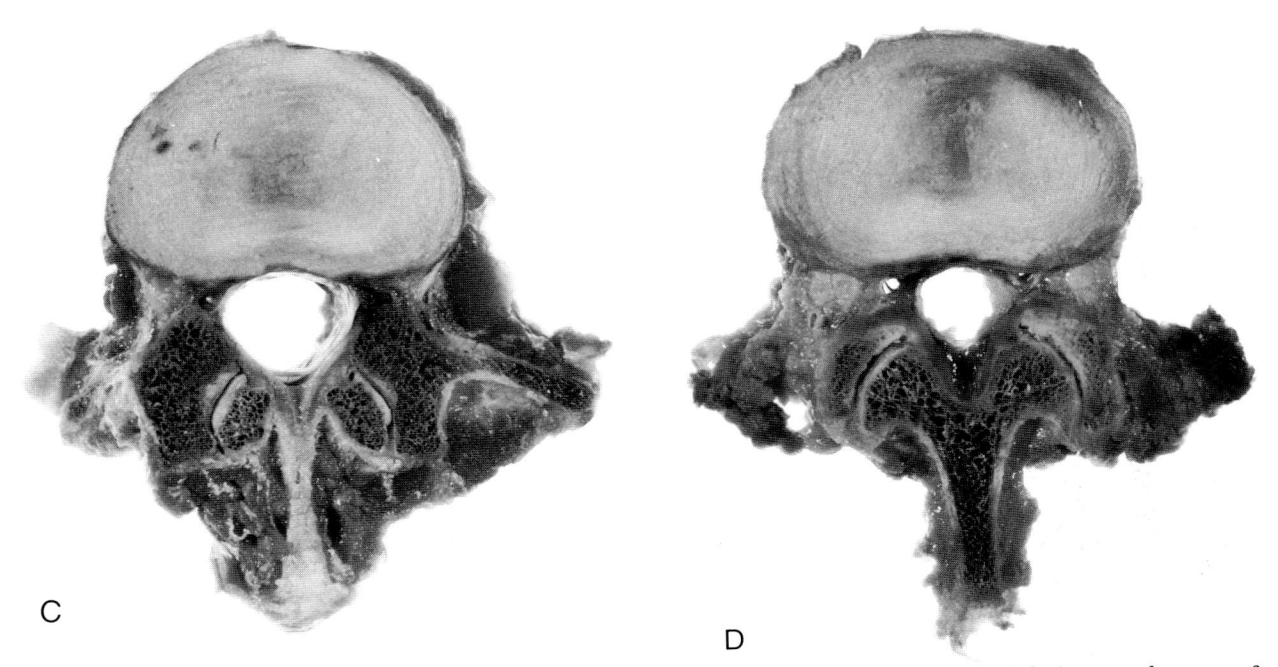

Fig. 3-9 (Continued). (C) Developmental stenosis. In macroscopic transverse section at L3–4, note the size of the normal central canal. (D) The same specimen at L4–5. At this level the central canal is small, segmental developmental stenosis has occurred. (C, D) from Kirkaldy-Willis WH, Heithoff KB, Bowen CVA, Shannon R: Pathological anatomy of lumbar spondylosis and stenosis correlated with the CT scan. Radiographic Evaluation of the Spine. Edited by Post MJD. New York, Masson, 1980 (Figure continues).

new bone formation underneath the fusion may narrow the spinal canal (Fig. 3-9F). In *Paget's disease* enlargement of a vertebral body may cause stenosis. In *fluorosis,* commonly encountered in some parts of India, new bone formation within the spinal canal may compromise the cauda equina.

A COMBINATION OF FACTORS

Nerve entrapment may be caused by only one of the lesions discussed above but quite often two or more causes operate together to have a more pronounced effect. Three examples are disk herniation with degenerative stenosis, disk herniation with developmental stenosis, and disk herniation with both degenerative and developmental stenosis.

VENOUS HYPERTENSION

Throughout this chapter we have been concerned mainly with the way in which one or another kind of lesion causes pain by entrapping spinal nerves and those of the cauda equina. Previous authors have demonstrated experimentally that degenerative changes in the spine are often accompanied by venous hypertension in bone adjacent to a joint. Such hypertension may produce pain by causing pressure on small nerves in bone, annulus fibrosus, or ligaments. It may interfere with the circulation of the spinal nerves or those

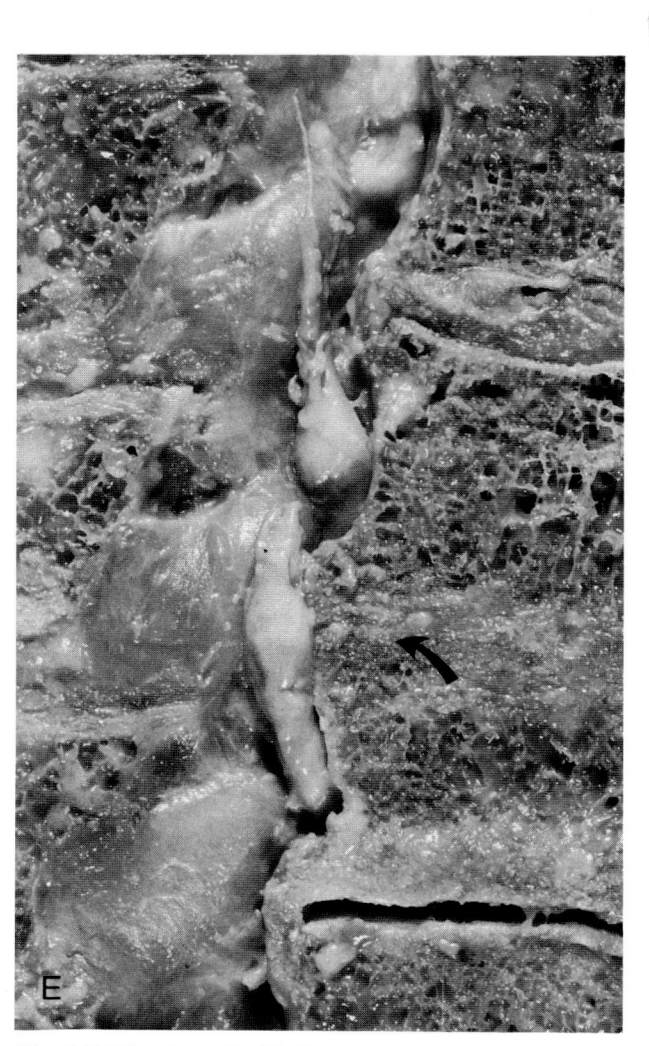

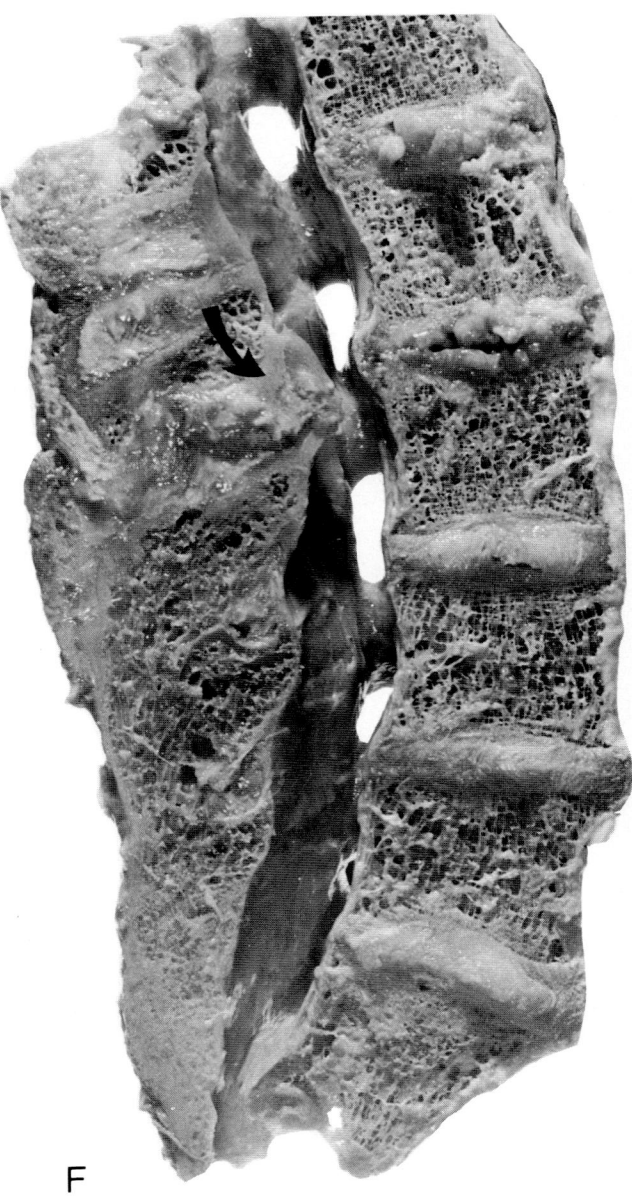

Fig. 3-9 (Continued). (E) Post-traumatic stenosis. Macroscopic sagittal section shows two lumbar vertebral bodies that are fused as a result of previous trauma with fracture. New bone formation at the site of the fusion has narrowed the central canal (arrow). (F) Post-fusion stenosis. Microscopic sagittal section of a lumbar spine with a posterior fusion done 20 years previously. A solid posterior mass of bone is present from L3 to the sacrum. The disks in front are well preserved. At the L2–3 level the disk is disrupted and the posterior facet joints are enlarged to produce central stenosis (arrow). ((F) from Kirkaldy-Willis WH, Wedge JH, Yong-Hing K, Reilly J: Pathology and pathogenesis of lumbar spondylosis and stenosis. Spine 3:319, 1978).

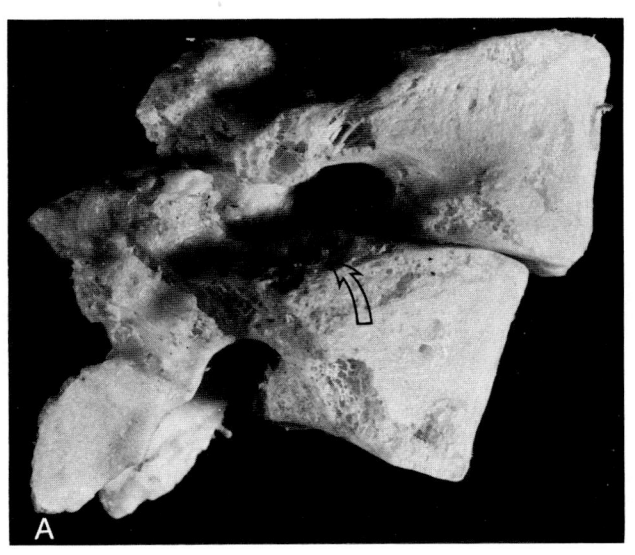

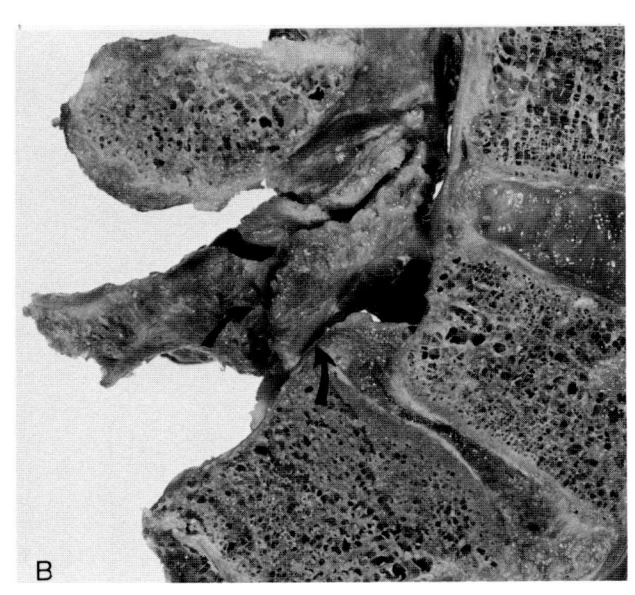

Fig. 3-10. Spondylolisthesis and other lesions. (A) Degenerative spondylolisthesis. The upper vertebra (L4) has slipped forward on the lower (L5). The inferior facet of L4 is almost touching the back of the body of L5 (arrow) and the L5 nerve is entrapped at this level. (From Farfan HF, Reilly J, Yong-Hing K, MacKay RW, Kirkaldy-Willis, WH: Pathological anatomy of the lumbar spine. Disorders of the Lumbar Spine. Edited by Helfet AJ, Gruebel-Lee DM. Philadelphia, JB Lipincott, 1978) (B) Isthmic spondylolisthesis. In macroscopic sagittal section of lumbosacral spine, the defect in the pars interarticularis is clearly seen (left arrow). The L5 nerve is entrapped between the back of the sacrum and the bone of the pars just above the defect (right arrow). (Figure continues).

of the cauda equina. The bizarre sensations in the legs of a patient with spinal stenosis may be due in part to venous hypertension.

AN OVERALL VIEW

The whole picture of degenerative changes, the effect of developmental stenosis, and the effects of direct factors is shown in Figure 3-11. This demonstrates the way in which an enhancing factor—developmental stenosis—may accentuate the degenerative process and the way in which spondylolisthesis, trauma, Paget's disease, fluorosis and fusion may produce one-level or multilevel spinal stenosis.

SUMMARY

The pathology and pathogenesis of degenerative and other lesions in the lumbar spine are viewed in an overall perspective. This has two components: (1) three horizontal bars demonstrating the three phases—dysfunction, the unstable phase, and stabilization (Fig. 3-1)—and (2) three vertical columns setting out changes in the facets and in the disk, and the interaction of these two (Fig. 3-6). A composite picture is obtained by superimposing (1) on (2). This way of looking at changes in the lumbar spine will be employed again in later chapters as we consider diagnosis, prognosis, and treatment.

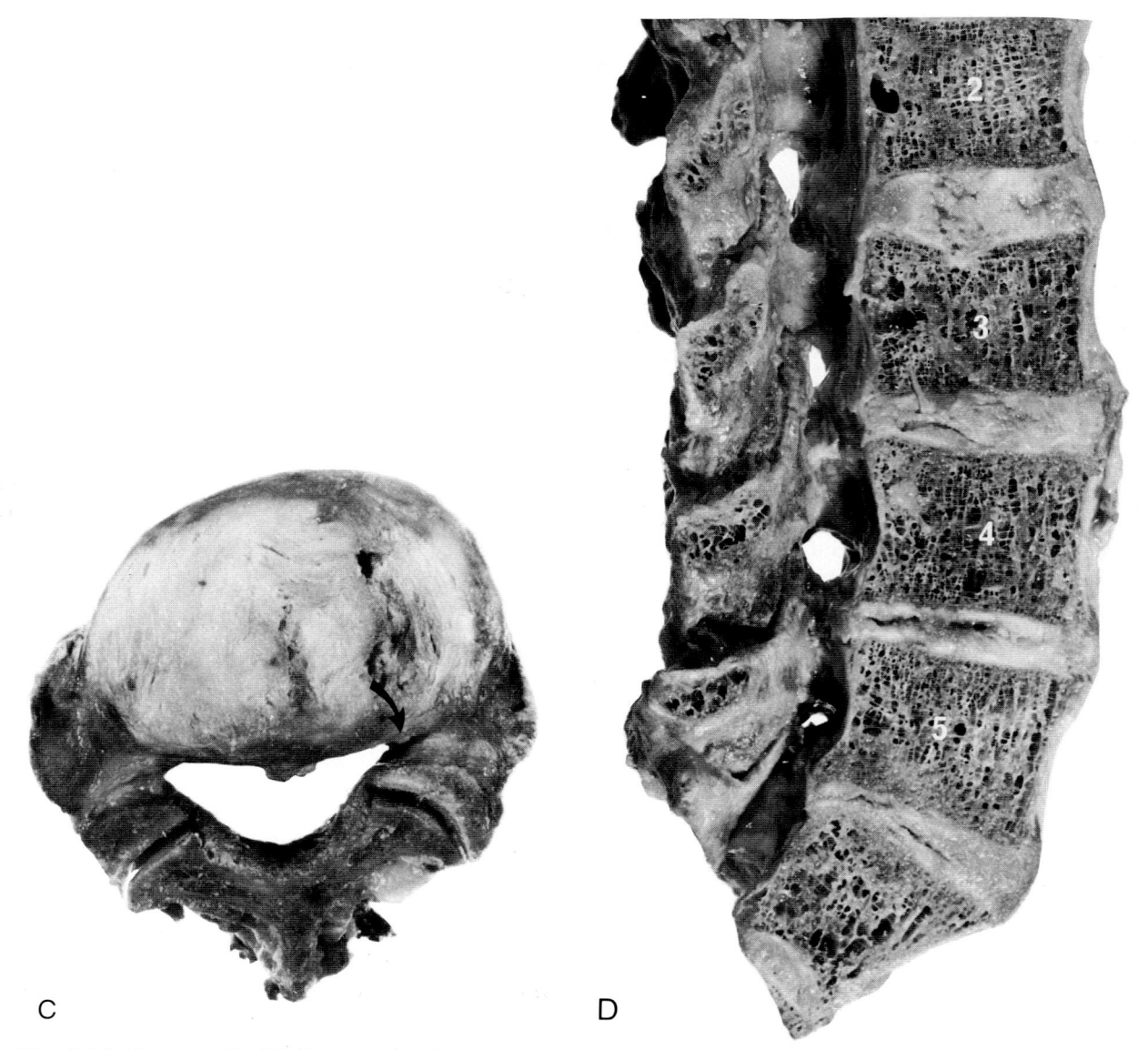

Fig. 3-10 (Continued). (C) Lesion of unknown origin. In macroscopic transverse section at the level of the L5–S1 disk, the vertebral body is asymmetrical in shape. The pedicle on the right (arrow) is shorter than that on the left. The left lamina is shorter than the right lamina. The changes may be developmental or may result from rotational trauma to the neural arch. (From Kirkaldy-Willis WH, Heithoff KB, Bowen CVA, Shannon R: Pathological anatomy of lumbar spondylosis and stenosis correlated with the CT Scan. Radiological evaluation of the Spine. Edited by Post MJD. New York, Masson, 1980.) (D) Sequential changes in the lumbar spine. Macroscopic sagittal section demonstrates an old fracture of the upper cartilage plate of L3 with herniation of the L2–3 nucleus pulposus into the body of L3 (a Schmorl's node). Early disk disruption is present at L3–4, and marked disruption at L4–5. At L5–S1 the disk has been resorbed. The L2–3, L3–4, and L5–S1 foramina are small.

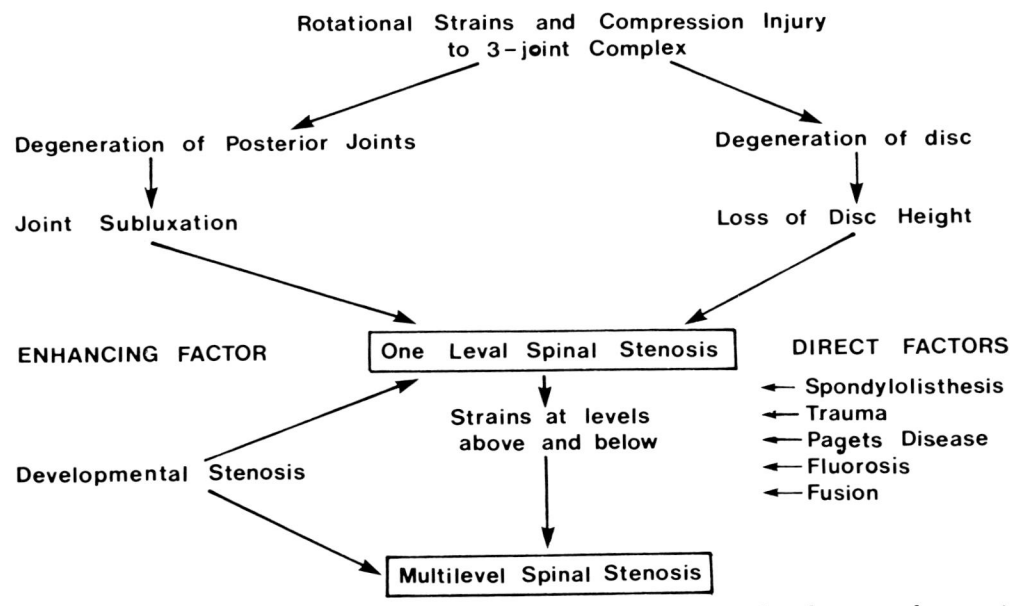

Fig. 3-11. Diagrammatic demonstration of how the enhancing factor (developmental stenosis) and direct factors (spondylolisthesis, trauma, Paget's disease, fluorosis, and spinal fusion) can cause spinal stenosis or supplement any underlying degenerative change.

REFERENCES

Pathology

1. Reilly J, Yong-Hing K, MacKay RW, Kirkaldy-Willis WH: Pathological anatomy of the lumbar spine, Disorders of the Lumbar Spine. Edited by Helfet AJ, Gruebel-Lee DM. Philadelphia, JB Lipincott, 1978
2. Kirkaldy-Willis WH, Wedge JH, Yong-Hing K, Reilly J: Pathology and pathogenesis of lumbar spondylosis and stenosis. Spine 3, No. 4: 319, 1978
3. Kirkaldy-Willis WH, Heithoff KB, Bowen CVA, Shannon R: Pathological anatomy of lumbar spondylosis and stenosis correlated with the CT scan, Radiologic Evaluation of the Spine. Edited by Post MJD. New York, Masson, 1980

Venous Hypertension

1. Arnoldi CC: Interosseous hypertension. Clin Orthop Related Res 115:30, 1976

4 The Perception of Pain

W. H. Kirkaldy-Willis

THE PROBLEM

The presenting symptom in nearly every patient with a mechanical or degenerative lesion in the lumbar spine is pain. Some patients have sensory or motor defects, in addition. It is important that the physician have some knowledge of the modern theory of pain and of how it can be applied to treat the patient.

All pain is real. We tend to think that when we can identify a lesion in the spine, the pain is "real" and that when we cannot do this, the pain is psychological. It is closer to the truth to say that in nearly all patients, pain has both psychological and physical aspects, that both are "real," and that sometimes one and sometimes the other predominates. At the present time, our knowledge of the way in which pain is perceived is mainly theoretical. Fortunately, we can use both fact and theory to alleviate a patient's pain.

It is reasonable for the clinician to enquire if the pain is mainly of physical origin, if it is chiefly of psychological origin (due to the personality of the patient), or if it results from a combination of physical and psychological causes.

Every patient with low back pain of physical origin undergoes a secondary change in personality. The patient with an acute low back strain or a disk herniation is under stress until the condition that produces the pain is resolved. This presents a relatively simple problem. Even here, the help of an experienced psychologist is often invaluable. The patient who has endured pain for months or years presents a much more difficult problem. This becomes still more difficult when the patient has had one, two, three, or more operations and still has pain. Each episode of pain and operative trauma affects not only the nerves supplying the joints and overlying muscles but also the entire nervous system and thus the entire personality of the patient.

Two further aspects of the problem must be considered. First, for psychological reasons the patient may present with a "chronic psychosomatic pain syndrome" that includes symptoms of low back pain among other symptoms. In this case the physician should seek help from the psychologist and allied personnel in a pain clinic. Second, as a result of long-standing back pain and several operations, the psychological and physical status of the patient may be so poor that it is beyond the power of the physician or surgeon to alleviate the pain. In this instance, it is better to tell the patient frankly that we are not clever enough to be of help. Assistance can be obtained from the psychologist, from the pain clinic, and sometimes, with careful selection, from neuro-augmentive surgery (see chapter 18).

THE GATE CONTROL THEORY OF PAIN

The Gate Control Theory was first propounded by Melzack and Wall in 1965.[1] It has since undergone some modification. Although still a theory it can be used in practice both to increase our understanding of the perception of pain, and to enable us to plan management of lesions of the lumbar spine in such a way that pain is inhibited.

Summation of Impulses

Pain is not perceived through direct stimulation of free nerve endings in the tissues supplied by small-diameter fibers that pass directly to a pain center in the brain. It is perceived because of the summation of impulses from both large(L)- and small(S)-diameter nerve fibers that activate transmission (T) cells in the dorsal horns of the spinal cord. When the threshold for pain is reached in the dorsal horn, impulses stimulate the T cells and this initiates the central transmission of pain (the action system). Impulses pass to the reticular formation in the brain stem, to the midbrain, and to the cerebral cortex, with resultant perception of pain. This summation of impulses may be accompanied by prolonged activity in the cells of the nervous system and by spread of pain to other body areas.

The Substantia Gelatinosa

The substantia gelatinosa (SG) is situated in the dorsal horns of the spinal cord. It contains cells that exert an inhibitory effect on the transmission of impulses leading to the perception of pain. Impulses passing along the large(L) fibers stimulate the SG cells and increase inhibition of pain. Impulses passing along the small(S) fibers decrease the inhibitory effect of the SG cells and facilitate central pain transmission.

The Gate

Activity in the SG cells closes or opens the gate. Impulses traveling along the L fibers close the gate. Those in the S fibers open the gate so that impulses that lead to pain perception can pass through.

Modulation of Pain Perception

The activity of the gate formed by the SG cells is modulated not only by impulses from the L and S fibers but also by descending feedback from the reticular system, the thalamus, and the cerebral cortex (Fig. 4-1).

PERIPHERAL MODULATION OF PAIN

Mechanoreceptors, encapsulated corpuscles supplied by large- and medium-sized nerve fibers, are found in the articular capsule, the ligaments, and the fat pads of the posterior joints. These fibers produce information about static joint position, pressure changes in the joints, joint movement (acceleration and deceleration), and stresses that develop in the joint at the extreme point of movement. We have already seen that stimulating L fibers tends to close the gate and inhibit pain perception.[4]

Pain receptors, free nerve endings and plexuses that are supplied by S fibers, are found in the articular capsule, the fat pads, the ligaments, and the walls of blood vessels. These receptors become activated by mechanical deformation of joint structures and by mechanical and chemical irritation. Stimulating the S fibers tends to open the gate and to enhance the perception of pain.

Inhibition of pain is increased by stimulating the mechanoreceptors (L fibers) in two ways: by movement and activity of muscles and joints and manipulation of the joints.

Pain is enhanced by inactivity and immobilization, by injury to peripheral nerves with loss of L fibers, and by degeneration of peripheral nerves with loss of L fibers.

The physician, therefore, can control pain considerably by therapy that promotes activity and movement. The tempo of such activity must not be so great that it produces pain. Manipulation tends to inhibit pain by stimulating the L fibers. On the other hand, immobilization either from inactivity or produced by segmental muscle hy-

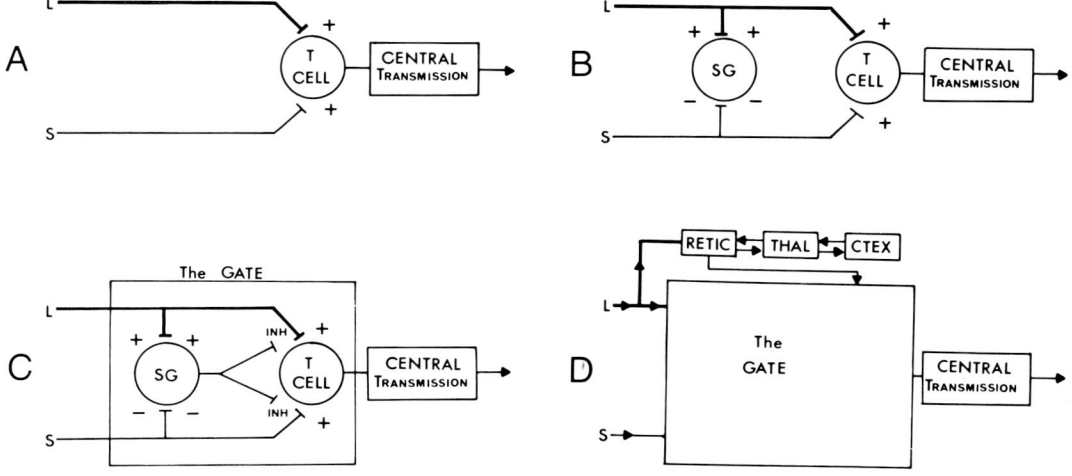

Fig. 4-1. The gate control theory (after Melzack and Wall). (A) Summation of impulses from large fibers (L) and small fibers (S). Excitatory effect (+) on transmission cell (T). (B) Addition of Substantia Gelatinosa (SG) cell. Impulses from large fibers (L) have an excitatory effect on the SG cell (+), whereas those from the small fibers (S) have an inhibitory effect (−). (C) Stimulating the SG cell produces an inhibitory effect (INH) on the T cell, and pain perception is decreased. (D) Impulses from large fibers (L) also ascend directly in the dorsal columns to the reticular formation (Retic), the thalamus (Thal), and the cerebral cortex (Ctex), which in turn feed back to modulate activity in the cells of the dorsal horn (the Gate).

pertonic contraction—often reflex to a posterior joint dysfunction—tends to enhance the perception of pain.

The painfree intervertebral three-joint complex is one in which normal movement and rhythm take place.

Treating a lesion of this complex necessitates a careful balance between activity and the avoidance of pain. As the lesion heals, the tempo of activity can be increased. Complete healing implies a return to normal activity and movement.

CENTRAL MODULATION OF PAIN

The reticular formation in the brain stem discharges impulses continually and exerts an inhibitory effect on pain by closing the gate in the SG via the reticulospinal tract. This inhibitory effect is augmented by the following:
1. Distracting attention from the site of pain
2. Concentrating on work or other activity
3. Sleep
4. Hypnosis
5. Emotional states that increase blood catecholamines
6. Drugs such as largactyl, valium, and morphine.

Reticular activity is depressed and pain is enhanced by (1) concentrating attention on the pain and (2) barbiturates.

The cerebral cortex regulates the activity of the reticular formation. Reticular activity is increased and the perception of pain is inhibited, via depression of cortical activity, by the following four factors: emotional tranquility, sleep, hyperventilation leading to hypocarbia, ingestion of large amounts of alcohol. The following emotions and substances depress reticular activity by increasing cortical activity: anxiety, uncertainty, and fear; Ingesting benzedrine, marijuana, and LSD; *small amounts of alcohol;* coffee and tea.

The Central Control Trigger. Melzack and Wall[1] postulate the existence of a central control trigger in the nervous system that activates the brain processes controlling the sensory input. In this way memory of previous experiences and response to pain impulses may affect the transmission of impulses from the action system.

The Central Biasing Mechanism. It is proposed that the reticular formation in the brain stem acts as a central biasing mechanism that exerts a tonic inhibitory influence on the transmission of impulses leading to pain perception at all levels. Thus, activity in the reticular formation tends to reduce pain perception.

Consideration of peripheral and central modulation of pain enables the physician to influence both the process of healing of a lumbar spine lesion and the inhibition of pain. The author is indebted to Leriche[2] for concepts expressed in his book *The Surgery of Pain,* to Melzack and Wall for their explanation of the Gate Control Theory of Pain[1] and to Sandoz[3] for his comments on reflex phenomena associated with spinal derangements and adjustments.

REFERRED PAIN AND RADICULAR PAIN

Referred pain is felt in an area far removed from the site of the lesion because the sensory pathways are distorted. MacKenzie proposed that continuous irritation of pain receptor systems in a particular tissue (i.e., posterior joint capsule) creates a state of hyperexcitability in related nerve cells in the dorsal horn of the spinal cord. Following this, afferent input from receptors in other segmentally related tissues gives rise to pain in these tissues. Referred pain from a lumbar posterior joint may be felt in the buttock, over the greater trochanter, down the back of the thigh to the knee, sometimes down the posterior or outer calf to the ankle, and rarely to the foot or toes. This type of pain can be reproduced by performing a posterior joint injection. When the tip of the needle reaches the joint capsule, the patient experiences pain, which varies greatly in its distribution from case to case. Referred pain is often associated with muscle hypertonus over the affected posterior joint. Peripheral tenderness to pressure over one or more distal areas in the limb may also be present.

Radicular pain is experienced in a dermatome, sclerotome, or myotome because of direct involvement of a lumbar spinal nerve. It is characterized by a detectable sensory, motor, or reflex deficit.

Clinically, these definitions are not always satisfactory because the diagnosis of referred pain is made by the exclusion of radicular pain. Leg pain in the absence of a neurological deficit is called referred. Leg pain in the presence of a neurological deficit is radicular. The difficulty arises in cases of early radicular pain when no neurological deficit has appeared as yet. Diminution of straight leg raising, a positive Lasegue test, a positive bowstring test, and tenderness over the sciatic notch are signs that suggest radicular involvement (see chapter 8). Relief of leg pain by infiltration of local anesthetic into the affected posterior joint indicates that the pain is referred.

The Arthrokinetic Reflex. A lesion in a posterior joint is often accompanied by sustained hypertonic contraction of overlying muscle. This hypertonus is segmental. It is secondary to the joint lesion, is mediated by an arthrokinetic reflex, and produces pain and tenderness in the muscle.

HOW THE PATIENT DESCRIBES PAIN

The Meaning of the Patient's Description. Much has been written about the way in which patients describe their pain. With the few exceptions discussed below, the writer has been disappointed at the lack of help obtained by asking the patient to describe the pain experienced. When pressed to describe the pain, the patient often replies, "I can't describe it but the pain that I have in my back and in my leg is unpleasant," or "makes my life miserable," or "is almost unbearable." The degree of pain felt seems more important than the kind of pain experienced.

Repeated Observation of the Patient. Repeated observation is essential and of great value to the physician. As the physician sees the patient on several occasions, he or she begins to sense the degree to which the patient is troubled by pain. Further help is obtained from the opinion of the psychologist (see chapter 6). Observing the way in which the patient responds to stress is also of value. The writer obtains a good deal of help from observing the reaction of the patient to a posterior joint injection (see chapter 8). It is only as the physician begins to know and understand the patient that he or she can assess the degree of pain of which the patient complains.

TYPES OF PAIN

Aching in the Legs. When the patient complains of leg pain, it is necessary to inquire whether this is in fact pain or aching. Aching in posterior thigh or calf is usually due to tightness of the hamstring or gastrocnemii muscles, a common feature of chronic low back pain, and is relieved by exercises to stretch these muscles.

Burning Pain. The distribution of this type of pain is often diffuse and vague. It does not usually conform to one or more dermatomes. It is sympathetic in origin. The sympathetic nervous system takes part in the innervation of the structures within the spinal canal via the recurrent nerve of Luschka and is stimulated in both arachnoiditis and postoperative fibrosis. The diffuse nature of the pain is due to the fact that sympathetic fibers run distally in the adventitia of the arteries rather than with the main nerves supplying the limb.

Unusual Sensations. In central spinal stenosis the blood supply to the nerves of the cauda equina is impaired. One result is the presence of abnormal sensations, bizarre in nature, that may affect the whole of one or both lower limbs. The patient may complain of an unpleasant feeling in the legs that is not pain but may be as disturbing as pain. He may say that the legs feel as though they do not belong to him. The legs may feel as though they are going to let the patient fall, they are made of rubber, or they were surrounded by a tight bandage. Before spinal stenosis was well recognized, the patient with these symptoms was thought to have a psychological problem. Now the presence of such abnormal sensations alerts the physician to the possibility of spinal stenosis.

THE APPRECIATION OF PAIN PERCEPTION

Pain perception takes place in four areas of the brain; the thalamus, the first level of perception; the postcentral cerebral cortex; the site at which the exact location and nature of pain is interpreted; the frontal cerebral cortex, the affective component—i.e., the area in which the experience of pain is associated with the site where it hurts—and the temporal cerebral cortex, the memory component—i.e., the site at which the memory of previous pain experience is stored.

As stated by Wyke,[4] pain is not a primary sensation such as vision or hearing but an abnormal emotional state produced by activating specific afferent pathways (the nociceptive system).

CONCLUSIONS

(1) Pain is a complex neurological phenomenon involving polysynaptic pathways that interact at several levels.
(2) Pain can be modulated both peripherally and centrally.
(3) The treatment of low back pain includes dealing with both the spinal lesion and the patient's pain.
(4) The physician can use his knowledge of the pain-modulating factors—peripheral, reticular, and cortical—to stimulate inhibition of pain.

REFERENCES

1. Melzack R, Wall PD: Pain mechanisms: a new theory. Science 150: 971, 1965
2. Leriche R: The Surgery of Pain. London, Ballière, Tindall, and Cox, 1939
3. Sandoz RW: Some reflex phenomena associated with spinal derangements and adjustments. Ann Swiss Chiropractors Assoc 7: 45, 1981
4. Wyke B: Neurological aspects of low back pain. The Lumbar Spine and Back Pain. Edited by Jayson M. New York, Grune & Stratton, 1976

Part II The Clinical Picture

5 Introduction

W. H. Kirkaldy-Willis

With the knowledge and understanding gained from the first part of this book we turn together now to consideration of the clinical picture. This is no easy task.

A SCIENTIFIC APPROACH

A nonscientific approach is all too common. It is tempting for the surgeon to say to himself, "This patient has a disk herniation, demonstrated by the myelogram or the CT scan. The lesion occupies space. An operation is required to remove the lump." Such an attitude is wrong for many reasons, in the first place because we know that 75% of disk herniations resolve and become symptom-free in 3 months with conservative care (Nachemson, personal communication). Another example—the surgeon reasons in this way. "This patient has had two disk explorations and a posterior fusion and still has severe low back pain. I will recommend an anterior-interbody fusion because I do not know what else to do and because a small percentage of such patients are relieved of their pain by this procedure."

There is no place in the management of low back pain for any approach other than one that starts by the physician using the most precise and scientific methods available to him. The approach should be as logical and well reasoned as possible.

The scientific approach demands the following of the physician or surgeon:
1. An exact and precise diagnosis of the clinical lesion
2. Knowledge of the nature, site, and level of the lesion
3. Assessment of the phase, Dysfunction, The Unstable Phase, or Stabilization, the framework in which the lesion occurs.
4. Understanding of the natural history of the disease process
5. Some comprehension of pathomechanics and pathology

The wise physician knows that in practice it is not always possible to be as scientific as he wishes to be. We make mistakes. We are often uncertain. This does not excuse us from failure to employ an outlook that is as highly scientific and factual as we can make it at this stage in our investigation (Table 5-1).

BEYOND SCIENCE

A Definition. We come to a point in our study of the patient at which perforce we are compelled to go beyond the realm of science into that of metaphysics. This means no more than that we

Table 5-1. Four Aspects of Diagnosis

Personality	Phase	Site and Nature of Lesion	Differential Diagnosis
The Past	Dysfunction	Posterior facets	Extrinsic lesions
Upbringing	Unstable	Sacroiliac joints	Congenital/developmental
Culture	Stabilization	Disk herniation	Trauma
Experiences		Lateral stenosis	Infections
The Present		Central stenosis	Rheumatoid
Intelligence		Spondylolisthesis	Neoplastic
Attitudes		Posterior muscles	Metabolic
Hopes, fears		Piriformis syndrome	Vascular
Satisfaction		Quadratus lumborum syndrome	
Resentment			
Disappointment			
Compensation			
Depression			
Hypochondriasis			
Hysteria			
The Future			
Goals			
Hopes			
Fears			

have to move into the realm beyond (meta)factual knowledge of the physical nature of things (physikos). The implication is that the physician moves on from the process of reasoning to one no less real but beyond and above that of reasoning with the mind. This is a natural transition but one that many of us fear to make.

The Early Stage. As we begin to give consideration to the personality of the patient suffering from low back pain, we are still in the realm of science. A psychological assessment starts by being scientific. It is nearly always qualitative rather than quantitative. As we try to measure the amount of the pain experienced we are mainly guessing.

The Metaphysical Realm. In their interaction the physician or surgeon and the patient soon move together into this realm. The transition takes place gradually but inexorably as the physician seeks to understand (1) the patient's past: his upbringing at home and at school, his cultural background, and any past experiences that color his reaction to pain; (2) what is going on in the patient's mind at the present time: his intelligence, his emotions, his hopes and fears, his satisfaction at home and at work, his feelings of resentment, his disappointments, his desire for compensation, his feelings of depression, and the presence or absence of hypochondriasis or hysteria; (3) the patient's attitude to the future: his goals, hopes, and fears.

The Effect of Personality on Pain Perception. The impact of personality has been considered to some extent in chapter 4. Each patient reacts differently to pain. Chronic pain has a marked and deep effect on every patient. The patient is not usually aware of this. During the course of several interviews the physician can begin to make a reasonable assessment.

Repeated Trauma and Multiple Operations. Each episode of trauma and each operation, in itself an episode of trauma, has profound effects on the patient's tolerance to pain. Recent research suggests that biochemical changes take place in the nervous system as a result of injury to a spinal nerve and that these extend far beyond the original site of trauma. It is likely that some of these reactions are mediated via the sympathetic nervous system.

The Process of Assessment. This process is initiated by the physician or surgeon. When managing a simple or straight-forward problem, he may well be able to complete the assessment of the patient's personality on his own. Simple measures render the patient free from pain in a short period of time. The patient's confidence is restored. With a little help he is back at home and at work and once again in the normal rhythm of life. In dealing with more complex or long-standing problems, help is sought from a psychologist who has an understanding of and interest in managing problems that arise in the patient with low back pain. This matter is dealt with in some detail in chapter 6.

It is essential that the physician and the psychologist sit down together to decide if the problem is mainly psychological and should be managed by the psychologist, if it is mainly physical and should be treated conservatively or by operation by the surgeon, or if it is a combined problem that requires help from both psychologist and surgeon. There are several other possibilities. (1) Objective data may clearly indicate that the results of an operation will be uncertain; nonetheless, sometimes it is right to take a chance and operate. (2) Surgery is maybe indicated from a physical standpoint, but for other reasons it appears unlikely to help the patient; in that case it is contraindicated. (3) The situation is so bad that the surgeon can do no more to help. The patient should be told this in a kindly, frank, and open way. (4) Neuro-augmentive surgery may offer a good chance of relief of pain. That subject is considered in chapter 18.

THE PHYSICIAN AND THE PATIENT

Rapport between physician and patient is built as a result of several interviews. During the course of these the physician tells the patient (1) what is wrong with his back, (2) how this can be put right, (3) the chances of success, (4) the problems and difficulties that lie ahead, and (5) what the future holds. Will the patient return to a normal home life? Will he be able to return to previous work? Will he need to look for lighter work?

Be Good to Your Back and It Will Be Good to You. It is essential for the patient to learn, through an understanding of his condition and through trust in his physician, to work first with the doctor and then on his own to complete the cure for himself. At some stage, and probably more than once, the physician needs to say, "I cannot cure your back pain. I can help you with advice, with various methods of treatment, possibly by an operation. It is up to you, with my help, to cure yourself. I and others will show you how to do this. But you yourself will have to make a big effort."

Referral to Another Physician. None of us should be reluctant to refer a patient to another physician (1) when the nature of the problem is beyond our particular knowledge and skill—not infrequently I refer patients to the pain clinic, the neurologist, or the rheumatologist; (2) when we realize that the patient is not satisfied with our management of his case; and (3) when it has not been possible to build the necessary rapport with the patient.

Kindness and Toughness. It goes without saying that patients with low back pain need a great deal of kindly and sympathetic understanding from their physician. When the patient is not making the necessary effort to help himself, it is kind to be tough. The patient sometimes needs to be told quite frankly that he will not improve until he makes an attempt to follow instructions given in the Back Class, to lose weight, and to do exercises regularly. The patient in this category who returns to the physician complaining that the pain is as bad as ever needs to be told, "Your back is no better because you have not followed my instructions. Go away and carry out what I've told you."

The Value of the Truth. Sometimes the physician has great difficulty in telling the truth to the patient. An example will make this clear. The patient with severe arachnoiditis needs to be told, "This is the serious nature of your trouble. I myself can do no more to help you. Another operation will only make things worse. It is possible that the doctor in the pain clinic can help you or refer you to someone else who can. You may well have to put up with pain for the rest of your life."

On other occasions, for example, when the patient, not really suffering much pain, has returned seeking more compensation, it gets the physician off the hook to say, "You are receiving a reasonable amount of compensation. I am sorry that I am not clever enough to be of any further help to you."

Make Haste Slowly. Except in dealing with a rare condition, such as a central disk herniation at L5–S1 in the presence of an acute chorda equina syndrome, it is never wise to rush to operation. Even when the surgeon considers that an operation will be necessary, it is wise to lead the patient slowly to this decision. The following approach is a good one, "I will try to help you without performing surgery. If at any time you feel that you cannot bear the pain any longer or that the treatment you are having is unbearable, tell me so, and if you ask me, I will be prepared to operate then." The onus of the decision is on the patient.

THE PATIENT'S RESOURCES

Each of us has resources for healing within the body. Every doctor is well aware of this but patients are often quite unconscious of this important fact. It is relatively easy for them to understand that the cells of the body are active in healing a cut finger or in fighting an infection. It is more difficult to get across to them that they have resources in the body to heal a lesion in the low back. For example, the patient who is contented and relaxed, who has confidence in the physician, and who can smile and laugh will get well more quickly than one who is anxious and afraid. An important part of the doctor's task is to help the patient to mobilize these inner resources. In doing this he may work with the patient himself, may seek help from the family and friends, may ask the psychologist for help, may get the social worker on the job, or when appropriate, talk to the minister, rabbi, or priest of the patient's church and ask for his help with the patient.[1]

THE PAIN DRAWING

Psychological assessment of the patient is considered at some length in chapter 6. It is not possible to do this type of assessment in more than a small percentage of patients.

Table 5-2. Scoring Sheet for Pain Drawing

Writing anywhere	1
Unphysiological pain pattern	1
Unphysiological sensory change	1
More than one type of pain	1
Both upper and lower areas of body involved	1
Markings outside body	1
Unspecified symbols	1

Score: 1 = Normal. 5 or more = Very bad.
Courtesy of L. L. Wiltse.

Pain Drawing. All patients are required to complete a pain drawing on their first visit to our clinic. The drawing can be done and assessed quickly. It gives a good deal of valuable information about both physical and psychological problems and enables the physician or surgeon to decide which patients should be referred for a full psychological assessment. The clinician uses the scoring sheet drawn up by Wiltse (personal communication) (Table 5-2).

The Posterior Joint Syndrome. Figure 5-1 is a pain drawing made by a patient with a posterior joint syndrome. The distribution of pain is characteristic. Only one type of pain is recorded. The score is 0.

The Sacroiliac Syndrome. Figure 5-2 is from a patient with the sacroiliac syndrome. Stabbing pain in buttock, posterior thigh, and groin is one characteristic picture for this condition. Numbness along the lateral calf is also recorded. The score is 1.

An L5–S1 Disk Herniation. Figure 5-3 gives the classical distribution of pain and numbness resulting from a herniation at the L5–S1 level. The score is 1.

The above pain drawings describe the distribution of pain from mechanical causes.

Pain of Mechanical and Psychological Origin. Figure 5-4 is a drawing made by a patient who 1 year previously had a diskotomy for an L5–S1 disk herniation. The pain pattern is not physiological; the sensory change is not physiological; more than one type of painful sensation is recorded; both the upper trunk and the legs are involved. The score is 4. The pain has a marked psychological overlay.

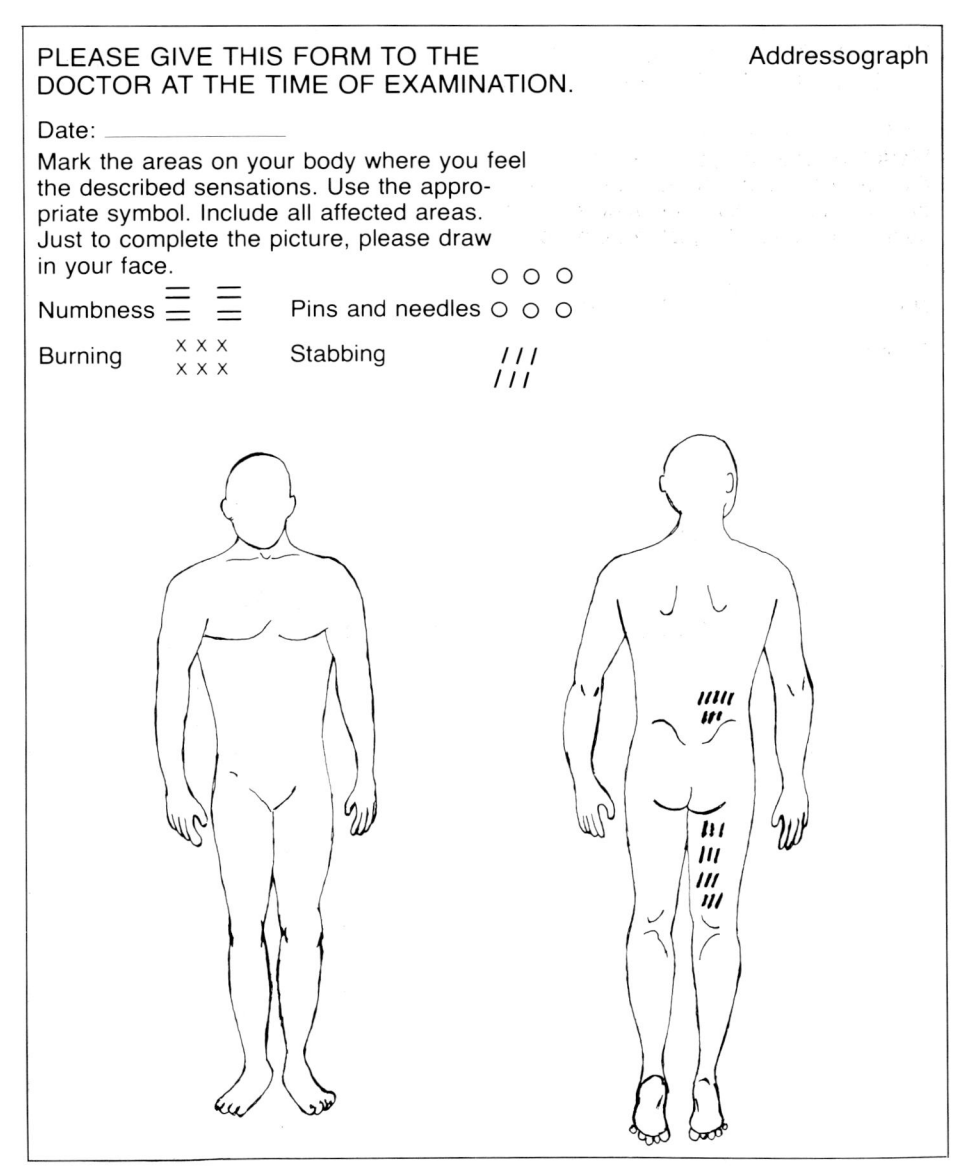

Fig. 5-1. Pain drawing by a patient with posterior joint syndrome. (After Mooney V and Robertson J: The facet syndrome. Clin Orthop 115: 149, 1976.)

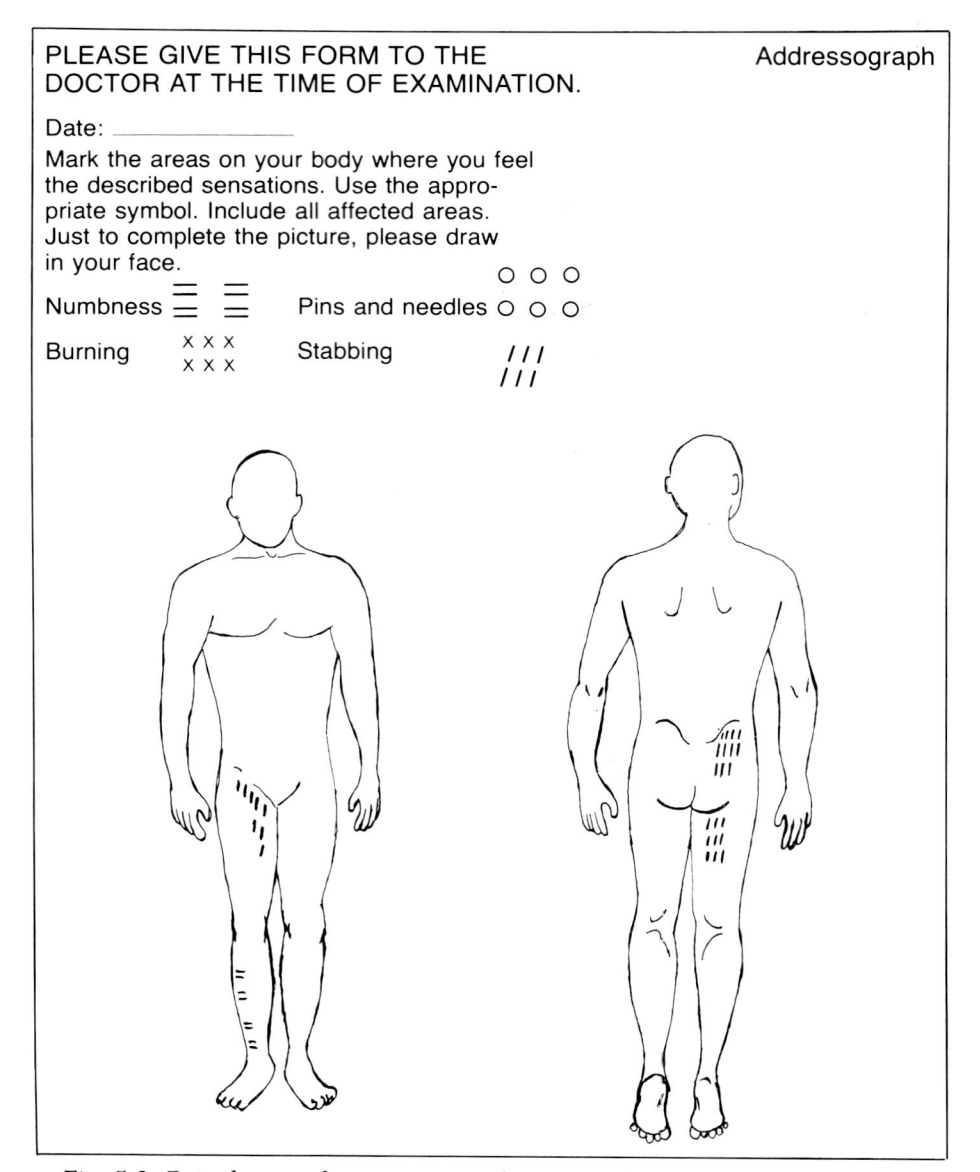

Fig. 5-2. Pain drawing by a patient with sacroiliac syndrome. (After Mooney V and Robertson J: The facet syndrome. Clin Orthop 115: 149, 1976.)

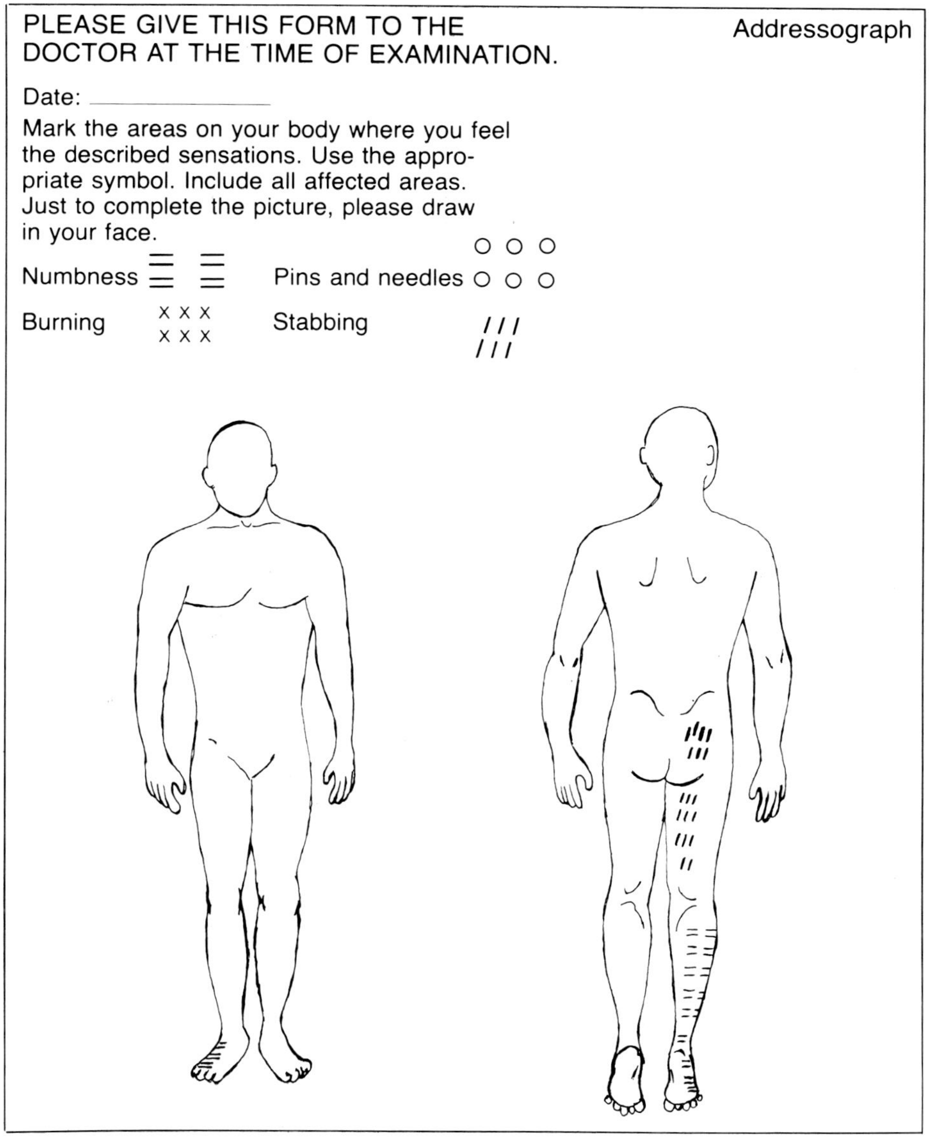

Fig. 5-3. Pain drawing by a patient with an L5–S1 disk herniation. (After Mooney V and Robertson J: The facet syndrome. Clin Orthop 115: 149, 1976.)

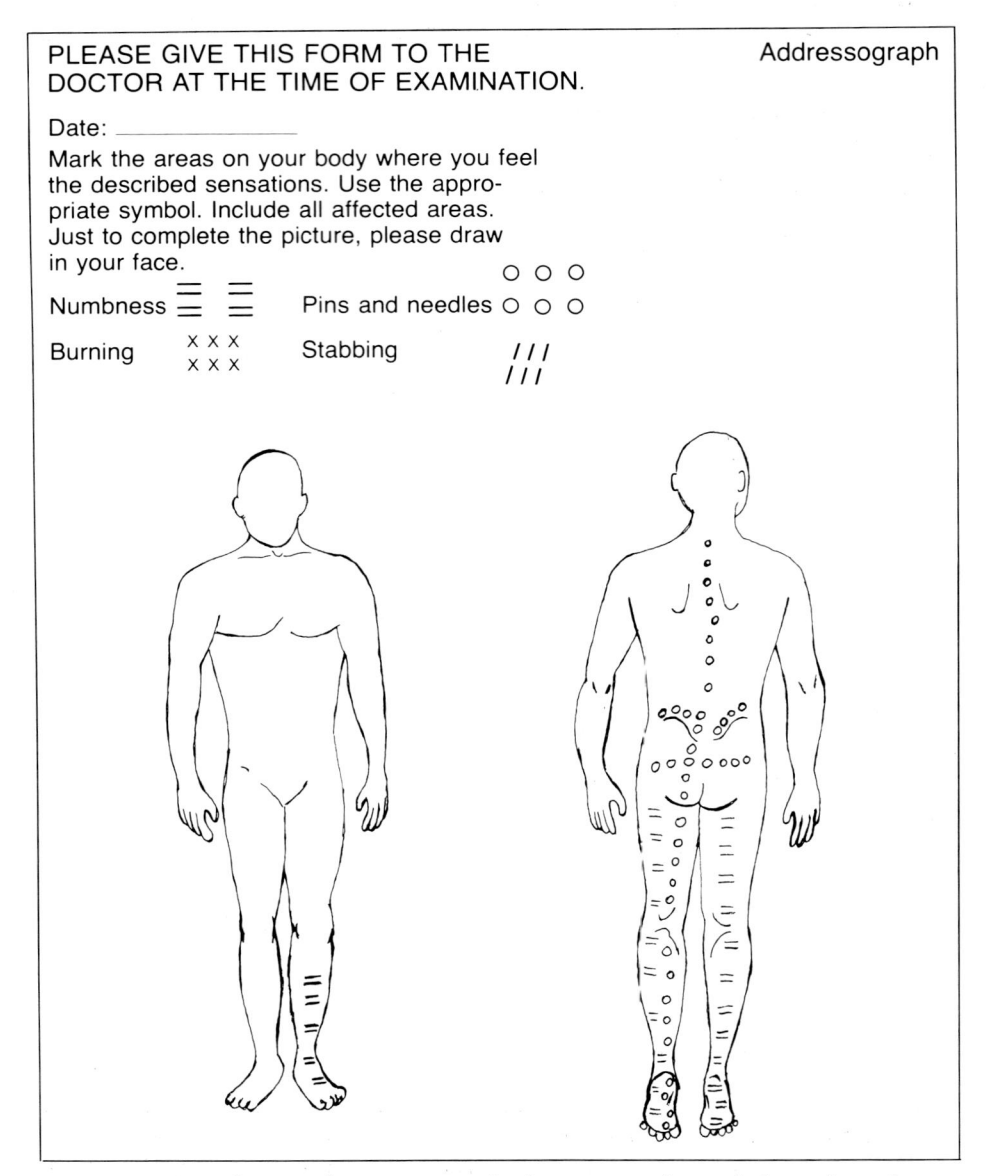

Fig. 5-4. Pain drawing by a patient who has pain with psychological overlay following a disk herniation. (After Mooney V and Robertson J: The facet syndrome. Clin Orthop 115: 149, 1976.)

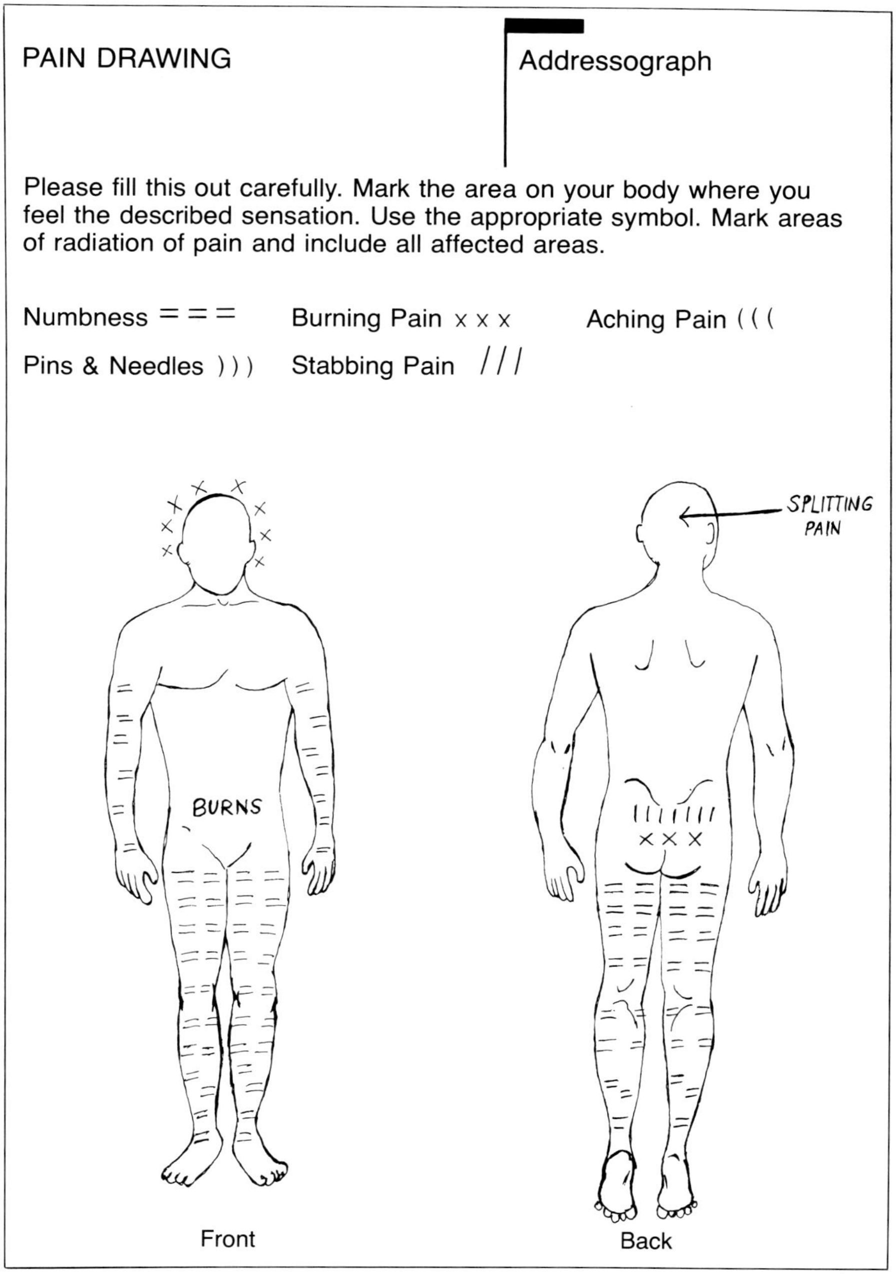

PAIN DRAWING

Addressograph

Please fill this out carefully. Mark the area on your body where you feel the described sensation. Use the appropriate symbol. Mark areas of radiation of pain and include all affected areas.

Numbness = = =   Burning Pain x x x   Aching Pain (((

Pins & Needles)))   Stabbing Pain / / /

SPLITTING PAIN

BURNS

Front   Back

Fig. 5-5. Pain drawing by a patient with symptoms that are almost entirely psychological in origin. (After Mooney V and Robertson J: The facet syndrome. Clin Orthop 115: 149, 1976.)

Pain of Psychological Origin. Figure 5-5 is a drawing by a patient whose symptoms are almost entirely psychological. The pain pattern and the sensory change are both nonphysiological. The chart contains writing. Both upper and lower limbs are involved. There are markings outside the body. The score is 5. The patient requires help from a psychologist in a pain clinic.

REFERENCES

1. Cassel EJ: The nature of suffering and the goals of medicine. New Engl J Med 306: 639, 1982
2. Mooney V, Robertson J: The facet syndrome. Clin Orthop 115: 149, 1976

6 Psychological Assessment

A. J. R. Cameron
L. F. Shepel

Psychological factors may markedly affect the way people experience and express pain.[1] The mounting evidence supporting this proposition has caused greater attention to be paid to the psychological assessment and management of pain patients.

Our objective in this chapter is to describe psychological assessment procedures that may be useful in evaluating patients with back pain. We have tried to describe our approach in concrete, practical terms in the hope that physicians and surgeons will find some useful suggestions for screening and referring patients, and develop a clearer understanding of how a psychologist might assess patients who are referred for evaluation.

THE PURPOSE OF THE PSYCHOLOGICAL ASSESSMENT

The purpose of the evaluation is to understand the patient's problem from a social and psychological perspective. Chronic back problems often result in secondary personal difficulties; conversely, psychological factors may give rise to or exacerbate complaints of pain and disability.[2] In the interests of formulating a sound, comprehensive treatment plan, it is useful to know how the back problem has affected the person's life or if psychological factors may be compounding the presenting complaint. *The ultimate objective, always, is to find ways to work with the patient or family to reduce distress and disability.*

Avoid Diagnostic Labels. Terms such as "hysterical," "hypochondriacal," and "regressed" often result in miscommunication, since their meaning is vague and they tend to engender negative perceptions of the patient and a sense of pessimism regarding the prognosis. Rather than falling back on such terms, it is important to identify as specifically as possible the environmental, behavioral, cognitive, and emotional factors that are relevant to the problem and its amelioration.

Distinguishing between "organic" and "functional" problems is of dubious value from the present point of view. Physical and psychological difficulties are not mutually exclusive. Nor can one type of difficulty be inferred from the presumed absence of the other. Regardless of the results of physical investigations, it seems prudent to try to understand what social or psychological difficulties (if any) exist, and how these might be resolved.

INDICATIONS FOR PSYCHOLOGICAL ASSESSMENT

In most settings it is neither feasible nor necessary to conduct a formal, complete psychological assessment of all patients who have back pain.

It seems reasonable to consider referral with patients who meet any of the following criteria:
1. Evidence of significant psychological distress (e.g., anxiety, depression, irritability)
2. Evidence of a stressful life situation; e.g., a major life change such as bereavement or occupational change or the presence of chronic tensions such as notable vocational or marital dissatisfaction
3. Complaints that appear disproportionate to organic findings
4. Social isolation
5. Evidence of drug abuse
6. A problem that is chronic or becoming so

Patients meeting one or more of these criteria may have complex problems and warrant careful evaluation including, perhaps, a referral for a formal psychological assessment.

THE REFERRAL PROCESS

The way the referral is conducted can dramatically affect the quality of the evaluation. Patients who are comfortable and confident about participating in the assessment are likely to be more candid than those who are defensive and wary. A careful referral process increases the probability that the patient will cooperate.

The basic problem is that pain patients quite understandably (and usually quite correctly) believe that their problems have a physical basis. The relevance of a psychological referral is unclear to the patient. So is its meaning. The patient may infer that the referring physician or surgeon believes that the problem is somehow less than real or that the patient is psychologically unstable. If so, the patient is almost certain to be quite guarded with the psychologist. The defensiveness may be expressed in the form of reticence, hostility, or a Pollyanna presentation, with the patient trying to project an image of robust psychological health by denying even mundane difficulties. The likely result is that the psychologist develops an incomplete or distorted view of the patient and his circumstances.

Clinical experience suggests that the following guidelines may help to circumvent or reduce defensiveness among patients who are referred to a psychologist.

1. Acknowledge the legitimacy of the problem. Patients are less likely to be defensive if they know that the referral does not imply that they are suspected of malingering or exaggerating. They may be reassured by unequivocal recognition that the pain is considered real. It is usually easy for physicians to give this reassurance, and for patients to accept it, when there are significant physical findings. The credibility of the verbal reassurance may be enhanced if the psychological referral is scheduled concurrently with ongoing physical investigations.

Potential problems arise when complaints seem disproportionate to organic findings. Even then, reassurance that the physician recognizes the genuine distress of the patient appears to be in order in most instances. For these patients usually do appear to be experiencing pain, whatever the origin. In any case, since we lack both objective measures of pain and a definitive understanding of pain mechanisms, the patient's self-report cannot be dismissed lightly regardless of hard findings.

2. Provide a positive rationale for the referral. If the patient misconstrues the psychologist as an adversary who is likely to discredit him or his problem, it is difficult for the psychologist to win his confidence. It is important that the psychologist be introduced as an ally who is concerned with finding solutions to problems rather than with passing judgment on the patient or the problem. For instance, if surgery is planned, it might be noted that to ensure the best possible result, it is important to investigate secondary difficulties that may have arisen because of the pain and to make sure that they are understood and dealt with appropriately. If surgery is not contemplated, the psychologist may be presented as someone who is often able to help patients find ways to ease discomfort and reestablish normal activities. The rationale should be honest and positive, should reflect respect for the legitimacy of the problem, and should make sense to the patient.

3. Inform other staff members of the general rationale. Persons other than the referring doctor often influence the patient's perception of the psychological referral. Skeptical patients may ask different clinical and clerical staff members about the consultation. If everyone offers a similar reassuring rationale, the patient is likely to be put at ease. But if explanations conflict or some staff members seem uncomfortable or evasive (because they don't know how to respond), the patient may become increasingly wary. It is therefore helpful if all staff members who have contact with patients are prepared to discuss the referral with the patient in an informed, matter-of-fact, reassuring way.

4. Let the patient know that the referral is routine. In some settings, psychological evaluations are routine. If the assessment is routine, the patient may be reassured by knowing this. Of course, if the referral is not at all routine, the patient should not be misled into believing it is: such deception is not only distasteful but is also readily detected through conversations with other patients and staff and may undermine trust. For the same reason, a statement that the referral is routine should be qualified as appropriate (e.g., "I routinely refer patients who have longstanding, perplexing problems like yours to make sure we don't overlook anything that might be helpful.")

5. Personalize discussion of the referral. Personalized discussion can both help to explain the referral and contribute to a comfortable, friendly tone. Three types of personalized comments may be useful.

First, the referring doctor might talk in a hypothetical way about his or her own probable reactions to a problem similar to the patient's. For instance, in suggesting that chronic pain often creates secondary personal problems, the doctor might say something like this: "A problem like you've been living with almost always wears a person down. I know that if I had to live with the sort of difficulty you've had, for as long as you've had it, it would certainly create a strain and take a toll." This sort of statement may help to normalize psychological or interpersonal problems associated with pain.

Second, the psychologist may be described in a personal way. Apprehensions may be reduced if the psychologist can be described as a helpful, friendly sort of person. (It is to be hoped that the psychologist has *some* redeeming personal qualities that can be mentioned!) If most patients have found that they enjoyed their contacts with the psychologist, it wouldn't hurt to note that.

Third, it may help to describe briefly specific instances in which the psychologist was able to assist people who had problems similar to that of the patient. If it's convenient, or if a patient is especially wary, it may also be useful to arrange for the patient to talk with previous patients who benefitted from working with the psychologist.

6. Make it clear that the referral does not imply a transfer. If patients mistakenly believe that they are being "dumped," they are likely to be resentful. They may have a more positive attitude toward the psychological assessment if they understand clearly that the physician or surgeon will continue to arrange any further tests or consultations required to ensure a thorough physical investigation, and maintain contact and review the patient's records regularly to monitor developments and progress.

STRUCTURED TESTS AND QUESTIONNAIRES

Minnesota Multiphasic Personality Inventory (MMPI)

The MMPI is the psychological test most commonly used to assess pain patients. It consists of some 550 true/false questions and yields scores on 10 clinical scales. Although all scales may be diagnostically useful, scales 1 and 3—also known as the Hypochondriasis (Hs) and Hysteria (Hy) scales, respectively—are particularly noteworthy. A high score on scale 1 indicates that the patient has reported experiencing a wide range of somatic complaints involving various physical functions and body areas. A high score on scale 3 results when the patient has reported some combination of physical complaints, superior adjustment, and sadness and lack of satisfaction with life.[3]

The MMPI as a Predictor of Treatment Response. High pretreatment scores on MMPI scales 1 and 3 have been associated with poor response to surgical procedures[4-6] and conservative treatment[7] (only scale 1 scores were predictive in the latter study). Pretreatment scores on a number of MMPI scales have been found to correlate with response to anesthesiologic and psychiatric interventions.[8] Results of these studies suggest that the MMPI may be useful in helping to identify patients who have a poor prognosis in response to a variety of common treatments.

A Note of Caution in Using the MMPI. It is prudent to use the MMPI cautiously. In some studies, no significant relationship was found between pretreatment MMPI scores and response to surgical[9] and rehabilitative[10] treatment. Moreover, in studies where a statistically significant association has been found between MMPI scores and treatment response, the relationship has sometimes been so modest as to be of limited clinical value.[5] As a final caveat, it is noteworthy that empirical study of the "Low Back Pain" and "Dorsal" scales (derived from the MMPI) has raised serious doubts about the validity of these particular scales.[11-13]

Practical Issues in Using the MMPI. There are practical as well as empirical grounds for using the MMPI judiciously. Patients sometimes resent taking the test. Some are overwhelmed by its length. (Although preliminary evidence suggests that shorter versions of the MMPI may be useful for assessing back patients,[14] additional investigations, especially prospective treatment outcome studies, are required to evaluate the predictive validity of these abbreviated tests.) Other patients object to the MMPI because, as a general psychiatric screening test, it includes questions about serious psychiatric symptoms that are usually irrelevant to the patient's situation; these questions may imply that the assessor believes the patient to have gross psychological problems. Still other patients are offended at being asked to spend time answering questions that may seem trivial, intrusive, or redundant.

Hence, the test must be introduced in a sensitive way so that negative reactions are minimized or circumvented. Part of the introduction may emphasize that the test helps us understand in a more precise way how the patient is feeling both physically and psychologically. We often note, for instance, that depression is common among people with chronic pain and that the test provides a standardized way of measuring the degree of depression. If the patient seems to resent a psychological evaluation, it may be best to omit the MMPI or to postpone it until rapport is established.

Serious misinterpretation of test results may occur. *The profile must be interpreted by someone familiar with MMPI interpretation and current MMPI research.*

The MMPI as a Gross Screening Instrument. Elevations on scales 1 and 3 have been associated with less favorable response to common treatments, as noted above. Our evaluation of patients who have t-scores greater than 70 on either of these scales, or whose test profile is otherwise abnormal, is especially thorough. We assume that these people may be at above-average risk for poor response to physical treatments and we want to ensure that from a psychological point of view everything possible is done to secure a good outcome.

McGill Pain Questionnaire

The McGill questionnaire was developed by Melzack[15] to provide detailed information about both the intensity and the quality of pain. The central part of the questionnaire (Fig. 6-1) lists three classes of adjectives that may be used to describe pain: *sensory* adjectives focus on temporal, spatial, pressure, thermal, and other sensory qualities; *affective* adjectives refer to the emotional (tension, fear) and autonomic properties of the experience; *evaluative* words allow the patient to report the overall subjective intensity of the total pain experience.

The questionnaire yields scores (described in Melzack's paper) that provide a number of quantitative indexes of the patient's discomfort. These may be useful both for monitoring progress and for understanding in a more fine-grained way what the patient is experiencing.

THE INTERVIEW

The MMPI and other structured tests may help to identify patients whose problems are complicated by psychological factors. But they provide little information about what might be done to

What Does Your Pain Feel Like?

Some of the words I will read to you describe your *present* pain. Tell me which words best describe it. Leave out any word-group that is not suitable. Use only a single word in each appropriate group—the one that applies *best*.

1	2	3	4
1 Flickering	1 Jumping	1 Pricking	1 Sharp
2 Quivering	2 Flashing	2 Boring	2 Cutting
3 Pulsing	3 Shooting	3 Drilling	3 Lacerating
4 Throbbing		4 Stabbing	
5 Beating		5 Lancinating	
6 Pounding			

5	6	7	8
1 Pinching	1 Tugging	1 Hot	1 Tingling
2 Pressing	2 Pulling	2 Burning	2 Itchy
3 Gnawing	3 Wrenching	3 Scalding	3 Smarting
4 Cramping		4 Searing	4 Stinging
5 Crushing			

9	10	11	12
1 Dull	1 Tender	1 Tiring	1 Sickening
2 Sore	2 Taut	2 Exhausting	2 Suffocating
3 Hurting	3 Rasping		
4 Aching	4 Splitting		
5 Heavy			

13	14	15	16
1 Fearful	1 Punishing	1 Wretched	1 Annoying
2 Frightful	2 Gruelling	2 Blinding	2 Troublesome
3 Terrifying	3 Cruel		3 Miserable
	4 Vicious		4 Intense
	5 Killing		5 Unbearable

17	18	19	20
1 Spreading	1 Tight	1 Cool	1 Nagging
2 Radiating	2 Numb	2 Cold	2 Nauseating
3 Penetrating	3 Drawing	3 Freezing	3 Agonizing
4 Piercing	4 Squeezing		4 Dreadful
	5 Tearing		5 Torturing

Fig. 6-1. Adjective checklist section of the McGill Pain Questionnaire. Reprinted by permission of the publisher from Melzack R: The McGill Pain Questionnaire: major properties and scoring methods. Pain 1: 277, 1975 by Elsevier Science Publishing Company Inc.

resolve the problem. Information required to formulate a treatment plan is obtained by interviewing and observing the patient and, if possible, the family. We shall discuss interviewing and behavioral observations separately, although they may overlap considerably.

During the interview we try to get a *general* picture of patients and their circumstances. We want to know what their day-to-day lives are like, who are the significant people in their lives and what sort of relationships they have with them, what interests them, what they worry about, how they see themselves and others, what important experiences they've had, and what sorts of things they would like to accomplish in life.

We also want to get a very *specific* picture of the pain problem, and we'll limit the present discussion to this aspect of the interview. By the time the interview is complete, we want to know as much as we can about (1) the history of the problem from the point of view of the patient, (2) situational fluctuations in pain, (3) secondary problems that have arisen because of the pain, (4) how the patient expresses pain, (5) how others react to the patient's pain and disability, (6) what effect the patient believes the problem is having on others,

(7) if the patient derives important benefits from having pain and disability, (8) how the patient thinks about the problem, (9) patterns of medication use, (10) the patient's mood, (11) what the patient has tried to do to alleviate the pain, and (12) if the patient would have any interest in working with a psychologist. We'll comment briefly on each of these issues in turn.

Problem History. Beginning the interview by asking about the history of the problem helps put patients at ease by allowing them to start with material that is usually well rehearsed and not emotionally charged. It also helps to establish a clear sense that we are interested in focusing on the pain problem and its resolution and are not conducting a psychiatrically oriented interview.

It is important to note discrepancies between the patent's report and the written record. Misunderstandings may give rise to unnecessary worry. We also note comments the patient makes about care received in the past; this information clarifies the patient's preferences and may therefore enable current staff to relate to the patient more effectively. Complaints or concerns about current care are solicited and the patient is encouraged to let us know if we are doing things that are annoying.

Situational Fluctuations. Under what conditions is the pain better or worse? What activities or situations are avoided because of pain? Under what circumstances is the pain either reduced or largely ignored because of compelling diversions? Has the patient explored ways to minimize the impact of situations that trigger pain (e.g., by experimenting with different positions if sexual intercourse is painful)?

Most patients report that pain fluctuates with activity. Few indicate spontaneously that pain varies with mood or stress. To elicit such information we note that many patients find that their mood affects their ability to tolerate pain, and we encourage the patient to discuss fluctuations in *pain tolerance* as a function of mood or external stresses. We are careful to avoid implying that the negative mood or stress is the presumed primary cause of the pain.

Secondary Problems. "What effects has the pain had on you and your relationships?" This open-ended question helps to establish which effects are most salient for the patient. Common problems include difficulties at work (including household chores), sleep disturbance, tension (irritability, "bad nerves"), depression, strained family relationships, financial worries, disruption of sexual interest and activities, and restriction of recreational pursuits. If the patient omits any of these areas, we make specific inquiries.

Problems attributed to pain are explored in detail to determine if they are in fact secondary problems. It is crucial to know, for instance, how things were before the pain began. This is diagnostically significant since one might expect secondary problems to dissipate spontaneously in many (though not all) cases if the back problem can be resolved. However, if the patient attributes an independent problem (e.g., chronic relationship difficulties, primary depression) to the back problem, one would not expect this "secondary" problem to be relieved through physical treatment.

Expression of Pain. Pain may be expressed in many ways. These include verbal reporting, complaining, crying, taking medication, sighing, grimacing, reclining, rubbing the affected area, limping, and inactivity. It is useful to know how the patient expresses pain and how patterns of expression vary across situations.

The way the patient expresses pain may have either adaptive or maladaptive consequences. For instance, a person who attempts to be stoical and inhibit any acknowledgment of pain may be seen as inexplicably "moody" by others: in this case, letting others know about the problem may help to avoid misunderstanding and strained relationships. Conversely, a patient who exhibits persistent, theatrical pain displays may elicit resentment and/or excessive nurturance that undermines the patient's independence. If a person must live with a chronic or recurrent problem, the quality of the person's life will be determined to a considerable extent by the adaptiveness of the pain expression.

Reactions of Others. Ideally, families and co-workers should make necessary allowances for the patient's pain and disability while doing everything possible to encourage independence and normal activities. Difficulties arise if others become (1) resentful, impatient, and antagonistic; (2) excessively solicitous in a way that keeps attention focussed on the pain and discourages independence; or (3) overbearing or condescending in encouraging the patient's progress. Many patients are reluctant to say negative things about the significant people in their lives, and sensitivity is required to elicit candid information.

Effects of the Problem on Others. Does the patient's back problem create serious difficulties for others? Patients sometimes have a sense of guilt that their problem causes hardship for others. Their specific concerns may or may not be realistic. If they are unfounded, it is important to clarify this. If it appears that others are indeed affected as adversely as the patient imagines, attention can be focussed on attempting to reduce these problems.

Benefits from Pain. Patients may receive psychological or financial benefits from pain or disability. Such benefits can represent impediments to rehabilitation. However, identification of payoffs for pain is a difficult, complex process.

The basic diagnostic problem stems from the fact that back problems almost always result in some life changes that *could* be construed as beneficial from the patient's point of view. For instance, back problems commonly result in sympathetic attention, decreased vocational responsibility, and financial compensation. Even people who normally get all the attention they want, sincerely enjoy their work, and are unquestionably highly motivated to get back to normal find themselves receiving such "benefits." Hence the simple observation that the presenting problem results in "benefits" does not justify a conclusion that the patient is relying on the back problem to secure psychological or financial advantages.

On the other hand, it would seem naive to overlook the possibility that such benefits might undermine the patient's response to treatment. It seems prudent to investigate very carefully those patients who have been dissatisfied with their work or personal lives. The person who has been dissatisfied but has lacked the skill or courage to make changes may discover that the back problem makes it possible to alter or avoid unpleasant vocational or personal situations.

To say that the symptoms may be yielding important benefits does not necessarily imply that the patient is deliberately manipulative. Consider, for instance, a man who has felt progressively inadequate in his work and in his sexual relationship. He develops a back problem and finds that he has a legitimate reason to avoid both work and sex. This man may be less likely to resume work and sexual activity on his own initiative than another patient who has the same organic problem but who thrives on his work and thoroughly enjoys sexual relations. It is not that the first man consciously decides to keep complaining of pain to avoid stressful activities; he is just less likely than the second man to disregard continuing discomfort, because he lacks the zest for living that pulls the second man back into a normal routine.

In a situation like this, a key diagnostic task is to determine the feasibility of helping the patient find solutions to the background problems. If our hypothetical man is able to find ways to improve vocational satisfaction and to establish a gratifying, comfortable sexual relationship with his wife, one would expect his prognosis to be improved.

The Patient's Thoughts about the Problem. The way the patient thinks about the problem may influence the degree of subjective discomfort and "pain behavior." We try to get an idea of the extent to which the patient is *preoccupied* with pain and related problems. A number of indicators suggest preoccupation. Patients may acknowledge that the problem is so bad that they often have difficulty getting their minds off it. Or they may demonstrate preoccupation by continually bringing conversations back to their complaints. Elevation on MMPI scale 1 and evidence that the patient's life is largely devoid of satisfying, absorbing activities suggest indirectly that preoccupation may be a problem.

It is also instructive to notice how patients *label* their pain. There is evidence that the same aversive stimulus may be experienced as more or less painful depending on how it has been labeled.[16] It seems plausible to hypothesize that patients who have developed a habit of regularly thinking and talking about their pain as "excruciating," "unbearable," etc., may thereby exacerbate their discomfort. This is not to deny that some pain is indeed excruciatingly intense but merely to suggest that loose usage of such extreme labels may magnify perceptions of the pain.

Finally, we try to determine if patients have

specific *fears or misconceptions.* Fears of cancer and progressive degenerative conditions are the most common fears we see in patients with back pain. Such fears may be engendered or intensified by diagnostic investigations: patients going for tests in Nuclear Medicine, for instance, have sometimes inferred that a diagnosis of cancer was being considered.

Patients with catastrophic fears may be reluctant to voice them. They may be inhibited by a foreboding sense that a feared diagnosis will be confirmed if investigated or by a concern about appearing hypochondriacal. If patients are simply asked what they think is causing their pain, they often merely repeat opinions of physicians as if these opinions are their own. And, indeed, they may genuinely believe that these explanations are rational. However, this does not necessarily mean that they do not at the same time harbor fears that something more sinister is wrong. To overcome inhibitions about reporting catastrophic fears, it may be useful to say something like this: "Sometimes the people we see have private fears about what is wrong with them. If you have any nagging fears in the back of your mind, even fears you've hesitated to express because you know they're probably groundless, it's important that we know about them. Some of the people who come to us have been worrying needlessly for a long time and have found it helpful to bring their concerns out in the open so they could be discussed with the doctors on our team."

Medication Use. It is important to identify patients who are overusing analgesic medications. We also explore the use of psychotropic drugs. Some patients take substantial amounts of either analgesics or psychoactive drugs in response to problems (e.g., irritability, tension, depression, insomnia) that may be relieved, partially if not wholly, through psychological means.

Mood. Pain patients are sometimes depressed. Although the relationship between pain and depression is not clearly understood and is undoubtedly complex, it has been suggested that pain sometimes may be a manifestation of "atypical" or "masked" depression.[17-19] A recent study revealed that pain patients (most had back pain) were more likely than controls both to be diagnosed as depressed and to have a family history of depressive disorders.[20] Among pain patients with no demonstrable physical pathology, 30% were both diagnosed as depressed and found to have a family history of depression. Although this was a small study (20 pain patients) and interviews were not conducted blind, it suggests that depression may be a central problem of some patients presenting with pain. There has been speculation that pathophysiological changes associated with depression might contribute to the development of back problems.[21] Whether a primary or secondary problem, depression may require direct treatment.

The diagnosis of depression is described in detail elsewhere.[22] In brief, it is noteworthy that some patients who deny depression are manifestly depressed according to psychiatric criteria; conversely, not all who describe themselves as depressed would be diagnosed as clinically depressed using the same criteria. Therefore, it is hazardous to rely solely on the patient's self-reported mood (although this is obviously important) in assessing depression. Other commonly used indicators of depression include elevation on scale 2 (Depression) of the MMPI and psychiatric criteria; the following list of indicators is abbreviated from the Research Diagnostic Criteria for Major Depressive Disorders:[23]

1. Increased or poor appetite; weight gain or loss (change of at least .5 kg/week for several weeks or 4.5 kg/year, not dieting)
2. Sleep difficulty, including too much
3. Reduced energy, tiredness
4. Psychomotor retardation or agitation
5. Loss of interest or pleasure in sex, social contact, or other usual activities
6. Self-reproach, excessive guilt
7. Diminished capacity to concentrate or think—e.g., indecisiveness, slowed thinking
8. Recurring thoughts of death or suicide; any suicidal behavior

Full psychiatric diagnostic criteria are described by Spitzer and his colleagues.[23]

In addition to assessing depression, it is important to consider the extent to which the person may be experiencing stress or anxiety. Patients may report being anxious (edgy, jumpy, nervous, highstrung, worried, etc.), experiencing chronic tensions, or undergoing major adjustments in their lives. Physical agitation or evidence of notable muscle tension is also noteworthy.

It is assumed that negative mood reduces pain tolerance. Depression and anxiety may also contribute directly to the sense of subjective distress that the patient labels pain.

The Patient's Attempt to Cope with Pain. Most patients attempt to reduce their pain and attendant problems in a variety of ways. It is informative to explore the range of strategies they use. Some have extensive repertoires of coping behaviors, while others rely almost wholly on activity restriction, medication, and medical or chiropractic treatments. It is important to identify patients who lack personal strategies for reducing discomfort and instances where patients may have prematurely given up a potentially useful strategy; e.g., some patients report unsuccessful attempts at self-relaxation (see chapter 17), but inquiry suggests that training in or application of relaxation procedures is inadequate.

Interest in Working with a Psychologist. Not all patients whom we think might benefit from working with a psychologist are prepared to do so. Practical restrictions or personal reservations that would preclude psychological treatment need to be investigated before such treatment is recommended.

Interviewing the Family. Whenever possible, interviews with family members or others who know the patient well are conducted with the patient's knowledge and permission. It is easier for others to provide independent opinions and points of view if they are interviewed alone. We solicit their observations and impressions regarding the problem and its effect on both the patient and other family members. Apparent discrepancies between accounts given by the patient and others need to be explored carefully; it can be misleading to discount either version out of hand.

BEHAVIORAL DATA

Specific information about the patient's behavior patterns is extremely informative. Fordyce[24] has published a number of very simple record forms that yield detailed information about the patient's activity level (Fig. 6-2). Developing a treatment plan and monitoring treatment progress may be greatly facilitated by having patients maintain such records during evaluation periods.

Behavioral tests may be undertaken to establish the patient's tolerance for normal activities. For example, if a patient complains that walking is painful, it is helpful to determine exactly how long or how far the person can walk under various conditions (e.g., walking continuously, pausing for brief rests). This information is of practical value for planning a treatment program, establishing concrete treatment goals and evaluating treatment progress.

Simple behavioral experiments may also be conducted to examine the extent to which the patient's pain-related behaviors are responsive to environmental changes. For instance, the patient's expressions of pain might be monitored during staff-initiated conversations that focus on pleasant topics having nothing to do with the patient's distress. If one can show that pain expression is reliably less frequent under the influence of such commonly available distracting activities, it suggests that the patient might benefit from a treatment plan that promotes increased involvement in diverting activities. In an analogous way, it is possible to conduct similar experiments designed to identify environmental factors (e.g., conversations focusing on pain, disability, and hardships) that may increase pain expression in order to pinpoint conditions that the patient and family should attempt to reduce (e.g., unnecessary conversations about pain). Evidence that pain expression fluctuates depending on such environmental shifts does not, of course, rule out an organic basis for the problem.

Fordyce's book[24] presents an extended discussion of the behavioral analysis of pain problems and includes many valuable practical clinical suggestions.

THE UPSHOT OF THE ASSESSMENT

It would be nice if psychologists could predict with confidence each patient's response to surgery or other physical treatments. Unfortunately, that is not possible. The results of the psychological

Please check each day which of the activities listed you engaged in.

Week of _____ , 19 ____

	MON	TUES	WED	THURS	FRI	SAT	SUN
1. VISITING							
Came to visit:							
Relative(s)							√
Others	√						
None							
Went out to visit:							
Relative(s)						√	
Others							
None							
2. OUTSIDE HOME TRIPS							
Sight-seeing excursion			√				
Movie, ballgame, concert, etc.							
Attended meeting							
Shopping					√		
Other							
None							
3. INSIDE HOME ACTIVITIES							
Calls made to relative(s) friends/neighbors				√			
Calls you received from relatives, friends, neighbors					√	√	
Reading							
Television							
Radio/records/tape							
Hobbies/handicrafts		√					
Others							
None							
4. WALKING QUOTA	√	√	√	√	√	√	√

Fig. 6-2. Activity diary. Adapted with permission of the publisher from Fordyce W: Behavioral Methods for Chronic Pain and Illness. St Louis, CV Mosby, 1976.

assessment may influence one's general level of optimism or pessimism about probable response to treatment. The MMPI research for instance, provides some evidence that gross predictions may be possible in at least some settings. But precise predictions are hazardous: some patients who seem to be high risks from a psychological point of view respond well; others whose cases seem straightforward have disappointing outcomes. The psychologist's findings may be taken into account by a surgeon who has to make a judgment about whether or not to proceed with surgery. But it is hard to imagine a case where surgery would be withheld on psychological grounds in the face of compelling physical indications for an operation.

In practice, we find our post-assessment discussions with the surgeon most valuable in formulating a treatment plan. These meetings provide an opportunity to integrate information and to develop a treatment strategy and rationale that can be shared with the patient.

If there is evidence of psychological difficulty, an appropriate treatment plan is formulated (in consultation with other members of the team) and presented to the patient for consideration. Common psychological treatment strategies are considered in chapter 17. In cases where indications for surgery are also present, the goal of the psychological treatment is to maximize the probability of a good surgical result. In the absence of remarkable physical findings, the goal is to do everything possible to resolve psychological difficulties, subjective discomfort, and physical disability in the hope that this, coupled with other rehabilitative efforts, will improve the quality of the patient's life and reduce distress.

ACKNOWLEDGMENT

We are grateful to Myles Genest, Donald Meichenbaum, Barr Taylor, Dennis Turk, and Carl von Baeyer for comments on previous drafts of this material.

REFERENCES

1. Melzack R: The Puzzle of Pain. Harmondsworth, Penguin, 1973
2. Mersky H, Boyd D: Emotional adjustment and chronic pain. Pain 5: 173, 1978
3. Marks PA, Seeman W: Actuarial Description of Abnormal Personality. Baltimore, Williams & Wilkins, 1963
4. Blumetti AE, Modesti LM: Psychological predictors of success or failure of surgical intervention for intractable back pain, Advances in Pain Research and Therapy, Vol. 1. Edited by Bonica JJ, Albe-Fessard D. New York, Raven Press, 1976
5. Pheasant HC, Gilbert D, Goldfarb J, Herron L: The MMPI as a predictor of outcome in low-back surgery. Spine 4: 78, 1979
6. Wiltse LL, Rocchio PD: Preoperative psychological tests as predictors of success of chemonucleolysis in the treatment of the low-back syndrome. J Bone Joint Surg 57A: 478, 1975
7. McCreary C, Turner J, Dawson E: The MMPI as a predictor of response to conservative treatment for low back pain. J Clin Psychol 35: 278, 1979
8. Strassberg DS, Reimherr F, Ward M, et al: The MMPI and chronic pain. J Consulting Clin Psychol 49: 220, 1981
9. Waring EM, Weisz GM, Bailey SI: Predictive factors in the treatment of low back pain by surgical intervention, Advances in Pain Research and Therapy, Vol. 1. Edited by Bonica JJ, Albe-Fessard D. New York, Raven Press, 1976
10. Cummings C, Evanski PM, Debenedetti MJ, et al: Use of the MMPI to predict outcome of treatment for chronic pain, Advances in Pain Research and Therapy, Vol. 3. Edited by Bonica JJ, New York, Raven Press, 1979
11. Rosen JC, Frymoyer JW, Clements JH: A further look at validity of the MMPI with low back patients. J Clin Psychol 36: 994, 1980
12. Towne WS, Tsushima WT: The use of the Low Back and Dorsal scales in the identification of functional low back patients. J Clin Psychol 34: 88, 1978
13. Tsushima WT, Towne WS: Clinical limitations of the Low Back scale. J Clin Psychol 35: 306, 1979
14. Turner J, McCreary C: Short forms of the MMPI with back pain patients. J Consulting Clin Psychol 46: 354, 1978
15. Melzack T: The McGill Pain Questionnaire: major properties and scoring methods. Pain 1: 277, 1975
16. Hall KRL, Stride E: The varying response to pain in psychiatric disorders. Br J Med Psychol 27: 48, 1954
17. Blumer D. Heilbronn M, Pedraza E, et al: New treatment of chronic pain with antidepressants. Presented at the 132nd Annual Meeting of the American Psychiatric Association, Chicago, IL, May 12–18, 1979
18. Engel GL: Psychogenic pain and the pain prone patient. Am J Med 26: 899, 1959
19. Lopez-Ibor JJ: Masked depressions. Br J Psychiatr 120: 245, 1972
20. Schaffer CB, Donlon PT, Bittle RM: Chronic pain and depression: a clinical and family history survey. Am J Psychiatr 137: 118, 1980
21. Levine ME: Depression, back pain, and disc protrusion: relationships and proposed psychophysiological mechanisms. Dis Nerv System 32: 41, 1971
22. Lewinsohn PM, Lee WML: Assessment of affective disorders, Behavioral Assessment of Adult Disorders. Edited by Barlow DH. New York, Guilford, 1981
23. Spitzer RL, Endicott J, Robins E: Research diagnostic criteria: rationale and reliability. Arch Gen Psychiatr 35: 773, 1978
24. Fordyce WE: Behavioral Methods for Chronic Pain and Illness. St Louis, CV Mosby, 1976

7 The Three Phases of the Spectrum of Degenerative Disease

W. H. Kirkaldy-Willis

The three phases of the degenerative process—Dysfunction, the Unstable Phase, Stabilization—are schematized in Figure 7-1. For clarity these three are separated into well-defined horizontal bars. In fact no such clear-cut distinction between them exists. The patient may pass gradually from one phase to the next. Following a recurrent episode of trauma the patient may pass from Dysfunction to the Unstable Phase. During recovery he may pass back to Dysfunction. As seen in chapter 1, the tendency over a period of years is that the patient's symptoms increase so that he passes from Dysfunction to the Unstable Phase and on to Stabilization, but this does not invariably occur.

DYSFUNCTION

The majority of patients seen in a low-back-pain clinic suffer from Dysfunction. During this phase the pathological changes are relatively minor and perhaps reversible. For this reason such changes are more difficult to demonstrate. The term Dysfunction implies that at one anatomic level (usually L4–5 or L5–S1) the three components of the joint are not functioning normally. The early pathological changes in the posterior facet joints and the disk are described and illustrated in chapter 3. Following injury these changes produce symptoms as discussed below. After recovery from injury the symptoms may cease. Further injury results in reappearance of symptoms.

Presentation

The presentation varies considerably. For convenience it can be divided into three types: rotational or compressive strain, sometimes due to a major but more often to a minor episode of trauma; pain that occurs after activity that is unusual for the patient—an example is the sedentary worker who gardens vigorously all weekend in early summer and some hours or 1 to 2 days later complains of severe low back pain of sudden onset for no clear reason; and recurrence of pain due to a very minor episode of trauma.

Mechanisms

The mechanisms involved are shown in Figure 7-2, a scheme modified from that of Paris.[7] The episode of trauma results in posterior joint (and annular) strain. Because of small capsular (and annular) tears, a small degree of joint subluxation takes place. The posterior joint synovium is injured, leading to synovitis. The posterior segmental muscles protect the joint by sustained hypertonic contraction. The muscle becomes ischemic and this causes more pain. Accumulation of metabolites in muscle further aggravates the pain

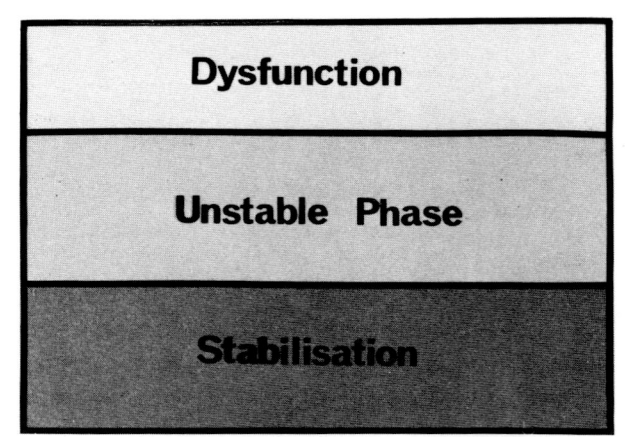

Fig. 7-1. The three stages (phases) of the degenerative process.

and sustains the hypertonic state of contraction. The posterior joints continue to be splinted and the minor subluxation is maintained. These changes later lead to fibrosis.

Symptoms

The symptoms are those of acute, subacute, or chronic low back pain. Pain is often localized to one area and to one side. Pain may be referred to the groin, to the region of the greater trochanter, and to the posterior thigh as far as the knee; it rarely passes below the knee. The pain is relieved by rest and made worse by movement. One or more particular movements "catch" the patient and aggravate the pain.

Signs

There are multiple signs. Tenderness to pressure is present, usually on one side and at one level over the sacrospinalis and multifidus muscle. The muscle at this site is in a state of sustained contraction (hypertonic). Lateral bending is abnormal; i.e., the patient bends more to one side than to the other (hypomobility). Muscle activity is abnormal. For example, normally the muscle on the right contracts when the patient bends to the left; however, this pattern may be altered. All movements are restricted, especially extension. Some degree of functional scoliosis, seen more clearly on forward flexion, may be present.

Palpation at the level of the lesion may demonstrate that one spinous process is out of line with the next.

Radiographic Changes

Anteroposterior stress radiographs demonstrate several abnormalities. Movement is decreased asymmetrically; i.e., the spine bends more to one side than to the other. The spinous processes may be out of line at one level. Normally, when the spine is bent laterally, the spinous processes rotate slightly to the side of bending. In Dysfunction the spinous processes may not move (rotate) to the side to which the patient has bent. Normally, with lateral bending the disk height is reduced on the concave side. In Dysfunction the space on the concave side may remain open.

Oblique views may show irregularity of posterior facets.

Lateral stress radiographs are rarely abnormal. In longstanding dysfunction they may reveal that small osteophytes are present at the anterior surface of the vertebral bodies and that the disk is slightly reduced in height. Figure 7-3 demonstrates radiographic changes seen in the anteroposterior view. Figure 7-3A shows a high riding

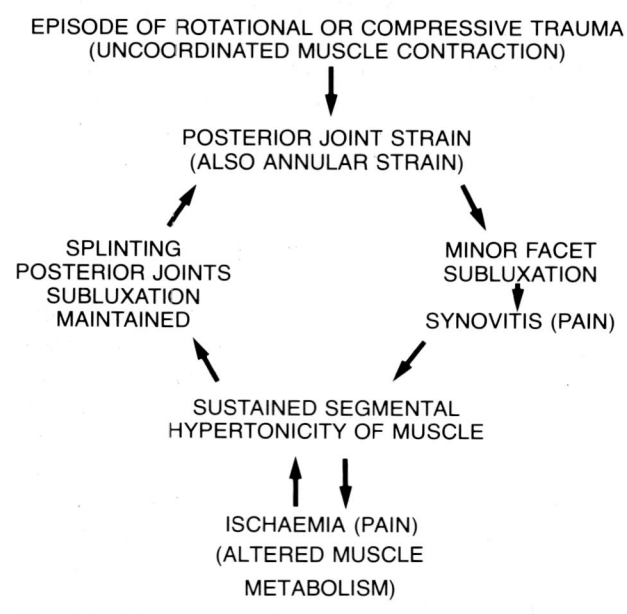

Fig. 7-2. Mechanics of Dysfunction. (Courtesy of S. V. Paris.)

The Three Phases of Degenerative Disease 77

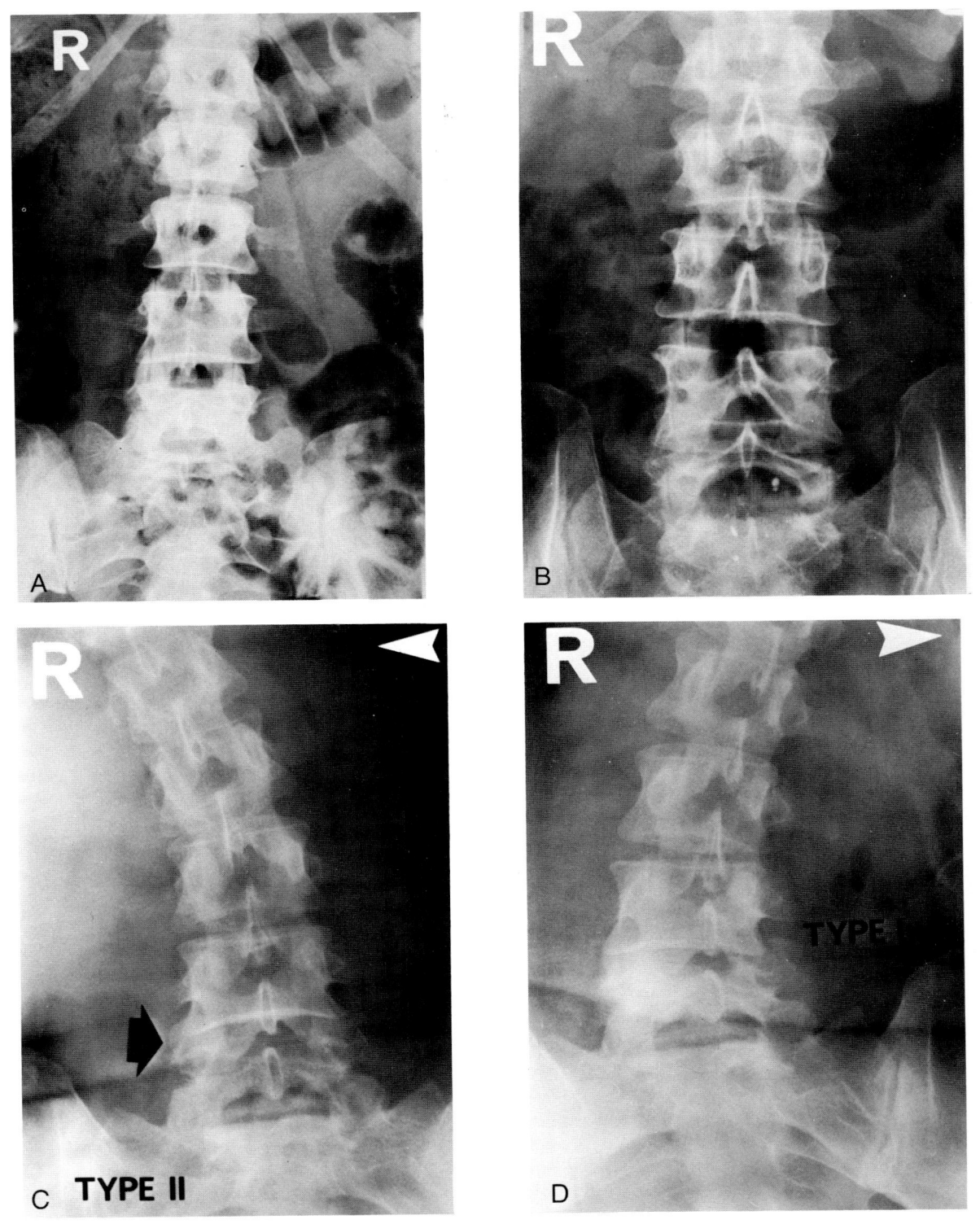

Fig. 7-3. (A) through (D). (Figure continues.)

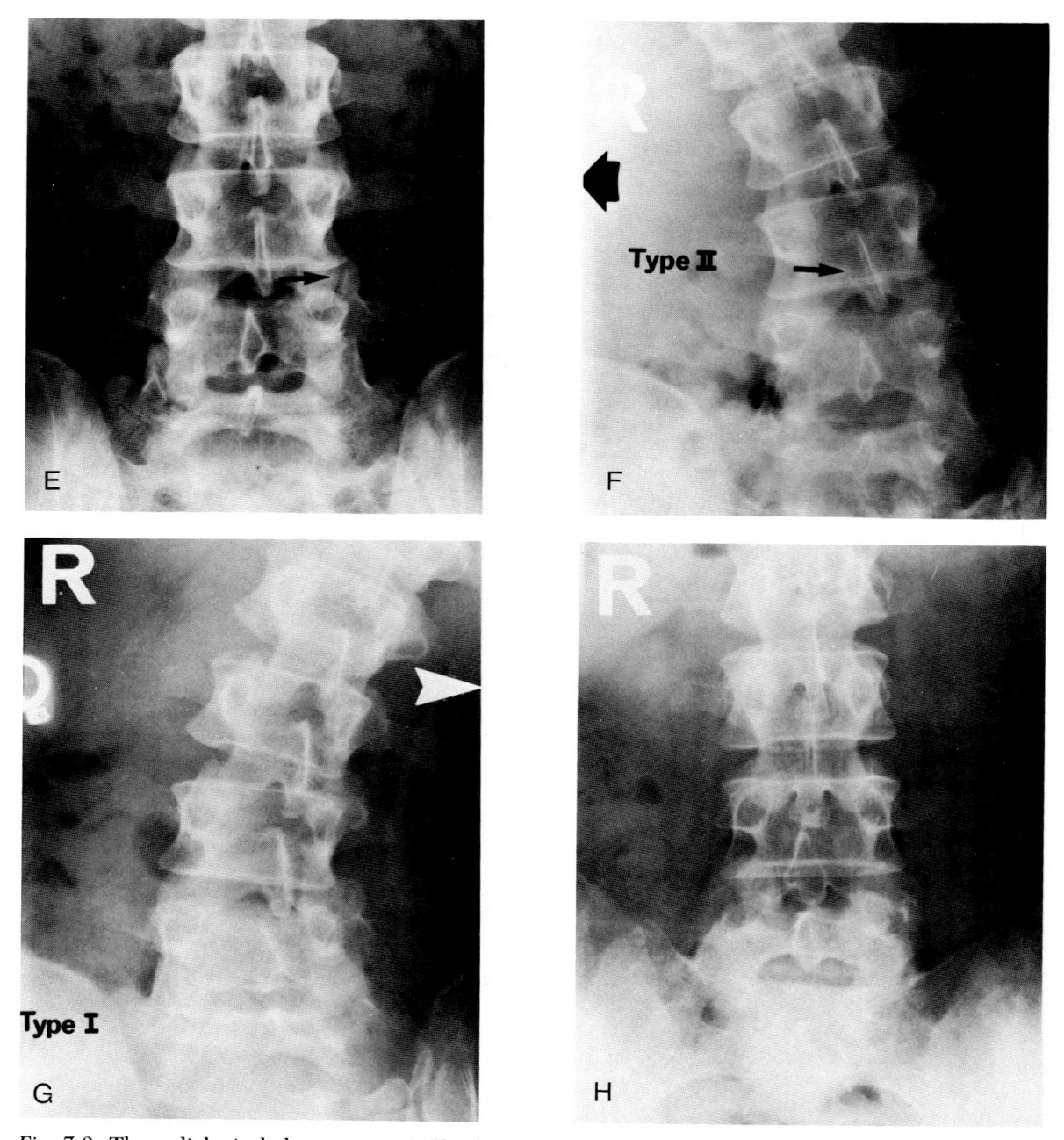

Fig. 7-3. The radiological changes seen in Dysfunction. (A) The L5 vertebra rides high. The intercrestal line passes through the middle of the L5 body. The L5–S1 joint is at risk. (B) The L5 vertebra is low in the pelvis. The intercrestal line passes through the upper part of the L4 body. The L4–5 joint is at risk. (C) When the spine is bent laterally to the right the spinous processes do not move in that direction. This lack of movement is characteristic of a Type II change (Dysfunction). (D) Radiograph from the same patient as in (C). When the spine is bent laterally to the left, the spinous processes move to the left. Such movement is normal and is called a Type I movement. (E) Standing erect (AP) view. The L4 spinous process (opposite the arrow) is to the left of that of L5. This indicates Dysfunction with rotation. (F) The same patient as in (E). When the spine is bent laterally to the right, the spinous process fails to move to the right. The L4 and L5 processes are malaligned. Dysfunction is confirmed. (G) The same patient as in (E) and (F). When the spine is bent laterally to the left, the spinous processes move normally to the left. They are normally aligned. (H) Standing erect AP view. L4 vertebra is slightly tilted on L5. (*Figure continues.*)

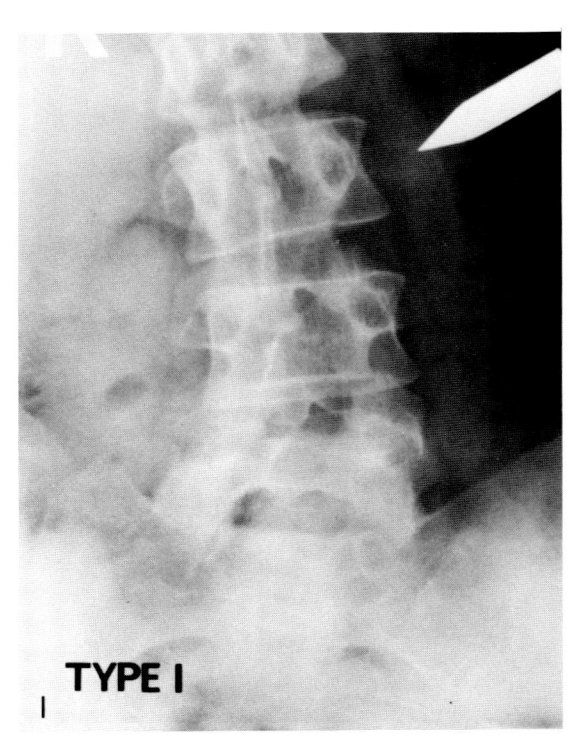

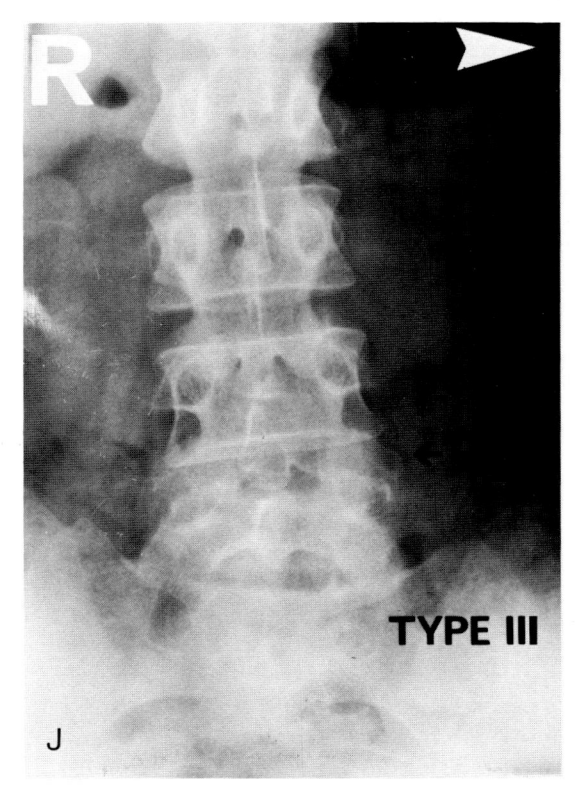

Fig. 7-3 (Continued). (I) The same patient as in (H). On lateral bending to the right the spinous processes moves to the right in a normal way (Type I). (J) The same patient as in (H) and (I). On attempted lateral bending to the left, the spine remains erect. The disk space opens on the left, a Type III change indicative of marked dysfunction.

L5 vertebra with the L5–S1 level at risk. Figure 7-3B shows a low riding L5 vertebra with the L4–5 level at risk. In normal lateral bending the disk closes on the concave side and the whole spine rotates so that the spinous processes shift to the concave side (Type I). During Dysfunction hypertonic muscles restrict rotation as the spine bends to the opposite side and may progress to the point at which the disk fails to close or even opens on the opposite side. Malalignment of spinous processes suggests rotational deformity, which can be confirmed by lateral bending views. These changes are demonstrated in Figures 7-3C through J. Table 7-1 sets out in tabular form the symptoms, signs, and radiographic changes found in Dysfunction.

Two problems arise. First, as we have seen in

Table 7-1. The Symptoms, Signs, and Radiological Changes Seen in Dysfunction

Symptoms
  Low back pain
    Often localized
    Sometimes referred
  Movement painful
Signs
  Local tenderness
  Muscle contracted
  Hypomobility
  Extension painful
  Neurological exam usually normal
Radiographs
  Abnormal decreased movement
  Spinous processes malaligned
  Irregular facets
  Early disk changes

discussing the pathology of low back pain (chapter 3), changes affecting the facet joints also affect the disk and vice versa. In Dysfunction the changes chiefly affect the facet joints, but small annular tears are also present. Sometimes a disk herniation is present as well. Therefore it is necessary to exclude this condition. This point will be discussed as we turn to consider herniation of the nucleus pulposus. Second, dysfunction at one level may complicate the Unstable Phase at another, usually lower, level as the lesion spreads to involve more than the original level.

THE UNSTABLE PHASE

With each successive episode of trauma, healing of capsular tears of the posterior joint and annular tears of the disk is less complete because the collagen of scar tissue is not as strong as normal collagen. The three parts of the joint complex are thus increasingly at risk. Early in Phase I the patient is more likely to develop recurrent Dysfunction. Toward the end of this phase it becomes likely that the patient will pass into Phase II. Throughout Phase II there is a tendency for the problem to recur and on each occasion the instability becomes more marked.

Presentation

The presentation may either be similar to that described above for Dysfunction or chronic and insidious without any recorded history of minor trauma.

Mechanisms

The mechanisms involved are twofold: a further episode of trauma and continuing stress. Either or both of these result in increased dysfunction. Progressive changes seen in the facet joints are degeneration of cartilage, stretching or attenuation of the capsule, and laxity of the capsule. Changes in the disk are coalescence of tears, loss of nuclear substance with internal disruption, and bulging of the annulus around the circumference of the disk. The result is detectable increased abnormal movement in the three-joint complex. The patient has entered the Unstable Phase (Fig. 7-4).

Symptoms

The symptoms may be no more than those seen in severe Dysfunction. The patient may complain that his back feels weak, that it feels as though it is going to give way, or that certain movements, coming upright again after bending forwards, produce a "catch" in his back.

Signs

The signs are twofold. Increased abnormal movement between one vertebra and the next may be detected by inspecting or palpating the spinous processes when the patient moves or lies on one side. A "catch," a sway, or a shift at one level may be observed as the patient returns to the standing position after bending forward. The patient may not be able to do this without supporting himself by placing his hands on knees or thighs.[2]

Radiographic Changes

Changes seen on X-ray confirm the diagnosis. Anteroposterior lateral bending radiographs may show that one vertebral body shifts to one side on the body below it—usually L4 or L5—and/or that a spinous process rotates on the one below, resulting in malalignment. This malalignment may be reduced on flexion to one side and increased on flexion to the other. One body may tilt abnormally on another.

Oblique views may demonstrate that the facet joints have opened and are malaligned.

Lateral radiographs in both flexion and extension frequently show increased movement. In degenerative spondylolisthesis the upper vertebra moves forward on the lower in flexion (because of erosion of the superior facets) and back toward the normal position in extension. More commonly a small degree of retrospondylolisthesis seen in

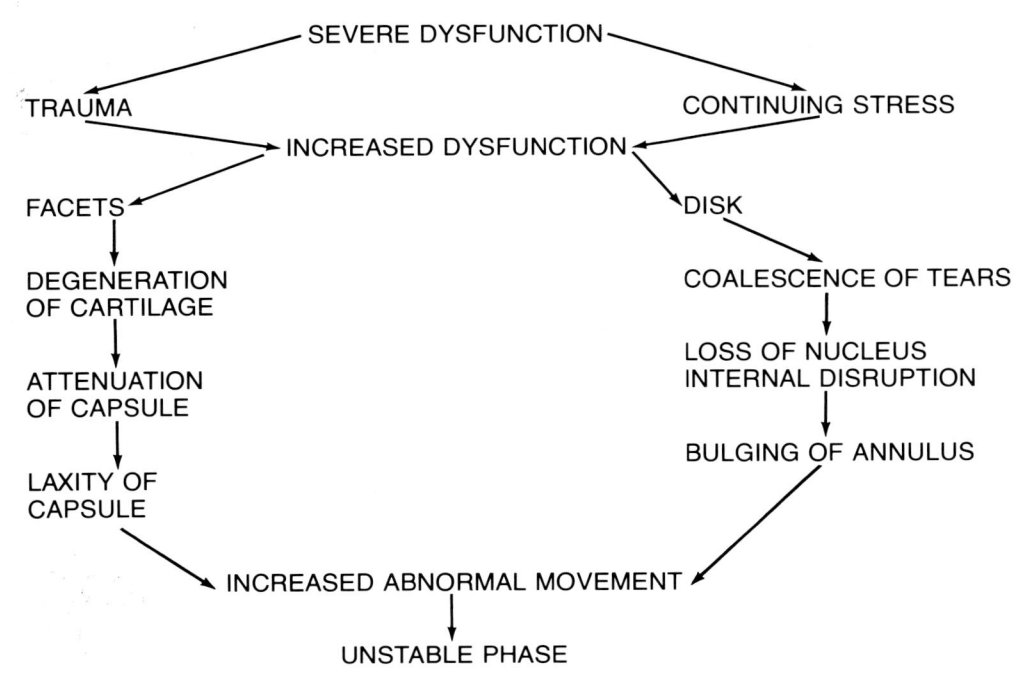

Fig. 7-4. Mechanisms of the Unstable Phase.

flexion becomes greater in extension. Extension may cause increased narrowing of the intervertebral foramen. The disk may open to an abnormal degree, at its anterior aspect during extension and at its posterior aspect during flexion. There may be an abrupt change in pedicle height at one level because one vertebra has rotated on another. CT scan images may show abnormal opening and closing of posterior joints on rotation to both left and right.

A summary of the clinical and radiological findings is shown in Table 7-2. Radiographs demonstrating some of the features of the Unstable Phase are shown in Figure 7-5.

Two points should be noted. First, in a patient with Instability at the L4–5 level concomitant Dysfunction may be present at the L3–4 or L5–S1 level. Second, the patient may shift from Phase II back to Phase I. For example, minor trauma may produce enough added capsular and annular laxity in a case of severe Dysfunction so that the physician can detect, clinically and radiologically, the presence of increased abnormal movement and place the patient in Phase II. Adequate treatment may result in sufficient healing by scar formation in the posterior joint capsule and the annulus so that the increased movement disappears and the patient is once again in Phase I. But the

Table 7-2. The Symptoms, Signs, and Radiological Changes Seen in the Unstable Stage

Symptoms
  Those of dysfunction
  Giving way of back: "catch" in back (on movement)
  Pain on coming to standing position after flexion
Signs
  Detection of abnormal movement (inspection, palpation)
  Observation of "catch," sway, or shift when coming erect after flexion
Radiographs
  Anteroposterior
    Lateral shift
    Rotation
    Abnormal tilt
    Malaligned spinous processes
  Oblique
    Opening facets
  Lateral
    Spondylolisthesis (in flexion)
    Retrospondylolisthesis (in extension)
    Narrowing foramen (in extension)
    Abnormal opening of disk
    Abrupt change in pedicle height
  CT changes

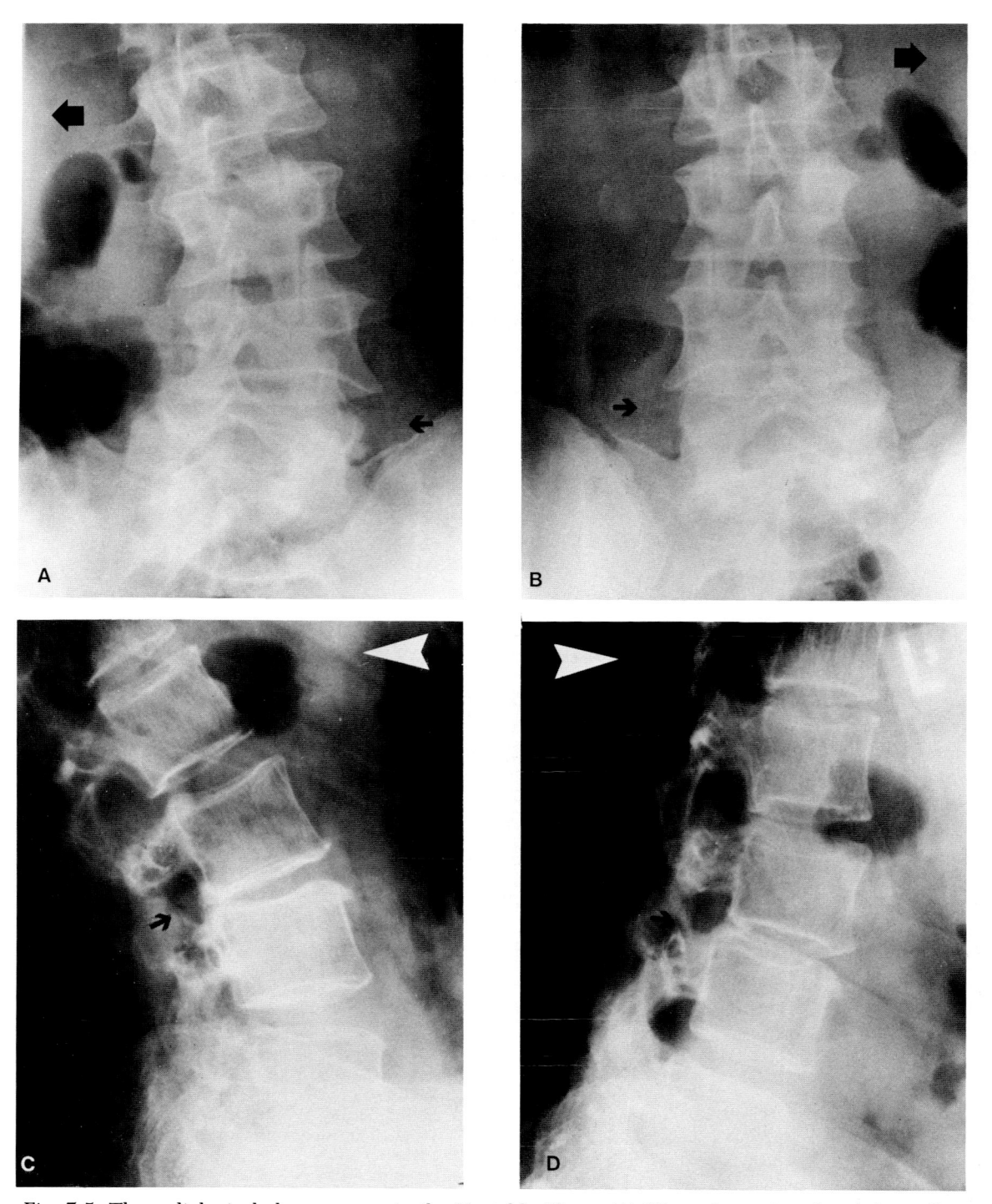

Fig. 7-5. The radiological changes seen in the Unstable Phase. (A) When the patient bends laterally to the right (viewer's left), the body of L4 moves laterally to the left relative to the body of L5 (arrow). (B) The same patient as in (A). On attempted lateral bending to the left (viewer's right), the spine remains erect. The body of L4 shifts to the right (arrow). Instability is seen at L4–5. (C) In this lateral view in extension the body of L3 is displaced slightly forward on that of L4 (arrow). (D) The same patient as in (C). In flexion the body of L3 is further displaced forward on that of L4 (arrow). Instability is due to degenerative spondylolisthesis. (Figure continues).

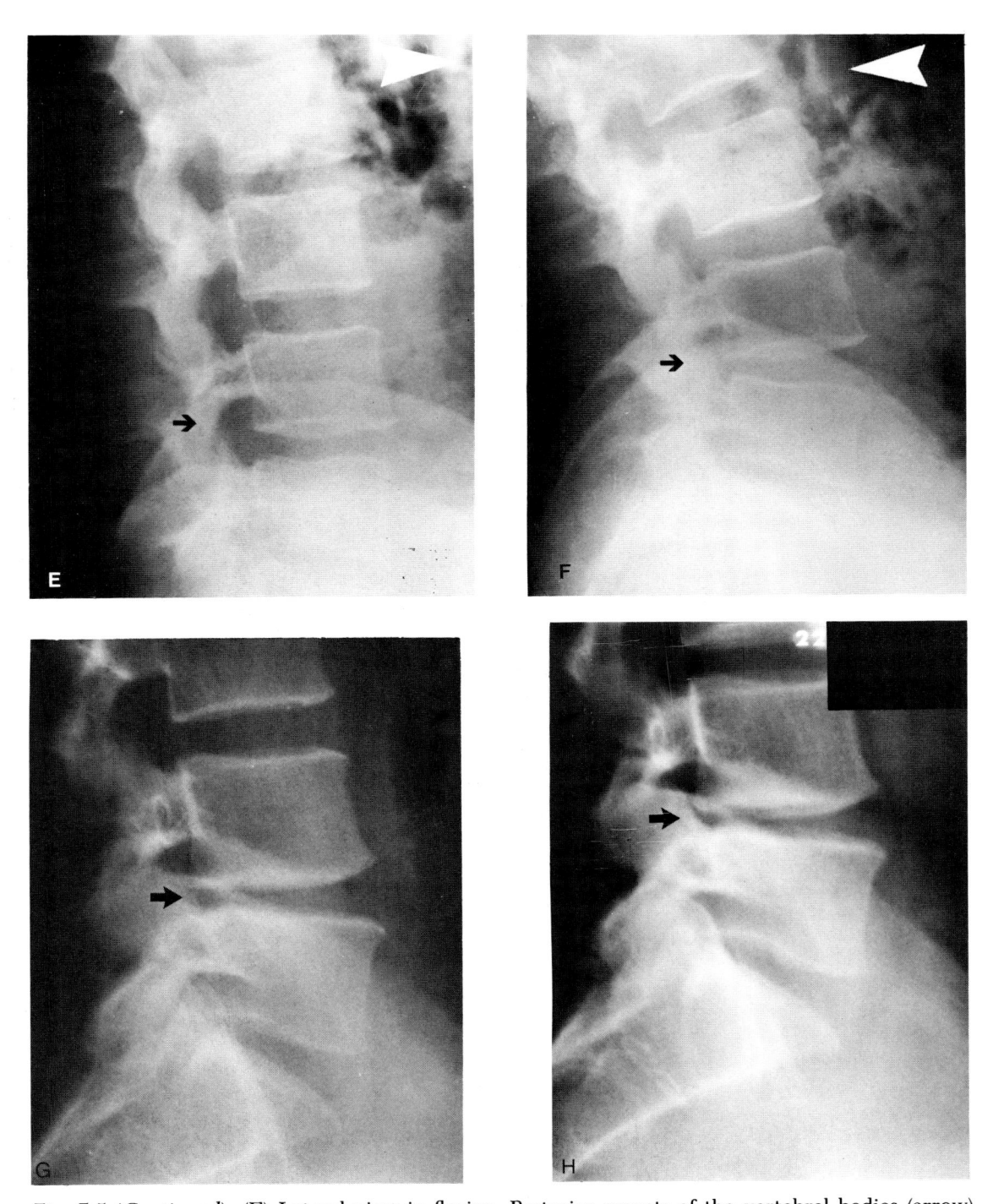

Fig. 7-5 (Continued). (E) Lateral view in flexion. Posterior aspects of the vertebral bodies (arrow) are aligned normally. (F) The same patient as in (E). In extension the body of L4 is displaced posteriorly on that of L5 (arrow). Retrospondylolisthesis is indicative of instability of minor degree. (G) Lateral view in flexion. The vertebral body of L4 is displaced posteriorly on that of L5 (arrow). (H) The same patient as in (G). In extension the body of L5 is further displaced posteriorly on that of L5. The anterior aspect of the L4–5 disk has opened. Marked retrospondylolisthesis indicates gross instability (Figure continues).

84 *Managing Low Back Pain • 7*

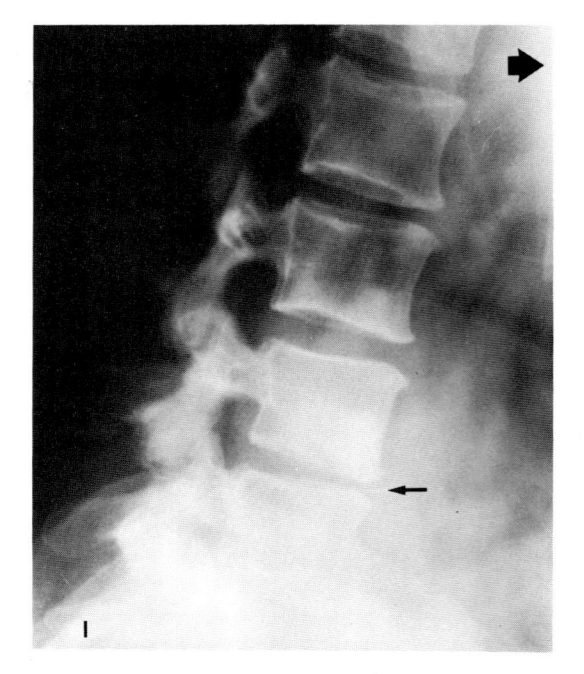

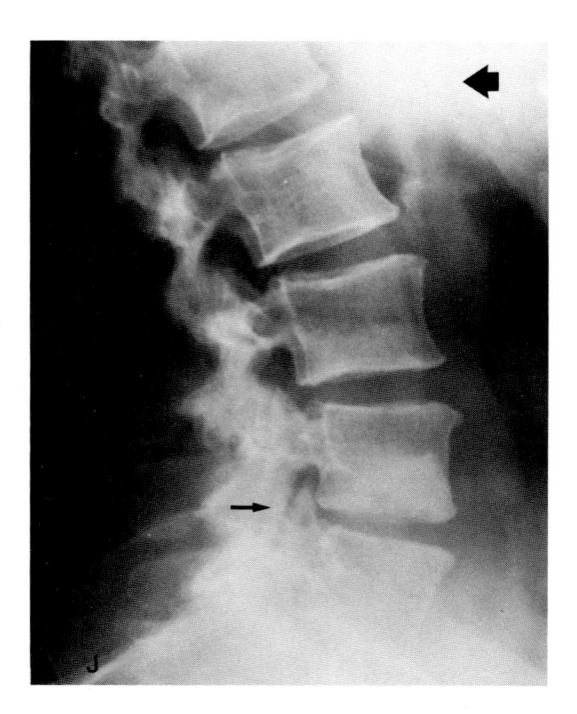

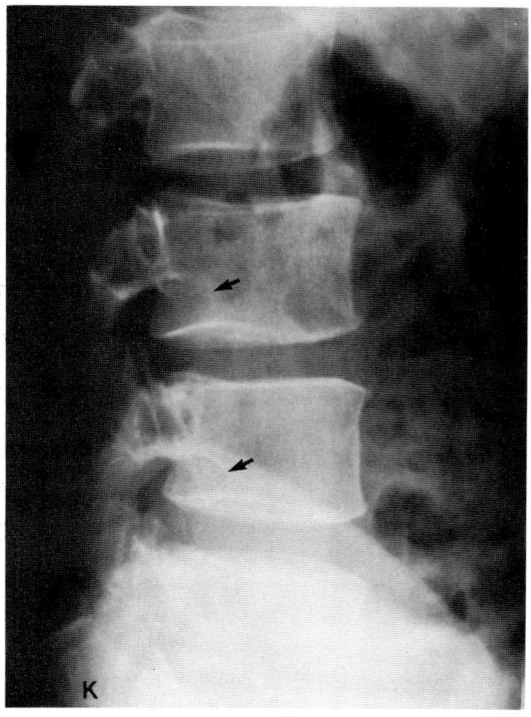

Fig. 7-5 (Continued). (I) Lateral view in flexion. Loss of disk height at L4–5 (arrow). On either side of the disk the anterior aspects of the bodies are closely approximated (Instability). (J) The same patient as in (I). In extension retrospondylolisthesis of L4 on L5 (arrow) is present. Thus signs of instability in both flexion and extension are present in this patient. (K) At the L3 and L4 levels abrupt loss of pedicle height (arrow) is apparent compared with that at L2 (above the arrow). At L3 and L4 the base of the pedicles lies over and not behind the vertebral bodies. This change is caused by rotation of L3 on L2 and indicates instability in this case. (Figure continues).

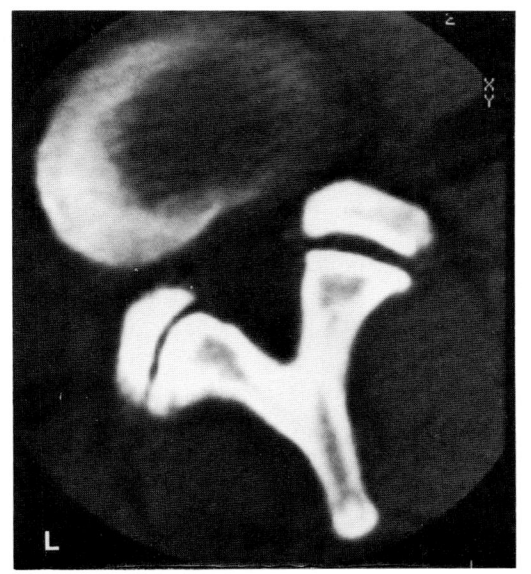

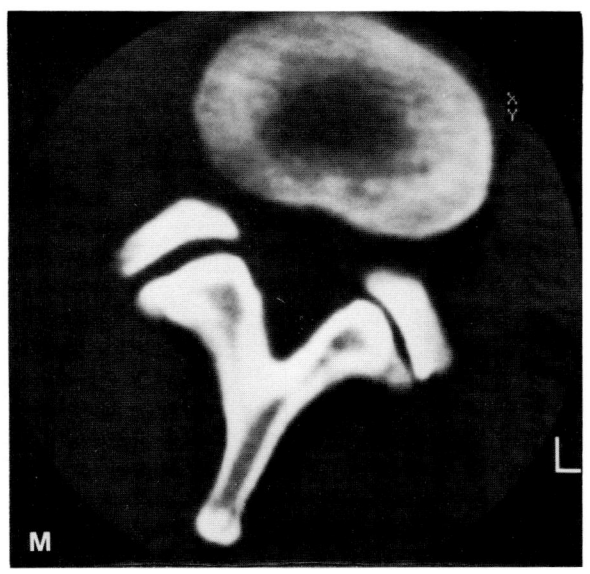

Fig. 7-5 (Continued). (L) CT scan at L4–5. When the spinous process rotates to the left, the left posterior joint opens widely. (M) CT scan of the same patient at L4–5. When the spinous process rotates to the right, the right posterior joint opens. Instability is seen at L4–5.

condition may be so severe that no treatment other than fusion can deal with the Instability.

STABILIZATION

The patient enters Phase III as a result of increasing stiffness of a spine that was previously unstable.

Presentation

Phase III disease presents in two ways. In the older patient, there is a long history of low back pain. Back pain is commonly associated with a degenerative scoliosis and abnormal muscle action. Leg pain is often the predominant feature. This will be discussed more fully when we consider central and lateral spinal stenosis. More rarely, in younger patients, the back pain decreases and leg pain is the most pronounced feature.

Mechanisms

Three mechanisms are at work. Stiffness of the posterior joints is increased because of destruction of articular cartilage, fibrosis within the joint, enlargement and locking of the facets, and periarticular fibrosis. Similar changes occur in the disk, with loss of nuclear material, approximation of vertebral bodies, destruction of the cartilage plates, fibrosis within the disk and osteophyte formation around the periphery of the disk. Occasionally a bony ankylosis joins two vertebrae together. These changes often cause entrapment of spinal nerves as discussed in Chapter 8 (Fig. 8-6).

Symptoms and Signs

Frequently low back pain that was severe over past years becomes less incapacitating. This in fact may be the commonest occurrence rather than the exception. Painful episodes may occur from time to time. These are often muscular in origin

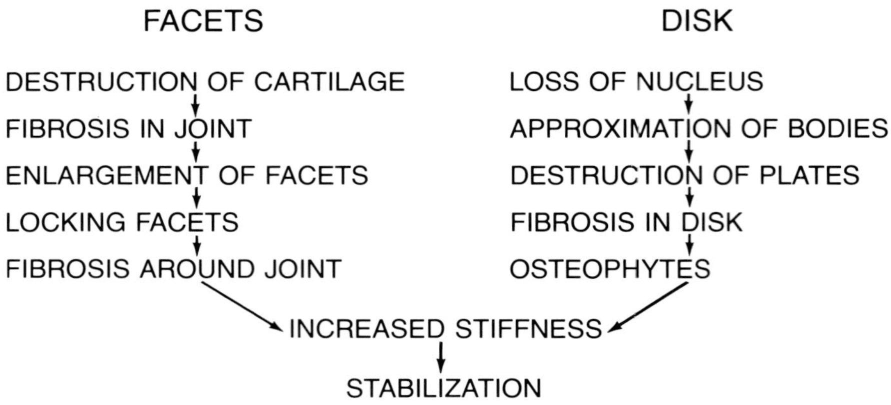

```
FACETS                                    DISK

DESTRUCTION OF CARTILAGE          LOSS OF NUCLEUS
         ↓                                ↓
FIBROSIS IN JOINT                 APPROXIMATION OF BODIES
         ↓                                ↓
ENLARGEMENT OF FACETS             DESTRUCTION OF PLATES
         ↓                                ↓
LOCKING FACETS                    FIBROSIS IN DISK
         ↓                                ↓
FIBROSIS AROUND JOINT             OSTEOPHYTES
                  ↘            ↙
                  INCREASED STIFFNESS
                         ↓
                    STABILIZATION
```

Fig. 7-6. Mechanisms of Stabilization.

and can be relieved by xylocaine (Lidocaine) injections and/or by a corset.

Signs

Commonly seen signs are tenderness to pressure over several areas; marked stiffness of the spine, with reduction of movement in all directions; and a scoliosis, often with a rotational component. Neurological signs indicating nerve entrapment are sometimes elicited.

Radiographic Changes

Radiographs show marked degenerative spondylosis at one or at several levels, with enlarged and irregular posterior facets, loss of disk height, osteophytes that arise from the vertebral bodies, marked loss of movement (anteroposterior and lateral stress radiographs), marked reduction in the size of the foramina, and scoliosis.

It is important to remember that, with few exceptions, during Phase III back pain is not usually a serious problem, but leg pain with altered sensation and muscle weakness may be severe when the spondylotic changes have produced stenosis. Rarely, the resulting scoliosis may cause severe back pain.

Table 7-3. The Signs, Symptoms, and Radiological Changes Seen in Stabilization

Symptoms
  Low back pain of decreasing severity
Signs
  Muscle tenderness
  Stiffness
  Reduced movement
  Scoliosis
Radiographs
  Enlarged facets
  Loss of disk height
  Osteophytes
  Small foramina
  Reduced movement
  Scoliosis

The clinical and radiological findings are presented in Table 7-3 and radiographs showing typical changes in Figure 7-7.

CONCLUSIONS

It is important to assess as accurately as possible the stage (Phase) reached in the spectrum of degenerative disease of the lumbar spine because the treatment differs depending on the phase. This will be discussed in a later chapter. In brief, it is likely that conservative measures will be adequate during Dysfunction; during the Unstable

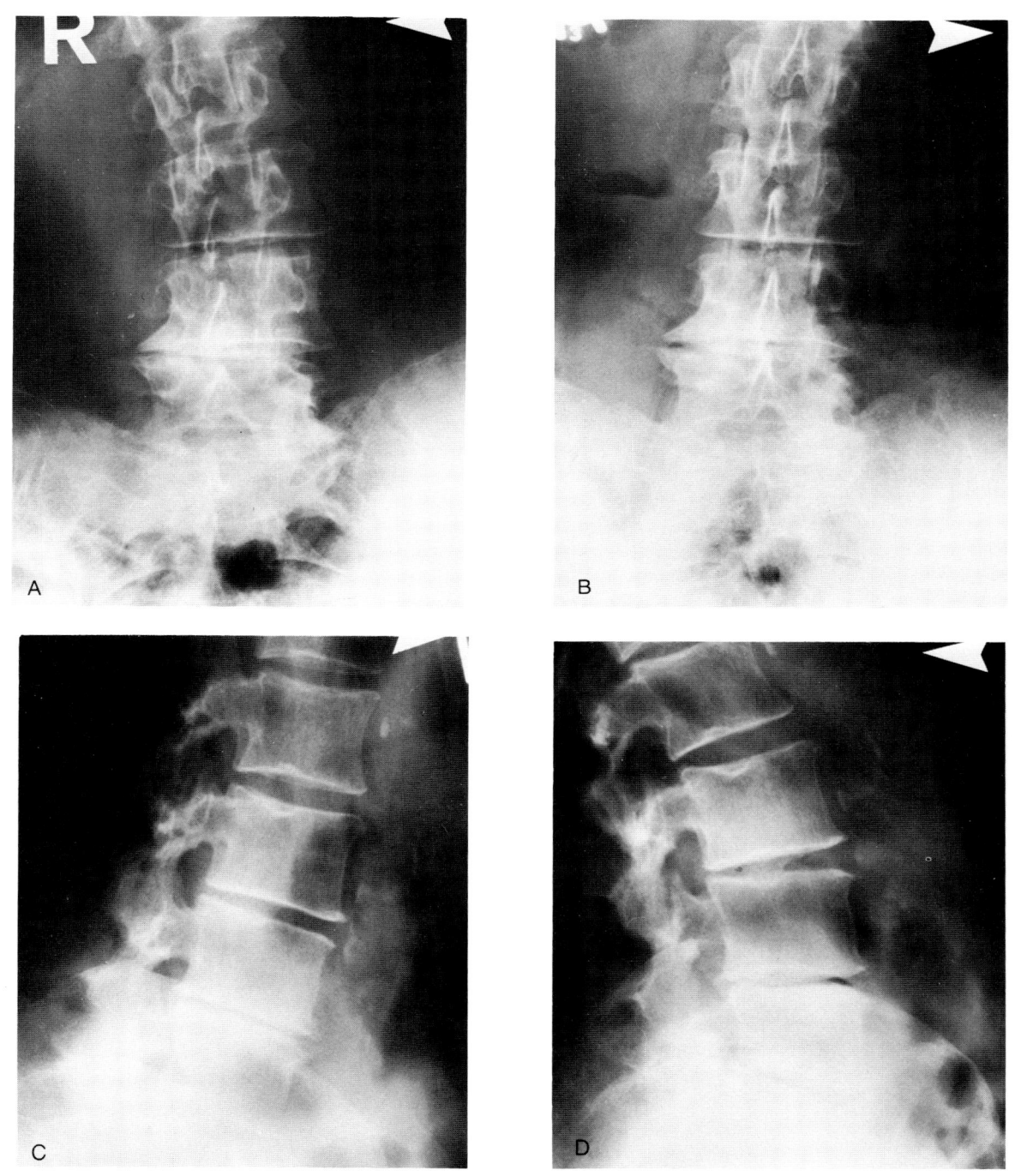

Fig. 7-7. The radiological changes seen in Phase III, Stabilization. (A) When the patient bends to the right, little or no movement of L4 on L5 or of L5 to the sacrum is evident. (B) The same patient as in (A). Lateral bending to the left also does not produce movement of L4 on L5 or of L5 on sacrum. (C) The same patient as in (A) and (B). This lateral view in flexion further confirms that no movement occurs at L4–5 or at L5–S1. (D) The same patient as in (A), (B), and (C). This lateral view in extension further confirms that no movement is present at the lower two levels. The degenerative changes in this patient's lower lumbar spine have advanced to the point of Stabilization. (Figure continues).

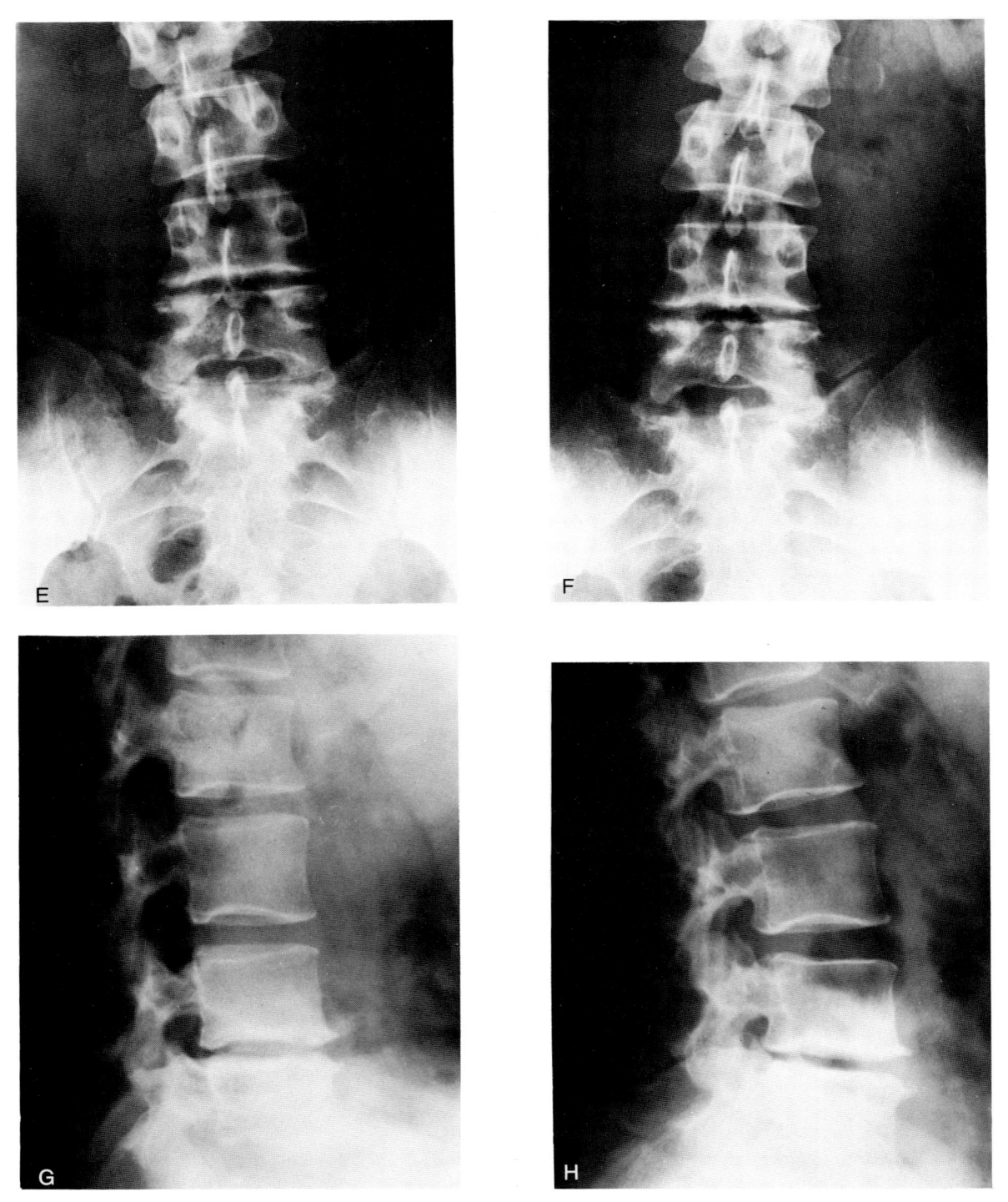

Fig. 7-7 (Continued). (E) Lateral bending to the right (viewer's left) demonstrates little or no movement at the L4–5 level. (F) The same patient as in (E). Lateral bending to the left (viewer's right) shows no movement at the L4–5 level. (G) The same patient as in (E) and (F). Lateral view in flexion shows that the L4–5 disk is markedly narrowed. (H) The same patient as in (E), (F), and (G). Lateral view in extension confirms the absence of movement at the L4–5 level. Stabilization at this level is due to advanced degenerative change.

Phase a decompression may be required to treat a disk herniation or central or lateral stenosis and a fusion may be necessary to treat instability; in the final phase (Stabilization) decompression may be indicated for central and/or lateral stenosis, but fusion is very seldom required.

ACKNOWLEDGMENTS

The author wishes to record his thanks to Dr. J. D. Cassidy for the illustrations of Dysfunction and to Dr. H. F. Farfan for his help with the definition of Instability.

SUGGESTED READING

1. Cassidy JD, Potter GE: Motion examination of the lumbar spine, J Manip Physiol Therapeut 2: 151, 1979
2. Frymoyer JW: The role of spinal fusion. Spine 6: 284, 1981
3. Helfet AI, Gruebel DM, Segmental Intervertebral Instability and Its Treatment: Disorders of the Lumbar Spine. Philadelphia, JD Lipincott, 1978
4. Hirsch C, Nachemson A: The reliability of lumbar disc surgery. Clin Orthop 29: 189, 1963
5. Kirkaldy-Willis WH, Farfan HF, Instability of the lumbar spine. Clin Orthop Rel Res, 165: 110, 1982
6. Nachemson A: The role of spinal fusion. Spine 6: 306, 1981
7. Paris SV: Personal communication

8 The Site and Nature of the Lesion

W. H. Kirkaldy-Willis

We turn now to consider the site and nature of specific clinical lesions. Table 8-1 demonstrates first the phase (the framework in which the lesion is seen) and then the lesion by name. Three points must be borne in mind. First, a specific lesion can be identified in more than one phase. For example a disk herniation may occur at the end of Phase I, during Phase II, and, rarely, during Phase III. Second, for clarity, lesions will be described as single discrete processes. Often more than one lesion is present at any given time. This we know from our study of pathology in chapter 3. For example, we shall describe the posterior facet syndrome and disk herniation separately. In practice, trauma to the facets is nearly always accompanied by trauma affecting the annulus. Compression injuries to the disk result in posterior facet degeneration at a later date. The condition called degenerative disk disease probably implies an equal amount of destruction of both facets and disk.

Third, one specific lesion may set the stage for the development of another. For example, the posterior facet syndrome may be complicated by the sacroiliac syndrome at a later date.[1] The clinical lesions will be considered in the following order:

1. Posterior facet syndrome
2. Sacroiliac joint syndrome
3. Herniation of the nucleus pulposus
4. Piriformis syndrome
5. Quadratus lumborum syndrome
6. Combined degenerative changes in posterior facet joint and disk
7. Lateral lumbar spinal nerve entrapment (lateral stenosis)
    (a) General considerations
    (b) During Phase II (Instability)
    (c) During Phase III (Stabilization)
8. Referred and radicular pain
9. Central spinal stenosis
10. Degenerative spondylolisthesis
11. Isthmic spondylolisthesis.

THE POSTERIOR FACET SYNDROME

The pathological lesions seen in the posterior facet joints have already been reviewed (chapter 3). The presentation of this syndrome, the mechanisms, involved, the symptoms and signs, and radiological changes have been discussed in chapter 7 under the heading Dysfunction and will not be repeated here. The presenting symptoms and signs during Phase I come chiefly from the posterior joints and the segmental muscles posterior to them. Symptoms arise from the posterior joints in several different ways.

Phase I, Dysfunction

In Phase I the patient may present with the symptoms and signs characteristic of the posterior facet syndrome or with a combination of the symptoms and signs of that syndrome and those

Table 8-1. Specific Clinical Lesions

Dysfunction	Posterior facet syndrome Sacroiliac joint syndrome Disk herniation Piriformis syndrome Quadratus syndrome
Unstable phase	Disk herniation Facet and disk degeneration Lateral stenosis Central stenosis
Stabilization	Lateral stenosis Central stenosis Multilevel stenosis Disk herniation

of a disk herniation. In the case of a central disk herniation the clinical findings may be masked by those arising from the facet syndrome. When the herniation is more lateral, a careful clinical examination and CT scan images make the diagnosis more obvious. In addition, the symptoms and signs of a posterior facet syndrome may be complicated by those of a sacroiliac sundrome (see below).[2,3]

Phase II, The Unstable Phase

During Phase II a part of the symptom complex arises from changes in the posterior joints and a part comes from pathology in the disk. As seen in chapter 3 the cause of instability is marked laxity of both the capsule of the posterior joints and the annulus fibrosus. As in Phase I most of the symtoms arise from changes in the facet joints to which, as seen in chapter 7, must be added the rather vague symptoms that suggest the presence of instability. Fortunately stress radiographs demonstrate the presence of increased abnormal movement in both posterior joints and disk.

Degenerative Disk Disease

The term "degenerative disk disease" is misleading. Degeneration of the annulus is present in Phase I. It is of minor degree until a disk herniation occurs. In Phase II the disk degeneration is of major degree, a sign that Instability is present. In Phase III degeneration of the disk (and of the posterior facet joints) is advanced. Thus radiological findings tell us whether we are dealing with a problem in Phase I, Phase II, or Phase III. It is this interpretation that matters when we turn to consider treatment.

Multiple Lesions

Recurrent rotational trauma most commonly affects the L4–5 joint. Frequently such a lesion spreads to an adjacent level at a later date. A simple example makes this clear. The initial trauma results in dysfunction at the L4–5 level. Recurrent trauma may produce increased dysfunction and eventually the patient enters the Unstable Phase. Further trauma may lead to dysfunction at the L3–4 level. In this instance we are dealing with posterior joint symptoms at two levels. To recognize this and to appreciate the different nature of the two lesions is vital in managing the problem.

THE SACROILIAC SYNDROME

Structure and Function of the Joint

The sacroiliac joint has well-developed cartilage surfaces, a synovial membrane, strong anterior and posterior ligaments, and a large internal sacroiliac ligament. After the fifth decade of life fibrosis takes place between the cartilage surfaces. By the sixth or seventh decade the joint has usually undergone fibrous ankylosis. Bony ankylosis is a rare phenomenon late in life. The joint surfaces can rotate 3 to 5° in the younger symptom-free patient. The joint has two functions: to provide elasticity to the pelvic ring and to serve as a buffer between the lumbosacral and the hip joints.[4]

Presentation

The syndrome presents with pain over one sacroiliac joint in the region of the posterior superior iliac spine. This may be accompanied by referred pain in the leg.

Mechanism

The mechanism of injury is not well understood. Until late in middle age a small amount of movement (3 to 5°) is usually present in the sacroiliac joint. After that age, movement is reduced by articular cartilage degeneration, by fibrosis, and rarely by bony ankylosis. It is possible that minor dysfunction in this joint leads to pain. It seems more reasonable to suppose that pain results from sustained contraction of muscle overlying the joint. This hypertonicity may accompany dysfunction in the sacroiliac or in the L4–5 or L5–S1 posterior joint.

Symptoms

Typical symptoms are pain over the back of the sacroiliac joint that varies in its degree of severity and referred pain in the groin, over the greater trochanter, down the back of the thigh to the knee, and, occasionally, down the lateral or posterior calf to ankle, foot, and toes.

Signs

The signs include tenderness on pressure over the posterior superior iliac spine, in the region of the sacroiliac joint, or in the buttock. Movement of the joint is usually reduced. Normally the joint moves by rotating in the sagittal plane. Restricted movement can be detected in two ways.

In the first, the patient stands with one hand resting to support himself on the couch. To examine the left joint the examiner places the thumb of his or her right hand over the spinous process of L5 and the thumb of his or her left hand over the left posterior superior iliac spine. The patient then flexes both left hip and left knee and lifts up the knee toward the chest. As this is done, the examiner can detect a small but definite amount of movement. Rotation in the joint causes the iliac spine to move downward in relation to the spinous process of L5. When the sacroiliac joint is "fixed," this movement of the iliac spine relative to the spinous process is reduced or absent.

Confirmation can be obtained by the second test. To examine the left joint the examiner places the right thumb over the apex of the sacrum and the left thumb over the ischial tuberosity. In a normal joint, flexing the left knee and hip and bringing the knee toward the chest causes the ischial tuberosity to move laterally away from the apex of the sacrum. When the joint is "fixed," the lateral movement does not take place (Fig. 8-1). The joint on the right is examined in a similar way.

Radiographic Changes

Usually no changes can be detected in the sacroiliac joint. Later in life small osteophytes can be seen at the lower margins of the joint. Radiographs do not assist the clinician to make the diagnosis but they do help to exclude other conditions such as early ankylosing spondylitis.

Comments

The sacroiliac syndrome is a well-defined syndrome. The physician who is cognizant of it and who looks for it will find that it is a commonly seen type of dysfunction. The exact nature of the lesion is not known. This syndrome usually responds well to manipulation or to injection of 1% lidocaine or 0.25% bupivacaine (Marcaine) into the joint or into the ligaments and fascia posterior to the joint. Often the same symptoms and signs are present with a posterior joint syndrome. Sometimes the pain in a patient with spondylolisthesis or in a patient who has had a fusion from L4 to the sacrum is caused by the sacroiliac syndrome and responds to treatment for it. Awareness that the syndrome exists, detecting its presence, and instituting the appropriate treatment enable the physician to relieve the pain in many patients who have previously responded poorly to treatment for what were thought to be other low back lesions.

HERNIATION OF THE NUCLEUS PULPOSUS

Introduction

Herniation of the nucleus pulposus can be of two kinds. A localised protrusion into the spinal canal, known as a "disk protrusion," may be present. The annular fibers are thinned, allowing nuclear material to move posteriorly, but are not completely ruptured. Alternatively, the posterior

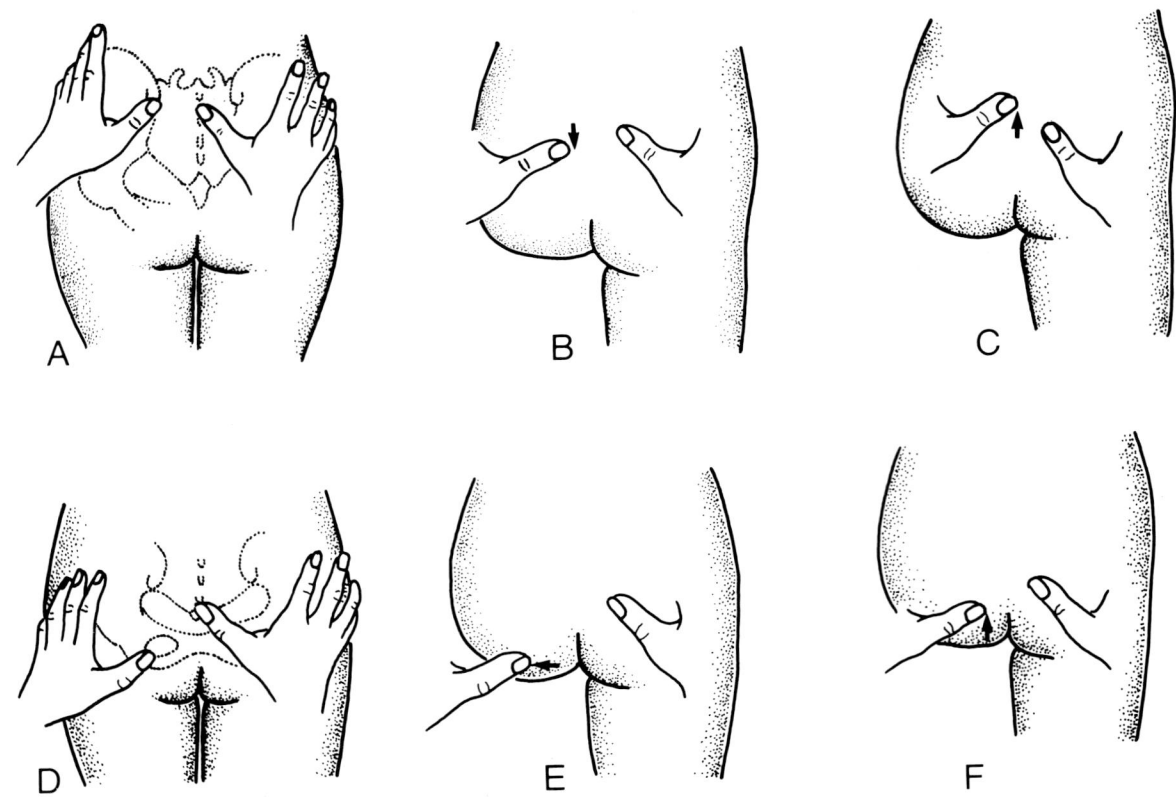

Fig. 8-1. Tests to demonstrate left sacroiliac fixation. Tests for upper part of joint in (A), (B), and (C) and for lower part in (D), (E), and (F). A. The examiner places the left thumb on the posterior superior iliac spine and the right thumb over one of the sacral spinous processes. B. When movement is normal, the examiner's left thumb moves downward as the patient raises the left leg. C. When the joint is fixed, the examiner's left thumb moves upward as the patient raises the left leg. D. The examiner places the left thumb over the ischial tuberosity and the right thumb over the apex of the sacrum. E. When movement is normal, the examiner's left thumb moves laterally as the patient raises the left leg. F. When the joint is fixed, the examiner's left thumb moves slightly upward as the patient raises the left leg.

annulus may be completely ruptured, which allows the nucleus to extrude into the canal. This is called an "extrusion" of the disk. The circumferential bulging of the annulus right around the disk, which is seen in Phase II, is not a herniation and must not be confused with it. The place of the disk herniation in the overall scheme of degeneration is discussed in chapter 3. This lesion occurs most often at the end of Phase I or early in Phase II. Later in Phase II loss of nuclear material results in lower pressures in the disk and the likelihood of herniation is less. Rarely, for reasons not well understood a disk herniation occurs in Phase III.

Presentation

The patient, usually between the ages of 30 and 50 years, recounts pain in the back and leg after lifting or after twisting and moving a heavy object. The symptoms and signs of disk herniation at different levels are clearly outlined in Figure 8-2.

Mechanism

The most common mechanism of injury is a series of recurrent rotational injuries that produce circumferential and radial tears and finally, with

The Site and Nature of the Lesion

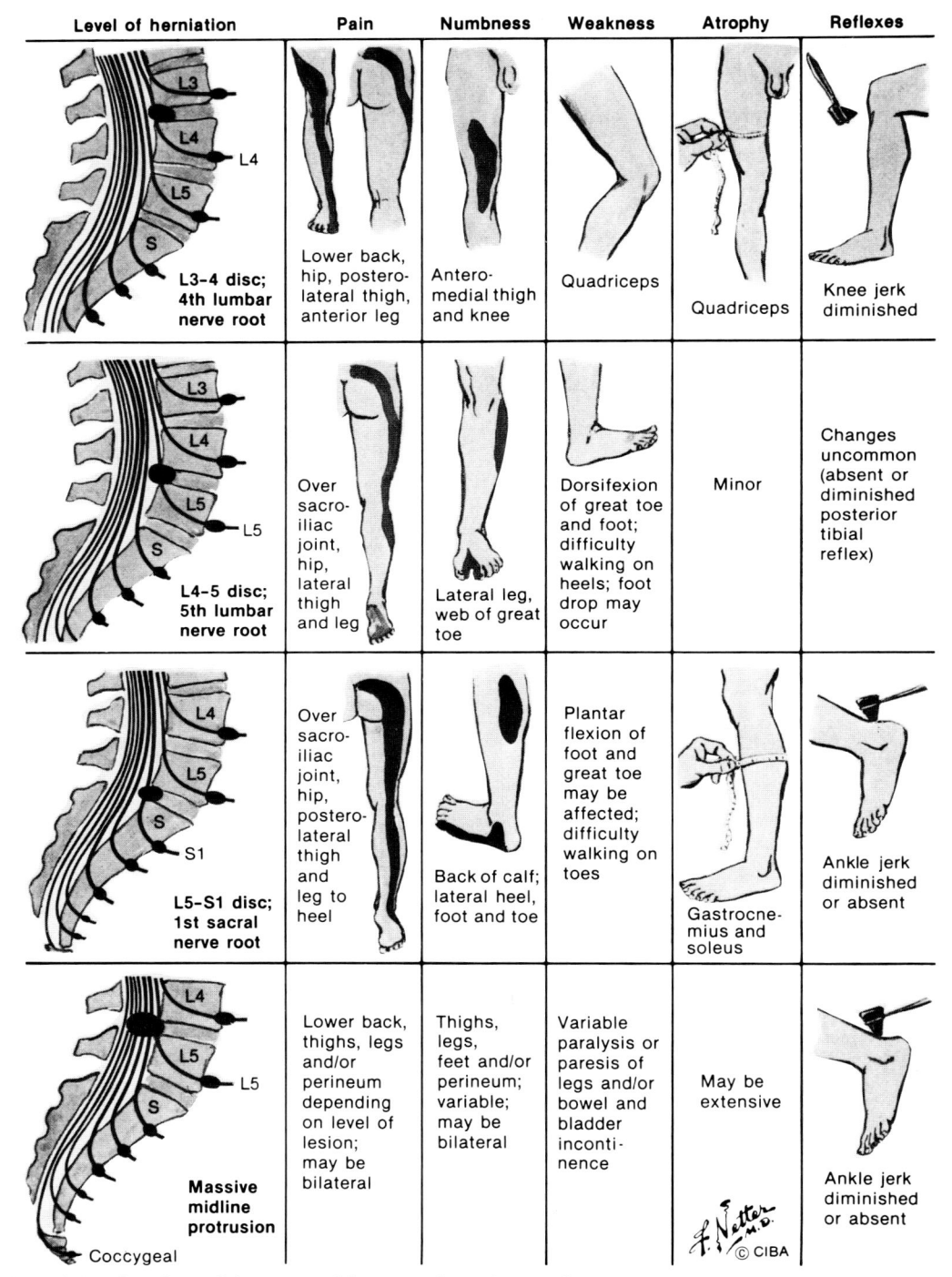

Level of herniation	Pain	Numbness	Weakness	Atrophy	Reflexes
L3-4 disc; 4th lumbar nerve root	Lower back, hip, postero-lateral thigh, anterior leg	Antero-medial thigh and knee	Quadriceps	Quadriceps	Knee jerk diminished
L4-5 disc; 5th lumbar nerve root	Over sacro-iliac joint, hip, lateral thigh and leg	Lateral leg, web of great toe	Dorsiflexion of great toe and foot; difficulty walking on heels; foot drop may occur	Minor	Changes uncommon (absent or diminished posterior tibial reflex)
L5-S1 disc; 1st sacral nerve root	Over sacro-iliac joint, hip, postero-lateral thigh and leg to heel	Back of calf; lateral heel, foot and toe	Plantar flexion of foot and great toe may be affected; difficulty walking on toes	Gastrocnemius and soleus	Ankle jerk diminished or absent
Massive midline protrusion	Lower back, thighs, legs and/or perineum depending on level of lesion; may be bilateral	Thighs, legs, feet and/or perineum; variable; may be bilateral	Variable paralysis or paresis of legs and/or bowel and bladder incontinence	May be extensive	Ankle jerk diminished or absent

Fig. 8-2. The clinical features of herniated nucleus pulposus. © 1980 Ciba Pharmaceutical Company, Division of CIBA-GEIGY Corporation. Reprinted with permission from Keim HA, Kirkaldy-Willis WH: Low Back Pain. Clin Symp 32: 6, 1980. Illustrated by Frank H. Netter, M.D. All rights reserved.

further trauma, a yielding of the annulus to produce a localized bulge. In some cases the annulus is completely ruptured. A severe compression injury with the spine flexed may cause a sudden rupture of the annulus.

Symptoms

The patient gives a history of attacks of low back pain over months or years. A relatively minor degree of trauma is followed by acute severe low back and leg pain. Often the back pain disappears with the onset of leg pain. The pain is made worse by forward bending, by coughing and by sneezing. It is relieved by rest with the patient recumbent and the knees flexed. In the case of a small midline protrusion no leg pain may be present. Occasionally the patient complains of muscle weakness, when this is of marked degree. Still more rarely there may be complaints of bladder and bowel dysfunction.

Signs

Commonly the physician can detect numbness over one dermatome (hypoesthesia). Muscle weakness of the quadriceps, of the dorsiflexors of ankles and toes, or of the plantarflexors may be present. The patient may not be able to pass urine or to defecate normally. Muscle atrophy of the quadriceps, of the gastrocnemii and soleus, or of the short toe extensors may be detected. The knee or ankle reflex may be absent or diminished. Straight leg raising is often markedly diminished. When the patient is able to stand, it is noted that the normal lumbar lordosis is lost. The back is straight. There may be a list to one or the other side. All movements are restricted. On attempted forward flexion, the list (a functional scoliosis) is increased. The Lasegue and bowstring tests are often positive. Performing the Lasegue test on one side may produce pain in the opposite (the affected) leg. With a small central herniation few signs may be present in the lower limb. In this case the presence of a list and diminished straight leg raising strongly suggest that a small central herniation is present[5] (see Fig. 13-8).

Radiographic Changes

No changes may be present. The lateral view may demonstrate slight reduction of disk height. The changes characteristic of the Unstable Phase may be seen.

Comments

It is relatively easy to distinguish between a posterior facet syndrome and a classical disk herniation. The patient with a small central herniation is difficult to diagnose. The presenting symptoms and signs may at a glance be those of a facet syndrome. The presence of a list and of marked diminution of straight leg raising strongly suggest that a disk herniation is present. Sometimes the lateral radiograph may reveal the presence of a small area of lucency adjacent to the upper or lower part of a vertebral body. This is a Schmorl's node and is caused by rupture of a cartilage plate with extrusion of disk material into the vertebral body. It usually does not produce symptoms.

THE PIRIFORMIS SYNDROME

Presentation and Mechanism

The syndrome presents as a minor twisting injury of one leg that occurs while the patient is in an awkward position or is lifting or carrying a weight. The incident is followed by severe buttock and sometimes leg pain.

The mechanism involves stretching and tearing of a number of the fibers of the muscle. Pain may persist for months unless the appropriate treatment is given. In some patients a part of the sciatic nerve passes through the substance of the muscle. Injury to the muscle may result in sciatic pain.

Symptoms

The symptoms include severe buttock pain that is deep-seated and may appear to be in the rectum or vagina. Pain may be referred down the back of the thigh to the knee, sometimes passing as far as the ankle, foot, or toes. Rarely, symptoms of nerve entrapment may be present.

Signs

Tenderness is present when the muscle medial to the greater trochanter is palpated. Pain on muscle contraction may be demonstrated by asking the patient to sit on the examining table with knees apart and ankles together and to resist the attempt of the physician to bring his knees together. On rectal or vaginal examination palpation of the muscle medial to the spine of the ischium produces marked tenderness and pain. The final conclusive test is a therapeutic one. Injecting a few milliliters of 1% lidocaine or 0.25% bupivacaine into the muscle medial to the ischial spine completely relieves the patient of his pain.

Radiographic Changes

Radiographs may demonstrate the presence of lumbar spondylosis, but this is not directly connected with the cause of the pain.

Comment

It is important to recognize the presentation of the piriformis syndrome and to distinguish it from other causes of low back and leg pain. Treatment by injecting a local anesthetic is simple and effective.[6]

THE QUADRATUS LUMBORUM SYNDROME

Presentation

The syndrome presents with pain between the 12 rib and iliac crest lateral to the erector spinae muscle mass. Usually there is no history of trauma.

Mechanism

The mechanism is not known. It has been suggested that strain to the muscle on one side results in rupturing a few fibers. Healing does not take place and pain persists.

Symptoms

Pain is present in the upper, middle, or lower part of the muscle lateral to the erector spinae muscle. Pain may be referred from the upper part of the muscle to the groin and inner thigh, from the middle part to the anterior thigh and inside of the knee, and from the lower part to the back of the thigh and inner calf.

Signs

Tenderness is present when the affected part of the muscle is palpated. Pain occurs when the muscle is stretched by being bent laterally to the contralateral side; it is abolished when 1% lidocaine or 0.25% bupivacaine is injected.

Radiographic Findings

Radiological examination is of no assistance in diagnosing this lesion.

Comment

Diagnosis is easy for the physician who is aware that the syndrome exists. It is important to consider and to exclude this cause of low back and referred leg pain.

COMBINED POSTERIOR FACET AND DISK DEGENERATION

As outlined in chapter 3, changes occurring in the posterior facets affect the disk and vice versa. Early changes produce Dysfunction. Progressive changes lead to the Unstable Phase. The result of these changes is often referred to vaguely as "degenerative disk disease." In the author's opinion it is better to think of this lesion as a combined degeneration of all three parts of the joint.

The symptoms and signs are those of the Unstable Phase.

The radiological changes seen in this phase have been described in chapter 7.

LATERAL LUMBAR SPINAL NERVE ENTRAPMENT (LATERAL STENOSIS)

Presentation

There are two types of presentation: that seen during Phase II (The Unstable Phase) and that seen in Phase III (Stabilization). The entrapment may be isolated, it may occur with a disk herniation, or it may follow diskectomy or chemonucleolysis. At this point the reader is advised to review the section on lateral entrapment (stenosis) in chapter 3 before proceeding further. The concept of lateral entrapment is difficult to master.

Mechanism

As shown in chapter 3, the mechanism involves progressive degenerative changes in both facets and disk, loss of disk height, subluxation of facets that allows the superior facet to move upward and forward on the inferior facet and impinge on the pedicle above, and narrowing of the intervertebral foramen and, still more important, of the lateral part of the nerve canal medial to the foramen (Fig. 8-3). The spinal nerve that exits at this level may be entrapped. Osteophytes that form on the medial edge of the superior facet may impinge on the nerve that exits one level lower and cause entrapment. Thus at L4–5 the L4 and/or the L5 nerves may be entrapped. At L5–S1 both the L5 and/or S1 nerves may be involved (Fig. 8-4).

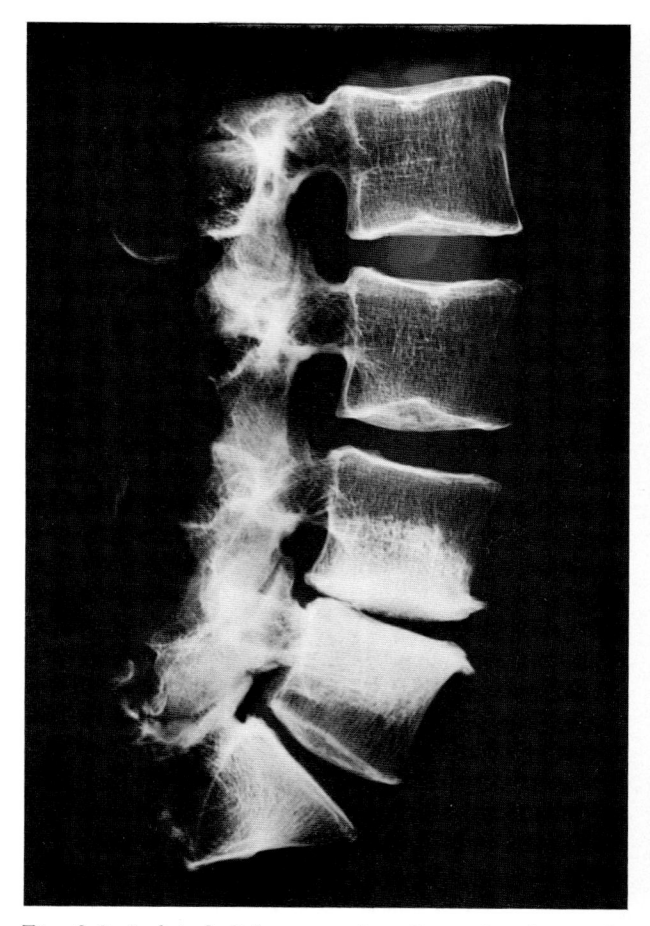

Fig. 8-3. Isolated disk resorption. Lateral radiograph of autopsy specimen of lumbar spine shows that marked resorption of the L4–5 disk has occurred. The vertebral bodies on either side are sclerotic. Retrospondylolisthesis of L4 on L5. The superior articular process of L5 is near the back of the body of L4, narrowing the foramen.

Entrapment during Phase II

This is a *recurrent* and *dynamic* type of entrapment. Instability of both disk and posterior facets allows abnormal increased movement both in rotation and in flexion–extension. With rotation the superior facet moves backward and forward, as the posterior joint opens and closes, and impinges on the spinal nerve. During extension the lateral canal is narrowed and the same kind of impingement occurs. Thus, the causes of this type of entrapment are twofold: structural changes narrow the lateral canal and recurrent dynamic narrowing occurs because the superior articular process moves back and forth (see chapter 3).

Entrapment during Phase III

By Phase III progressive degenerative changes have led to stabilizing the previously unstable segment. The deformity is fixed, often with some rotation. No movement occurs at the affected level. The changes are solely structural.

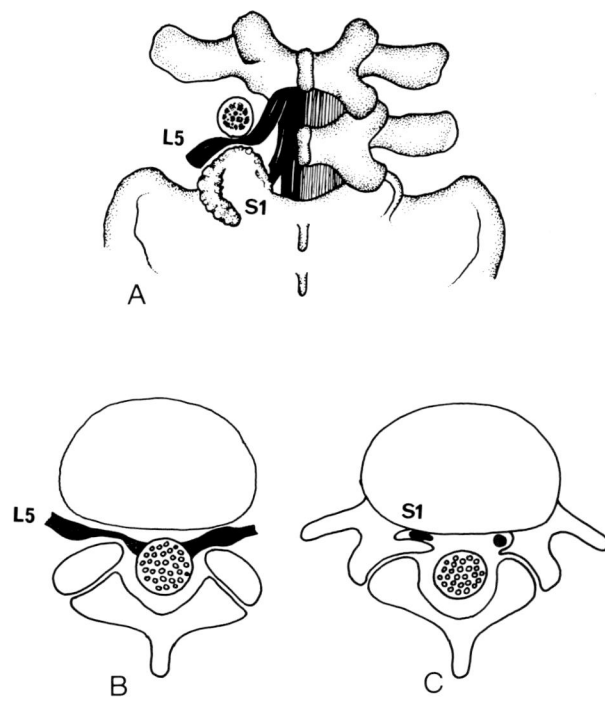

Fig. 8-4. Diagram demonstrating how two nerves are at risk at the L5–S1 level. A. The L5 nerve is entrapped between the pedicle of L5 and the superior facet of the sacrum, and the S1 nerve is entrapped between the enlarged superior facet of the sacrum and the back of the body of the sacrum. B. The cross-section shows entrapment of the L5 nerve between the upper part of the superior sacral facet and the back of the vertebral body of the sacrum on the left side. C. The cross-section reveals entrapment of the left S1 nerve in the narrow gutter at the base of the superior sacral facet.

Entrapment Symptoms in Phase II and Phase III

The patient may or may not complain of low back pain. The most common site of the pain is in the buttock, trochanteric region, and posterior thigh to the knee. Sometimes the pain passes further distally down the back of the calf (S1) or down the lateral aspect of the calf (L5) to the ankle and, occasionally, to the foot and toes. The patient may complain of altered sensation or hypoesthesia in the L5 or S1 dermatome. It should be appreciated, first, that these symptoms differ little from those of Phase I and those of a posterior facet syndrome

and, second, that the symptoms may be the same in both types of entrapment. In recurrent dynamic entrapment the symptoms may be intermittent.

Entrapment Signs in Phase II and Phase III

Movements of the lumbar spine are usually not much restricted. Straight-leg raising may be slightly reduced on the affected side. Neurological findings are usually normal. However, some blunting to touch and pin prick over the L4, L5, or S1 dermatome may be present. Loss of motor power and reflex changes are rare. The Lasegue and Bowstring tests may be positive (see below, referred and radicular pain).

Additional Signs Observed in the Unstable Phase

The signs indicative of Phase II may be elicited (see chapter 7, section on the Unstable Phase). Pain may be elicited with the patient in one of three positions (Fig. 8-5). First, the patient lies on his side with the painful leg on the couch. The examiner stands behind the patient, holds his chest and trunk with one hand, and rotates his pelvis forward toward the other side. This maneuver may move the lower superior facet toward the vertebral body and cause pain by creating pressure on the spinal nerve. The same test can be done with the patient standing. The examiner sits behind the patient and holds the pelvis to prevent movement. An assistant, standing in front of the patient, grasps the chest with both hands and rotates chest and upper trunk first to one side and then to the other. This movement may produce pain in the affected lower limb by shifting one superior articular process nearer to the back of the vertebral body above it. In a third test the patient lies on his face. With the left hand the examiner maintains gentle pressure on the back of the lumbar spine. With his right hand, he flexes both the patient's knees until the heels touch the buttocks. The hyperextension produced by this maneuver may result in leg pain that occurs because the lateral canal is narrowed by forward displacement of the superior articular process (Pheasant test). These tests are not always positive even when dynamic lateral stenosis is present.

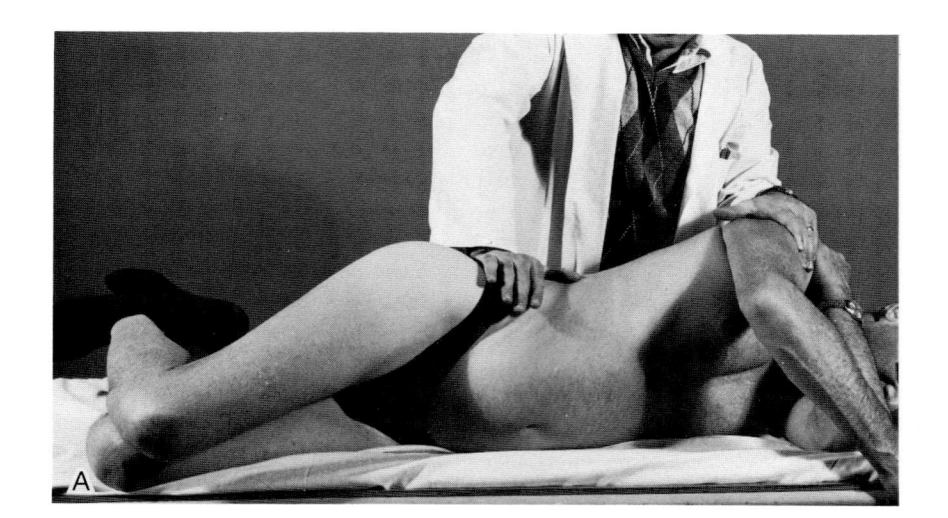

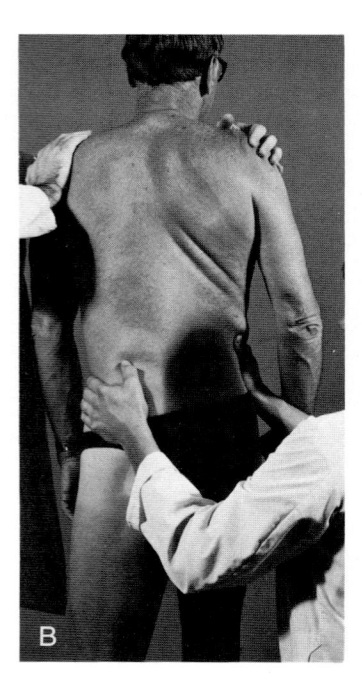

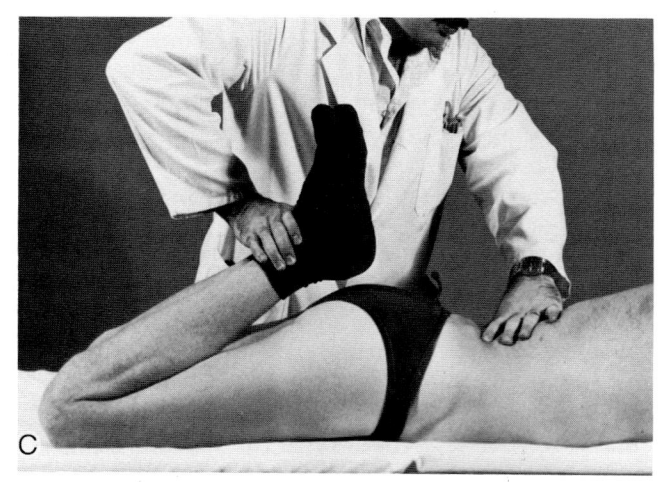

Fig. 8-5. Tests for dynamic lateral entrapment. A. The patient lies on his side with the painful side on the couch. The physician holds the patient's chest with the left hand and rotates the pelvis away from him with the opposite hand. This sometimes accentuates the leg pain. B. The patient stands erect. The physician holds the pelvis firmly. An assistant, standing in front of the patient, rotates the trunk first to one side, then to the other. This sometimes reproduces the leg pain. C. The patient lies prone. The examiner presses lightly over the lumbar spine with his left hand and flexes the knees and extends the hips with his right hand. This produces hyperextension and, in cases of central stenosis and of dynamic lateral stenosis may reproduce the leg pain (Pheasant test).

Radiographic Findings

The disk space at L4–5 or L5–S1 may be reduced in height and the vertebral bodies adjacent to the disk may be sclerotic (see Fig. 8–3). The foramen at one level may be smaller than normal. Lateral stress films may show that in extension the upper body moves backward on the lower (retrospondylolisthesis) and that the superior facet shifts toward the back of the vertebral body. The radiographic changes characteristic of the Unstable Phase may be seen in the dynamic type of lateral entrapment.

Comments

Lateral entrapment is a relatively common syndrome. The symptoms and signs are vague and merely suggest the presence of this lesion. The presence of the typical radiographic changes made the diagnosis more definite. CT scan images that make the diagnosis certain will be discussed in chapter 9 under the heading Diagnosis.[7]

REFERRED AND RADICULAR PAIN

It is convenient at this point to discuss the symptoms and signs that enable us to differentiate between referred and radicular pain.

Referred pain has the same distribution as the innervation of the affected posterior joint. With a lesion of the L4–5 joint the pain is of L4 and L5 distribution: down the back of the thigh and sometimes to the inner or outer calf. A lesion of the L5–S1 joint gives referred pain down the back of the thigh and sometimes down the back or outside of the calf, i.e., the L5 or S1 dermatomes. Subjective sensory changes in the L4, L5, or S1 dermatomes may be present. Motor and reflex changes are rare.

Radicular pain is due to irritation, inflammation, tension, or compression of the anterior division of a spinal nerve. Sensory, motor, and reflex changes are often present. Frequently, a definite reduction in straight leg raising is present. The Lasegue or Braggard test (dorsiflexion of the foot with maximum straight leg raising) is often positive. The Bowstring test (at maximum straight leg raising, the knee is flexed a few degrees and digital pressure is applied over the posterior tibial and lateral popliteal nerves at knee joint level) may produce pain and tenderness over one or other nerve. Tenderness may be present when pressure is applied over the sciatic notch. These simple tests often help the physician to differentiate between referred and radicular pain. They are particularly helpful in cases of lateral entrapment. They are not infallible. Further examinations such as the electromyogram will be described in chapter 9 under Diagnosis (Table 8-2).

CENTRAL SPINAL STENOSIS

Presentation

The condition most commonly presents as pain and altered sensation in one or both lower limbs. Occasionally motor weakness is the predominant symptom.

Mechanism

The posterior facets are enlarged and protrude in a medial and anterior direction so that the central canal is narrowed. Although it is the superior facets that narrow the lateral canals, the inferior facets are chiefly responsible for central canal narrowing. The presence of osteophytes at the back of the vertebral bodies and bulging of the annulus of the disk further narrow the canal. When preexisting developmental narrowing of the canal is present, a small disk herniation and/or some degree of central stenosis can produce severe symptoms. Pressure of these structures on the nerves of the cauda equina produces most of the symptoms and signs. Venous hypertension due to pressure on the veins of the cauda equina or the nerve roots perhaps is responsible for part of the clinical picture. Central stenosis is often accompanied by lateral canal stenosis at one or more levels. Starting at one level, usually L4–5, the spondylosis and stenosis can spread to involve several levels.

Table 8-2. Distinguishing Features of Low Back Syndromes

Syndrome	Back Pain	Leg Pain	Restriction of Movement	Restriction of S.L.R.	Nerve Compression Tests	Neurological Deficit
Posterior facet	Over joint	Referred (post. thigh)	Low back	Moderate	Negative	None
Sacroiliac	Over joint	Referred (anteropost. thigh)	Of joint	Rare	Negative	None
Herniation of nucleus pulposus	Often none	Post. thigh Post. lateral calf to toes	Low back	Marked	Positive	One level
Piriformis	Deep rectal, vaginal	Post. thigh	Hip rotation	Rare	Negative	None
Quadratus lumborum	Lateral to erector spinae	Groin Ant. thigh Post. thigh	Low back	Rare	Negative	None
Lateral stenosis	Often none	Buttock Trochanter Post. thigh Calf Ankle Toes	Rare	Moderate	Positive	Sometimes present
Central stenosis	Often not severe	Common Bizarre	Varies	Moderate	Positive	Multilevel

Symptoms

The clinical picture is bizarre. The usual presenting symptom is pain in one or both legs. It may involve one dermatome in one leg and a different dermatome in the other. It may involve the whole of one or even both legs. Its nature varies. Often, after walking three or four blocks the patient has to rest because of leg pain. After a few minutes rest the patient can walk the same distance again (neurogenic claudication). Pain in bed during the night is often relieved by walking round the room for a few minutes. This type of pain can be distinguished from that of vascular claudication by the fact that the patient can ride a stationary bicycle (with the lumbar spine in flexion) for several minutes without pain. In vascular claudication the patient quickly develops leg pain.

Sensory changes are common. The patient may complain of numbness in part or the whole of one or both lower limbs. He may say that the legs feel cold (when in fact they are not cold), that they do not belong to him, or that they feel as if made of rubber.

Muscle weakness is not commonly a presenting symptom though the patient may complain that he tires easily. Rarely, muscle weakness is severe.

Signs

Movements of the lumbar spine are only slightly restricted and only mildly painful. Sensory changes differ from those of a disk herniation. In the latter they are usually restricted to one dermatome. In central stenosis sensation may be diminished over several dermatomes in one or both lower limbs. The distribution may be different in one leg from that in the other. Alternatively, the whole of one leg may exhibit altered sensation.

Motor power may be diminished in the distribution of one or two motor nerves in one leg and that of different nerves in the other leg. For example the quadriceps may be weak on the left and the ankle dorsiflexors on the right. It is useful to test muscle power with the spine extended and the patient lying prone with knees flexed (Pheasant test). In this position motor weakness may be

Table 8-3. Differential Diagnosis of Central Spinal Stenosis

Vascular claudication
Diabetic neuropathy
Other peripheral neuropathies
Motor neurone disease
Multiple sclerosis
Other lesions of central nervous system
Spinal infections (acute, subacute, chronic)
Neoplasms (involving cauda equina, spinal nerves, or vertebrae)

Table 8-4. Classification of Spinal Stenosis

Congenital/developmental
Acquired
   Degenerative (central, lateral, both of these)
   Combined (with disk herniation, with developmental stenosis, with both)
   After laminectomy (scarring)
   After fusion (above the fusion, beneath the fusion)
   Trauma (early and late changes)
   Paget's disease
   Fluorosis

more marked. After testing for muscle power in both legs, it is useful to ask the patient to walk briskly for 5 minutes. Retesting after this may reveal increased muscle weakness. Occasionally, muscle weakness is so severe that the patient is unable to stand or walk.

Reflexes may be diminished or absent, the quadriceps on one side and the Achilles tendon reflex on the other. The overall picture is usually bizarre, but when the central stenosis involves only one level, the picture may resemble that of a disk herniation and may be mistaken for that (Tables 8-3, 8-4).

Radiographic Changes

Plain radiographs demonstrate enlarged posterior facets, approximation of one lamina to the next, decreased distances between the articular processes, diminished disk height, the presence of osteophytes that arise from vertebral bodies, and decreased size of the foramina. These changes are characteristic of spondylosis and are no more than suggestive of stenosis. Stress anteroposterior and lateral radiographs may reveal that instability is present (Fig. 8-6).

Comments

To the physician who is not aware of central spinal stenosis as a possible diagnosis, the symptoms may suggest a psychoneurosis, a desire for compensation, or a lack of desire to return to work. The physician who is aware that the syndrome exists will find the symptoms, signs, and radiographic changes strongly suggestive of the diagnosis. The diagnosis is made definite by myelography and by CT scan images (see below).[8,9]

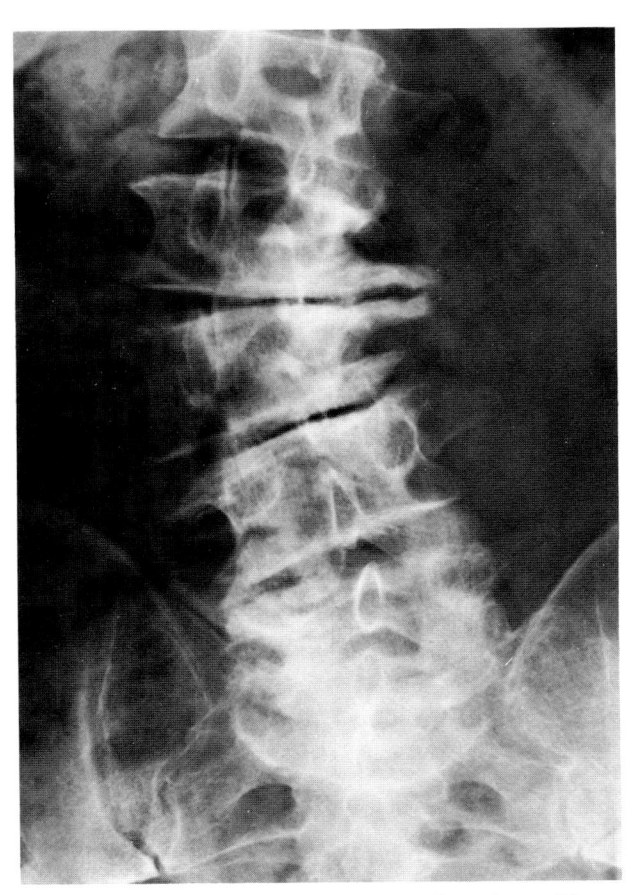

Fig. 8-6. Generalized spondylosis with scoliosis. The patient had symptoms and signs of compression of the L5 nerve on the right.

DEGENERATIVE SPONDYLOLISTHESIS

Presentation

The presentation is very similar to that seen in central spinal stenosis.

Mechanism

The mechanism involved is that of lumbar spondylosis, with marked erosion of posterior articular processes. In this respect degenerative spondylolisthesis differs from other types of spondylosis, which produce enlargement of articular processes. The disk yields and the inferior articular process moves forward as the superior process is continually more and more eroded. The upper vertebral body is displaced forward on the lower. The nerve that exits one level below the lesion is entrapped between the inferior articular process of the upper vertebra and the back of the body of the lower vertebra. At the L4–5 level the L5 nerve is entrapped between the inferior process of L4 and the body of L5. This lesion is most commonly seen at the L4–5 level but is sometimes encountered at the L3–4 or L5–S1 level. Rarely, a slip is seen at two or three levels (see chapter 3, Fig. 3-10A).

Symptoms and Signs

The symptoms are similar to those of central spinal stenosis.

The signs differ little from those seen in central stenosis. Examination of the lumbar spine may reveal that an upper spinous process is displaced forward on the process that is one below.

Radiographic Changes

Radiographs show the same changes as for spondylosis. An upper vertebral body has slipped forwards on the one below it. In the presence of instability, the upper vertebral body may be normally aligned on the lower in the lateral view in extension and displaced forward in the flexion view (Fig. 8-7).[10]

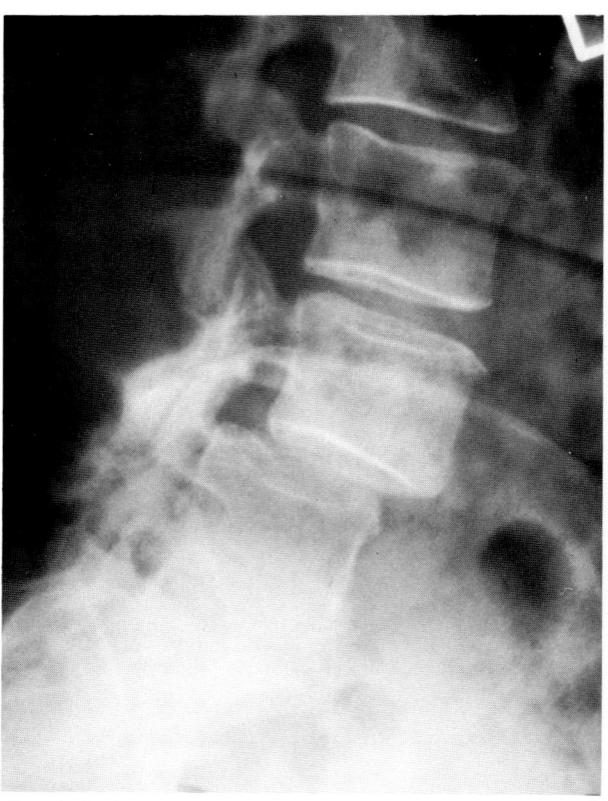

Fig. 8-7. Degenerative spondylolisthesis of the 4th on the 5th lumbar vertebra.

ISTHMIC SPONDYLOLISTHESIS

Presentation

The condition may present with low back pain alone, with a combination of low back and leg pain, or rarely, with leg pain alone.

Mechanism

The mechanism usually involves a fall onto the buttocks with the spine flexed. The result is a bilateral fracture of the pars interarticularis. It is thought that this usually occurs when the patient is between the ages of 6 and 12 years. Slowly, over subsequent years, the disk yields and the upper vertebra (usually L5) slips forward on the lower (usually S1). The slippage is graded as fol-

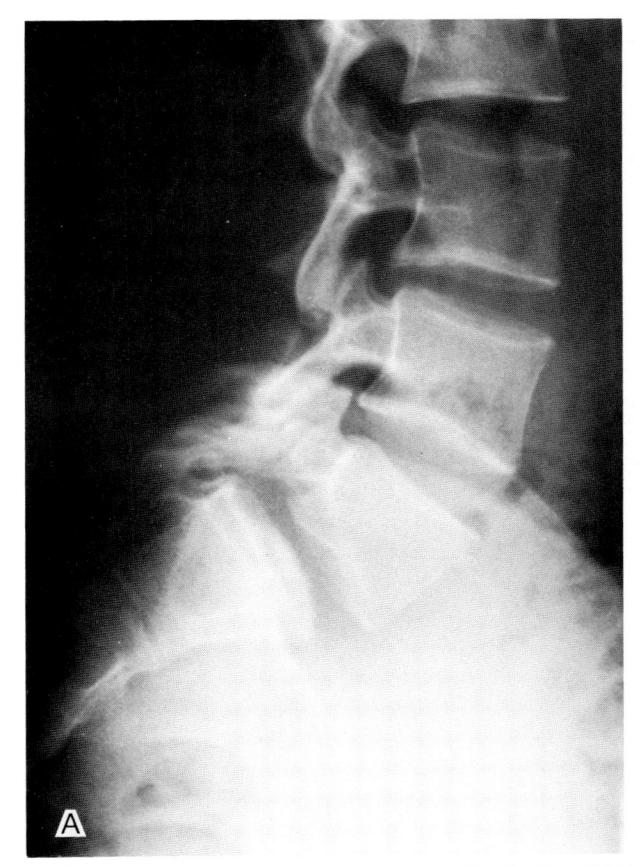

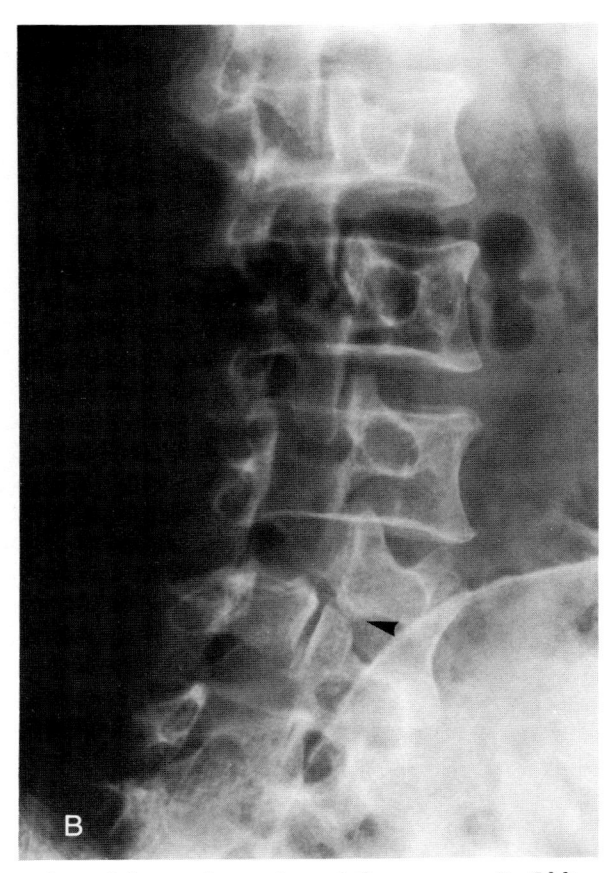

Fig. 8-8. Isthmic spondylolisthesis. A. The body of L5 has slipped forwards on that of the sacrum. B. Oblique radiograph in the same patient. A defect is seen in the pars interarticularis (arrow). (Figure continues).

lows: (1) first degree, less than one-third of the distance between the front and the back of the vertebral body; (2) between one-third and two-thirds of this distance; (3) more than two-thirds of this distance; and (4) spondyloptosis, slippage of one body completely forward on the body below with rotation through 90°. At the L5–S1 level, the L5 nerve is entrapped by forward displacement of that part of the pars interarticularis that lies immediately above the defect (the fracture) as it passes laterally to the L5–S1 foramen (see chapter 3, Fig. 3-10B).

Symptoms

Low back pain, leg pain, or both of these may be present. Occasionally, the leg pain is bilateral. In patients of any age pain may be sufficient to bring the patient to the physician. In children, adolescents, and young adults, the pain is commonly in the back alone. In older patients, often with superadded degenerative disease, the pain is usually in both back and leg. The leg pain is usually in the L5 nerve distribution.

Signs

Movement of the lumbar spine is painful, most marked in extension. Movements are slightly restricted, especially in extension. A step may be felt between the upper and lower spinous processes. When the slippage is at the L5–S1 level, the spinous process of L4 is felt anterior to that of L5. Straight leg raising may be slightly diminished. Sensation is diminished over the L5 dermatome. Muscle weakness occurs in the muscles sup-

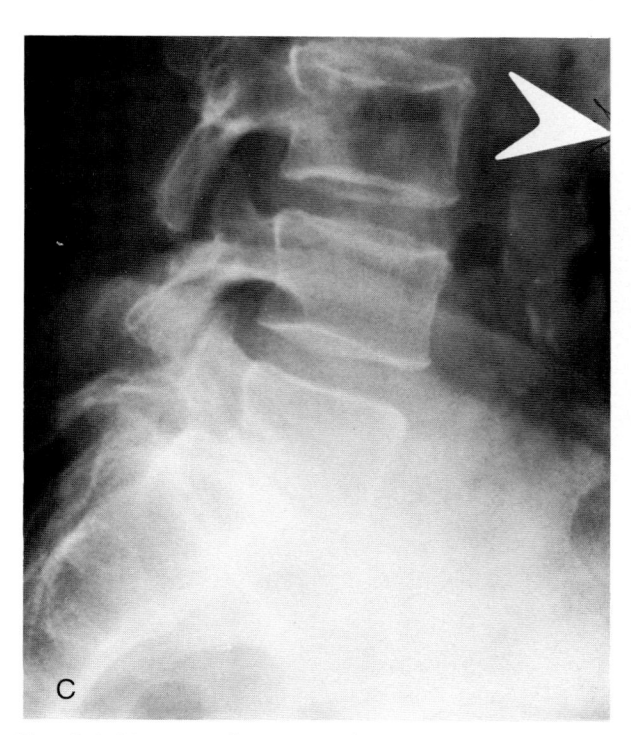

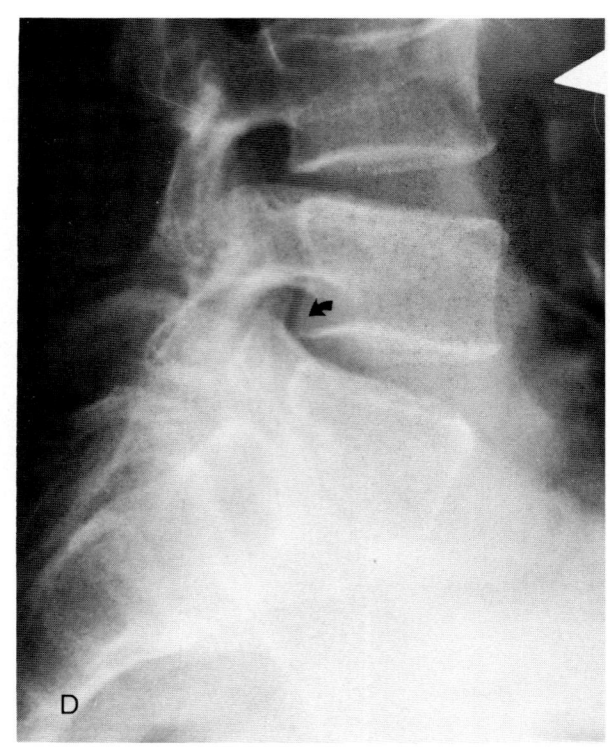

Fig. 8-8 (Continued). C. Another patient. Lateral view in flexion. Note the size of the L4–5 foramen. D. The same patient as in (C). In extension retrospondylolisthesis of L4 on L5 is present and the L4–5 foramen is very narrow. The isthmic spondylolisthesis at L5–S1 is complicated by instability at L4–5.

plied by the L5 nerve, the dorsiflexors of ankle and toes. In adolescents marked hamstring tightness may be present.

Radiographic Changes

The lateral view shows that the body of L5 is displaced forward on the sacrum. In the oblique view a fracture line (a defect) is demonstrated in the pars interarticularis. When there is instability flexion and extension lateral films sometimes show movement of L5 on the sacrum. (Fig. 8-8).

Comment

The radiographic findings are so obvious that the physician is tempted to explain the symptoms and signs on this basis in every patient. There are two pitfalls. The pain may be caused, not by the spondylolisthesis, but by a concomitant sacroiliac syndrome. It is therefore imperative to exclude this. It is advisable to treat the sacroiliac syndrome first. When such treatment does not relieve the pain, attention is given to management of the slippage. In spondylolisthesis strain is thrown on the posterior joints one level higher. This may cause pain and occasionally is responsible for lateral nerve entrapment at this higher level when there is instability at this level.

SUMMARY

In this chapter the different syndromes that are found in the three phases of the degenerative process are reviewed. We turn in the next chapter to consider the diagnostic procedures that are used to make as complete and accurate a diagnosis as possible.

REFERENCES

1. Kirkaldy-Willis WH, Hill R: A more precise diagnosis for low back pain. Spine 4: 102, 1979
2. Cassidy JD, Kirkaldy-Willis WH: The posterior facet joints in low back pain. Presented at the Annual Meeting of the International Society for the Study of the Lumbar Spine, Toronto, June, 1982
3. Mooney V, Robertson J: The facet syndrome. Clin Orthop 115: 149, 1976
4. Bowen V, Cassidy JD: Macroscopic and microscopic anatomy of the Sacroiliac joint from embryonic life until the eighth decade. Spine 6: 620, 1981
5. Keim H, Kirkaldy-Willis WH: Low back pain. Ciba Clin Symposia 32: 6, 1980
6. Pace JB: The piriform syndrome. West J Med 124: 435, 1976
7. Burton CV, Kirkaldy-Willis WH, Yong-Hing K, Heithoff KB: Causes of failure of surgery on the lumbar spine. Clin Orthop 157: 191, 1981
8. Kirkaldy-Willis WH, Paine KWE, Cauchoix J, McIvor GWD: Lumbar spinal stenosis. Clin Orthop 99: 30, 1974
9. Kirkaldy-Willis WH, McIvor GWD (Eds): Symposium on spinal stenosis. Clin Orthop 115, 1976
10. Wiltse LL, Kirkaldy-Willis WH, McIvor GWD: The treatment of spinal stenosis. Clin Orthop. 115, 83, 1976

9 Diagnosis

W. H. Kirkaldy-Willis
S. Tchang

INTRODUCTION

It is time now to consider how a complete and accurate diagnosis can be made. In doing this we have two different aspects of the problem in mind: the phase in which the lesion exists and the nature and site of the lesion. Before going further, the reader is advised to review the illustrations of radiographs in chapter 7.

For clarity we will describe one method by which the diagnosis can be made in a spinal unit. In the less severe cases (usually in Phase I, Dysfunction) the diagnosis is presumptive and the treatment is simple. Patients in this category make up 90% of the referrals to a bank clinic. Using this method time and expense are saved. An example serves to illustrate our approach.

The patient has been evaluated clinically and radiologically. A presumptive diagnosis of dysfunction that chiefly affects the posterior facet joints has been made. The treatment is to attend the Spine Education Programme, to wear a lightweight elastic supporting garment, and to undergo a course of five to ten manipulations. When this treatment regimen is successful, the patient's case is reviewed after 3 months. If treatment fails to relieve the symptoms, the patient is admitted to the hospital overnight for injection of 0.25% bupivacaine (Marcaine) into the posterior joints and overlying muscle. Relief of pain for only a few hours confirms that these joints are the chief source of the pain. However, long-lasting relief may be obtained. If the injections fail, the patient attends daily for 2 or 3 weeks as an outpatient for physiotherapy and occupational therapy. It is usually thought advisable to admit patients in whom this regimen fails to the hospital so that the nature of the lesion can be defined precisely. It is likely that the patient will require a CT scan, possibly a myelogram, and psychological evaluation.

This approach to diagnosis and treatment is not completely accurate. It does mean that 90% of patients can be relieved of their pain in a simple way at low cost. It allows the physician time to concentrate on other, more difficult problems. No patient is neglected. The patient with severe acute symptoms and signs or with a neurological deficit is admitted to the hospital quickly for diagnosis and treatment.

DIAGNOSTIC TECHNIQUES

Careful clinical examination and review of stress radiographs go far toward making the diagnosis. They are in fact essential. Later it is necessary to correlate clinical findings with those obtained from the myelogram or the CT scan (Table 9-1).

110 Managing Low Back Pain • 9

Table 9-1. Diagnostic Tests

Dysfunction
    Stress radiographs
    Effect of facet injection
    Effect of manipulation
Unstable phase
    Stress radiographs (to assess the phase)
    CT scan, myelogram, nerve blocks, E.M.G. (to diagnose the lesion)
Stabilization
    Stress radiographs (to assess the phase)
    CT scan, myelogram, nerve blocks, E.M.G. (to diagnose the lesion)

Injection of posterior joints is often most helpful. Our usual custom is first to inject (using 0.25% bupivacaine and fluoroscopic control) the joints at what is considered the affected level—usually L4–5. The patient then stands up, puts his back through a full range of movements, and tells the examiner whether or not he still has pain. If the first injection does not relieve the pain, another level—perhaps L5–S1—is injected. The patient tests the effect of this in the same way. If necessary, on rare occasions, the L3–4 joint may then be injected. This procedure makes it possible to identify the level of the lesion with certainty and to determine if the major source of pain lies in the facet joints.

Manipulation

Benefit from manipulation directed to a specific joint provides evidence of Dysfunction of that joint.

Myelography

Until recently, when patients had persistent leg pain, it was the custom in most centers to request a myelogram. Now that third and fourth generation high resolution CT scanners are available in many centers, this diagnostic tool bids high to replace myelography in most patients. Because the CT scan is not universally available, we will discuss myelography first.

In performing a myelogram, the water-soluble contrast medium metrizamide should be used. This medium is absorbed into the blood stream. Complications are few. Headaches, nausea, and vomiting are not as common or as persistent as after myelography done with an oil-based contrast medium. Cases in which the patient becomes disoriented or even psychotic for a few hours have been reported. Seizure is a rare complication following lumbar examination with metrizamide. Up to now no arachnoiditis has been reported in humans following metrizamide myelography.

A disk herniation within the confines of the central spinal canal is usually clearly demonstrated by an anterior or anterolateral defect in the contrast column at the disk space or by the cutting off of one nerve sheath. It is necessary to differentiate the defect caused by the presence of a herniation from that caused by the presence of spinal tumors. A myelographic defect caused by the presence of extradural tumors may simulate that caused by a disk herniation. However, the most common tumor in this group is metastasis, and it is invariably associated with bone destruction. Extradural neurofibroma produces characteristic bony erosion. Intradural tumors are confined within the dural sac, which is not displaced away from bony margins. Extradural abscess may present as an extradural mass, but usually the disk space is narrowed and destruction of the endplate of the adjacent vertebrae is evident. Myelography never demonstrates the presence of a disk herniation in the lateral nerve canal or lateral canal stenosis unless medial enlargement of the superior facet by an osteophyte is present.

Central spinal stenosis is clearly shown. In the degenerative type the canal is small and clover leaf or trefoil in shape because of medial protrusion of enlarged posterior articular processes and backward protrusion of osteophytic outgrowths from the back of the vertebral bodies. In the developmental type the central canal is small in both sagittal and coronal planes. In the combined type the observed changes demonstrate the features of both degenerative and developmental stenosis. The extent of the process—the number of segments involved—is also clearly delineated. It is useful during the course of the examination to ask the patient while he is standing to extend his lumbar spine as much as possible. Stenosis not evident in the neutral position may become evident with the spine extended, or stenosis already noted may become more marked (Figs. 9-1, 9-2).

The CT Scan

Computerized tomographic scanning is now widely used to diagnose lesions in the lumbar spine. At the start of our experience 5 years ago we soon became aware that for the first time we could see lateral canal stenosis and measure the degree to which it was present. We soon realized that in diagnosing central and lateral stenosis this was the best tool yet available. With the advent of high resolution scanning it is now possible to demonstrate soft tissue shadows. A high window setting is used for bony structures and a low one for soft tissues. With a cursor (a small white rectangle) placed over the soft tissue shadow, a mean density reading can be obtained. In this way the nature of the soft tissue can be assessed with reasonable accuracy. The mean density of disk material is the highest; fibrous tissue is next; then the densities of spinal nerves, of cauda equina, and fat follow in descending order. With the patient's trunk supine on the table and the pelvis rotated first to one side, then to the other using a small pillow or sandbag, it is possible to study the effect of rotation on the facets and lateral canals. The same can be done for flexion–extension movement.

Figures showing CT images illustrate the changes to be seen more clearly than any script. The following lesions are thus described: changes in the facet joints (Fig. 9-3A–F), changes due to disc herniation and fibrosis (Fig. 9-4A–F), changes due to central and lateral stenosis (Fig. 9-5A–F), further changes due to lateral stenosis (Fig. 9-6A–C) and changes seen after spinal fusion (Fig. 9-7A–F). A word of caution is necessary. Lesions or bony protuberances demonstrated in the myelogram or by the CT scan may not produce symptoms. It is essential to correlate the clinical symptoms and signs with myelographic and CT findings. In cases when doubt is present, a selective nerve block and/or electromyelography may be of assistance.

Selective Nerve Blocks

The rationale of this procedure is to identify the spinal nerve at the level of the symptoms. This is especially useful when images from the CT scan demonstrate lesions at two levels.

The Technique. For the L4 nerve at the L4–5 level, the skin is anesthetized under fluoroscopic control opposite the spinous process of L4, 5 to 6 cm from the midline, and a thin lumbar puncture needle is passed in the coronal plane angled at 45° toward the midline until contact is made with the transverse process of L4. The needle is withdrawn, reintroduced 1 cm caudal to the transverse process, and advanced toward the L4–5 foramen. When the needle reaches the L4 nerve, the patient experiences pain in the leg. It is important to ascertain if this is the pain that the patient has complained of. Injection of 1 to 2 ml of renographin demonstrates the tunnel of soft tissue in which the nerve runs laterally and caudally. At this point injecting 2 to 3 ml of 0.25% bupivacaine will abolish the pain. For the L5 nerve at the L5–S1 level the skin is anesthetized in the same way opposite the spinous process of L5 and the needle is advanced in the coronal plane and at 45° toward the midline. It is withdrawn slightly when it hits the transverse process of L5, introduced again to pass caudal to the process, and advanced until it contacts the L5 nerve at the L5–S1 foramen. To block the S1 nerve the needle is introduced posteriorly through the first sacral foramen and advanced to contact the anterior ramus. The remainder of the procedure is as described above.

The information obtained from this simple procedure gives no clue as to the nature of the lesion but does identify the level when this is in doubt.

Electromyography

Dr. J. R. Donat, neurologist at the University Hospital in Saskatoon, writes as follows:

"Electromyography is probably not necessary in patients with definite and well localized findings of radiculopathy on physical examination. It may occasionally confirm or help localize radiculopathy in patients with minimal findings or normal examination.

Routine nerve conduction studies are normal or show only non-specific findings in patients with radiculopathy. However, they help exclude other conditions such as a neuropathy which may confuse the diagnosis.

Electromyography per se may show fibrillation potentials and motor unit changes in dener-

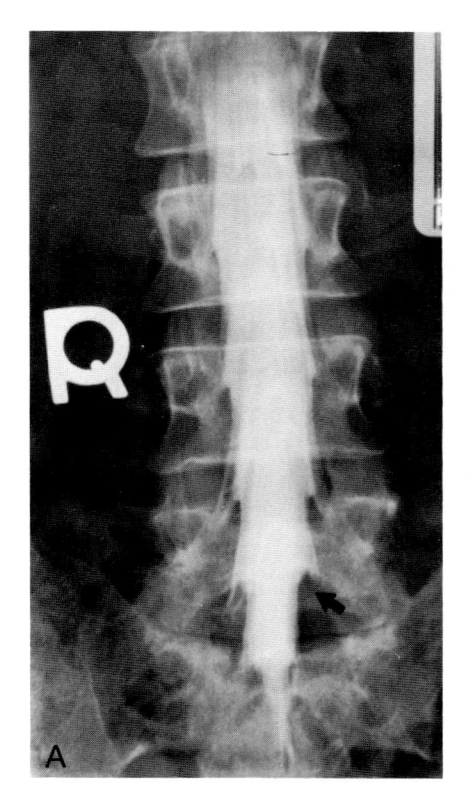

Fig. 9-1. (A) AP myelogram L5–S1 disk herniation on left. The S1 nerve sheath on the left is cut off (arrow). (B) AP and oblique myelograms showing L5–S1 disk herniation on right. There is a defect in the dye column (arrows). (C) AP myelogram showing one-level central degenerative stenosis at L4–5. The dye column is almost completely blocked at this level. (D) Lateral myelogram of the same patient. At the L4–5 level the dye column is indented anteriorly by a bulging disk (not a herniation) and posteriorly by the enlarged articular process. (E) AP myelogram. The column is almost completely interrupted at the L4–5 level because of marked one-level central stenosis, degenerative in type. (F) Lateral view of the same patient. The block at L4–5 is again seen. The AP diameter of the dye column is reduced in size; mild developmental stenosis is present.

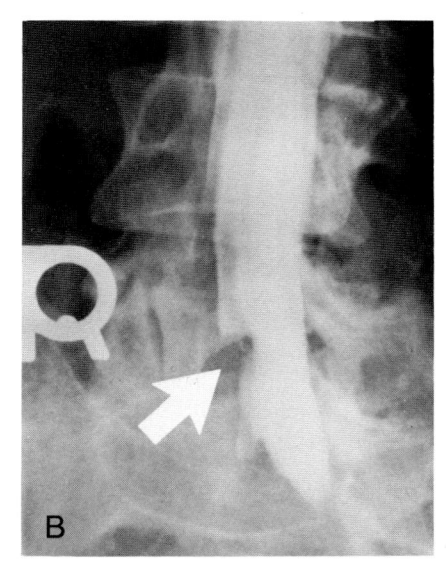

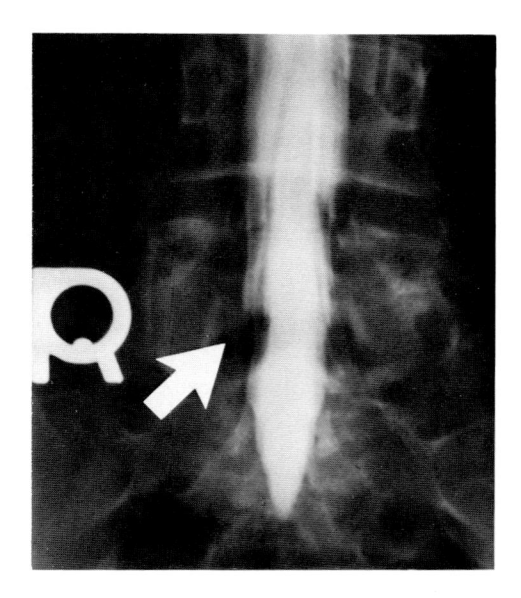

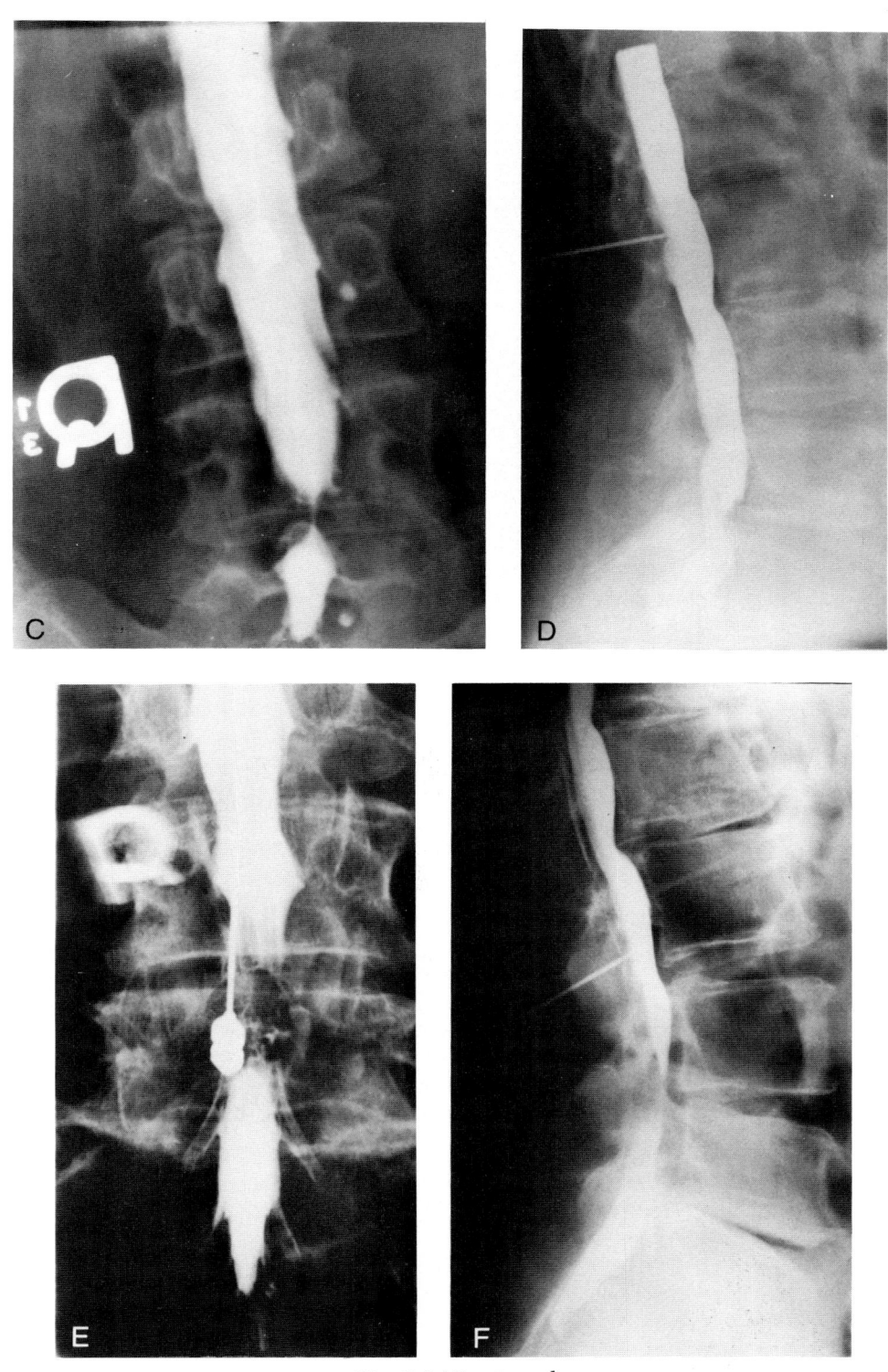

Fig. 9-1 (Continued).

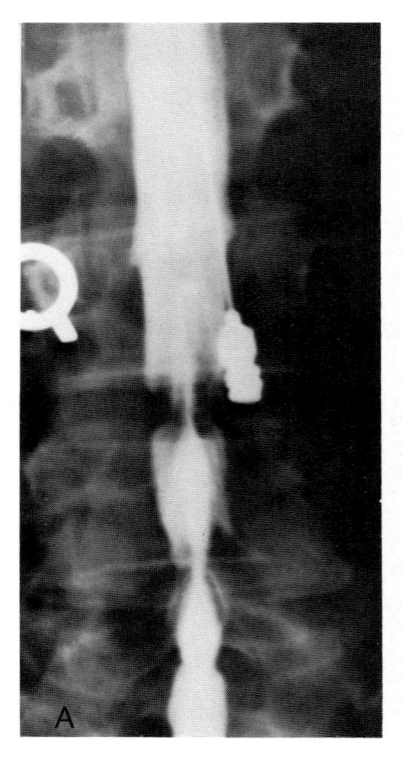

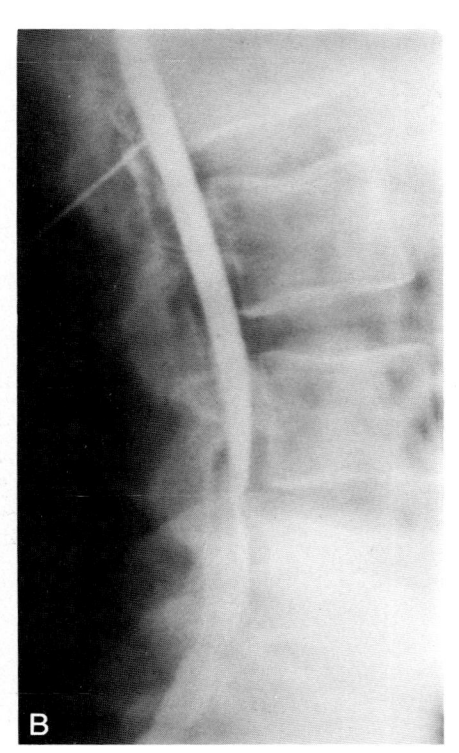

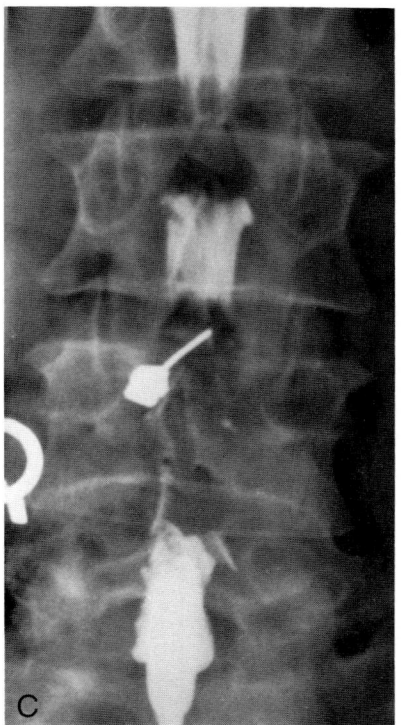

Fig. 9-2. (A) AP myelogram. Defects can be seen in the dye column at the L4–5 and L5–S1 levels, indicating the presence of degenerative central stenosis at two levels. (B) The same patient, lateral view. The AP diameter of the dye column is reduced. This suggests the presence of mild developmental stenosis. (C) AP myelogram. The dye column is interrupted at the L3–4, L4–5, and L5–S1 levels, indicating that very marked central degenerative stenosis is present at these three levels (Figure continues).

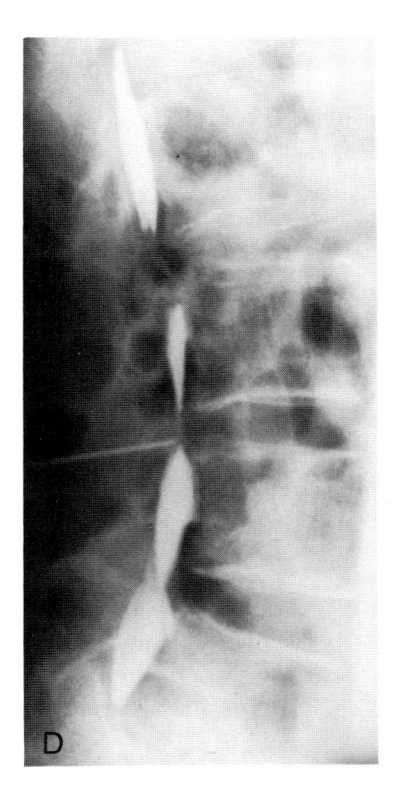

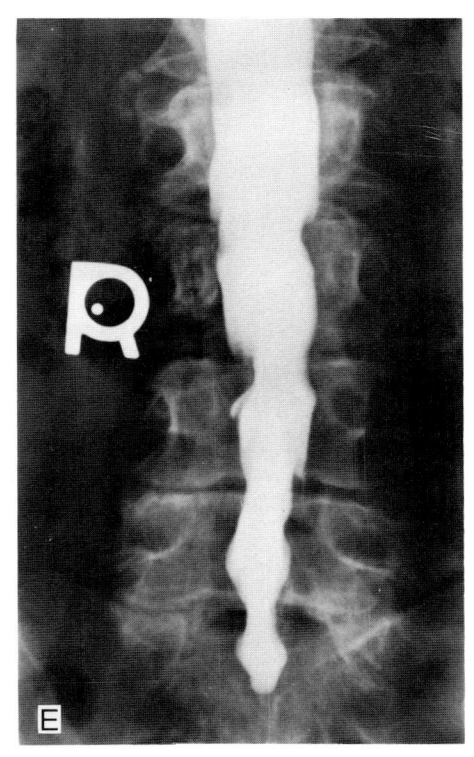

Fig. 9-2 (Continued). (D) The same patient, lateral view. The AP diameter of the dye column is markedly reduced. Developmental stenosis is complicated by degenerative stenosis. (E) AP myelogram. Marked irregularity of the dye column, which is narrow from L3–4 to the sacrum. (F) The same patient, lateral view. The dye column is indented anteriorly at every level by bulging of degenerated disks. At the lower levels the column is also indented posteriorly by enlarged articular processes. Multilevel degenerative central stenosis is present.

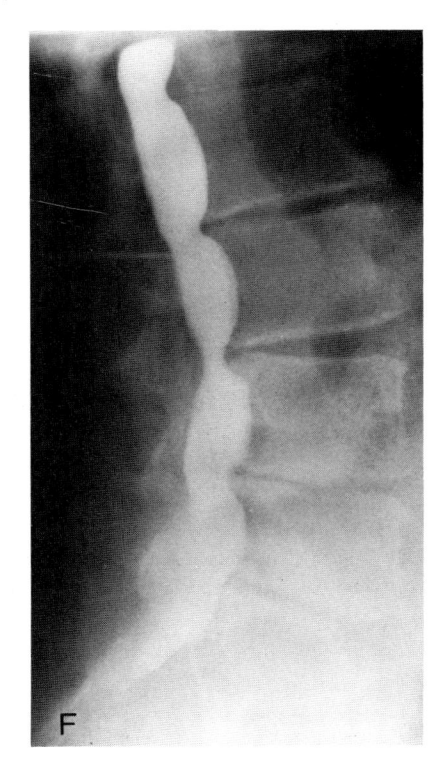

116   *Managing Low Back Pain • 9*

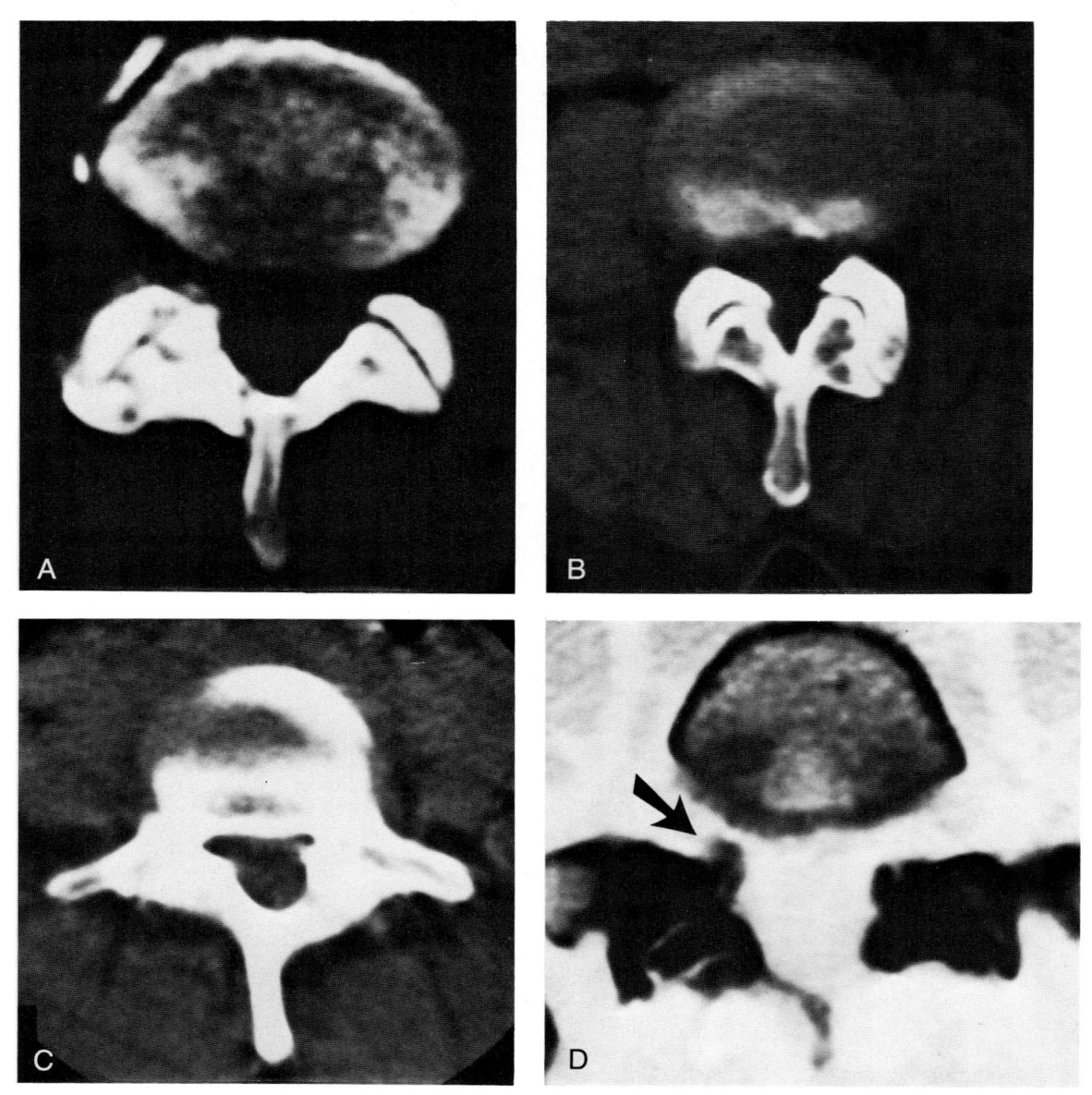

Fig. 9-3. (A) CT scan at the L4–5 level. On the right (viewer's left) the posterior facets are enlarged and fragmented. Marked posterior facet degeneration is present. (B) CT scan at the L4–5 level. Tropism of the facets is present. On the right (viewer's left) the facets are oblique. On the left they are more in the sagittal plane. (C) CT scan at the L4–5 level. The laminae are asymmetrical. The lamina on the right (viewer's left) is displaced forward relative to that on the left. The central canal is displaced to the left. (D) CT scan at the L5–S1 level. A large osteophyte arising from the anterior surface of the superior facet (arrow) has narrowed the right lateral canal (Figure continues).

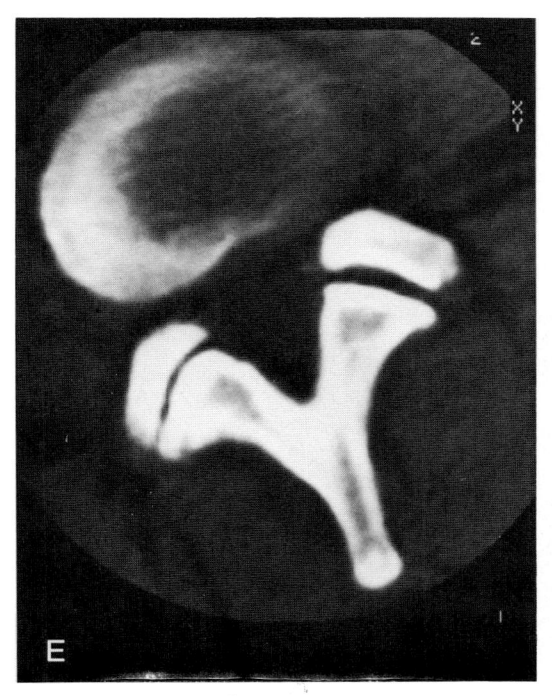

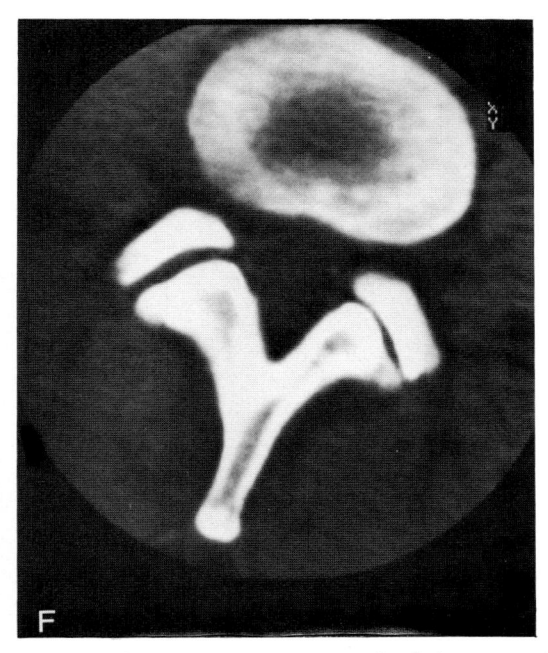

Fig. 9-3 (Continued). (E) CT scan at L4–5 with rotation. The posterior joint on the left (viewer's right) is open because of capsular laxity and the superior facet has moved forward to narrow the left lateral canal. (F) The same patient. Rotation in the opposite direction has opened the posterior joint on the right (viewer's left) and the right lateral canal is narrow. Instability at L4–5 with increased abnormal movement is present.

vated muscles. The distribution of abnormalities may help localize the lesion to a particular root. Denervation of para-spinal muscles confirms that the lesion involves nerve roots, but has little localizing value. Unfortunately, the EMG is negative in patients whose symptoms are due to irritation of dorsal roots.

Several new techniques for detecting lesions at sites proximal to those usually studied by routine nerve conduction methods are currently under investigation. These include the F-wave, H-reflex, and spinal evoked potentials.

The F-wave is a late response due to recurrent discharge of motor neurons following stimulation of their peripheral branches. Delay of F-waves evoked by stimulation of peroneal or posterior tibial nerves may suggest lesions of the L5 or S1 ventral roots. The H-reflex is the electrophysiological equivalent of the tendon reflex. Delay of the H-reflex recorded from the soleus muscle following stimulation of the tibial nerve at the knee may suggest a lesion of the S1 dorsal or ventral roots. Both these late responses are easily recorded with equipment generally available in EMG laboratories.

Spinal evoked potentials are recorded over the cauda equina or spinal cord following stimulation of peripheral nerves. This technique may be useful in detecting lesions of the L5 dorsal root which are not accompanied by weakness, reflex changes or EMG abnormalities. However, it requires computerized averaging of very large numbers of responses.

Clinical electromyography requires a great deal of skill and judgment. Undue confidence in equivocal or non-diagnostic abnormalities leads to frequent false positive diagnosis. The results of electromyography should always be considered in relation to the history, physical examination, and results of other investigations.

118   Managing Low Back Pain • 9

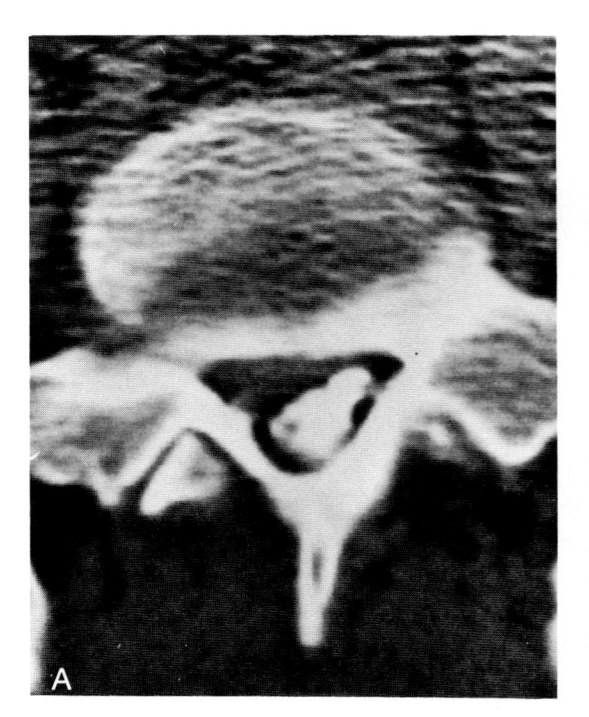

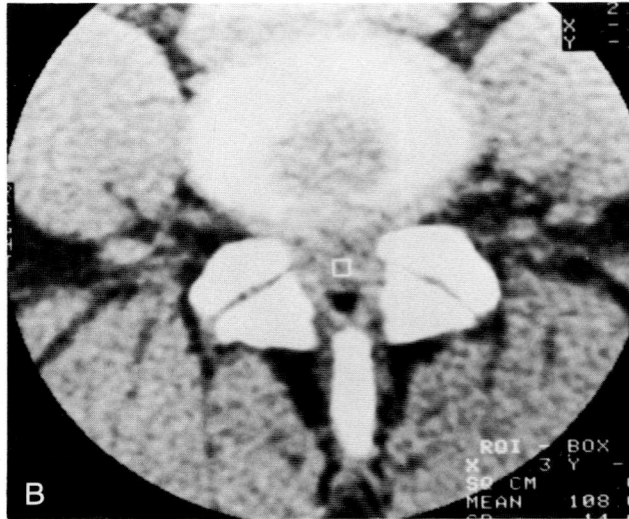

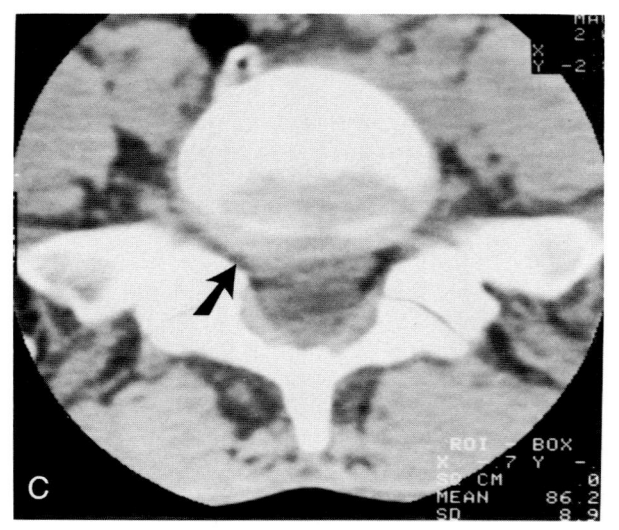

Fig. 9-4. (A) Disk herniation. Metrizamide myelogram followed by CT scan. At the L5–S1 level the dye is displaced posteriorly on the right by a disk herniation. (B) Disk herniation. Scan at L4–5. A large central disk herniation fills the central canal. The mean density of the shadow, as indicated by the white rectangle (the cursor), is 108, the density of a herniation. The mean density of the cauda equina would be much lower. (C) Disk herniation. CT scan at L5–S1. The soft tissue shadow of a disk herniation is seen on the right (arrow). The mean density is 86.2. (Figure continues).

Diagnosis **119**

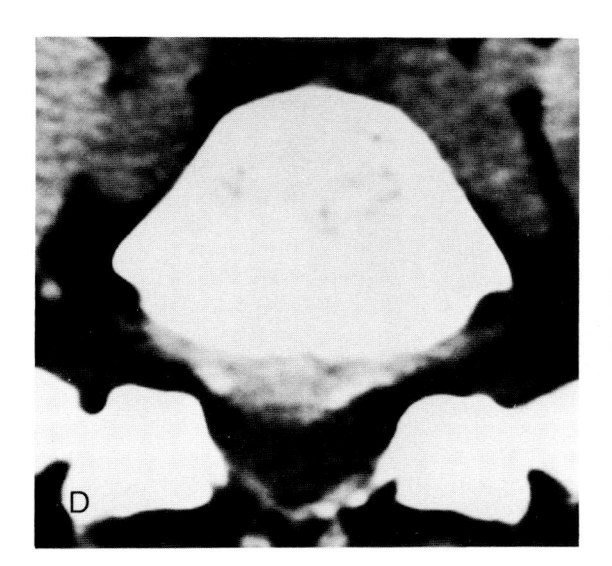

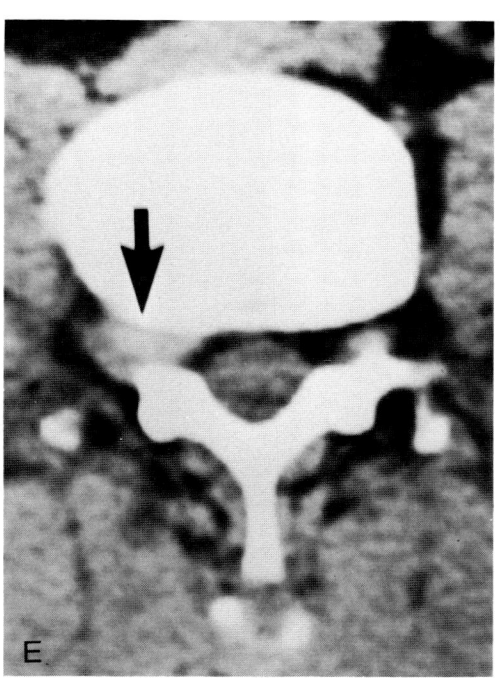

Fig. 9-4 (Continued). (D) Central disk herniation. CT scan at L5–S1. The soft tissue shadow of the central disk herniation is clearly seen. (E) Lateral disc herniation. CT scan at L4–5. The arrow points to a large soft tissue shadow on the right. This herniation would not be demonstrated in a myelogram. (F) Fibrosis. CT scan at L5–S1. The arrow points to a poorly defined soft tissue shadow. The mean density of this is 44.2, too low for a herniation, correct for scar tissue.

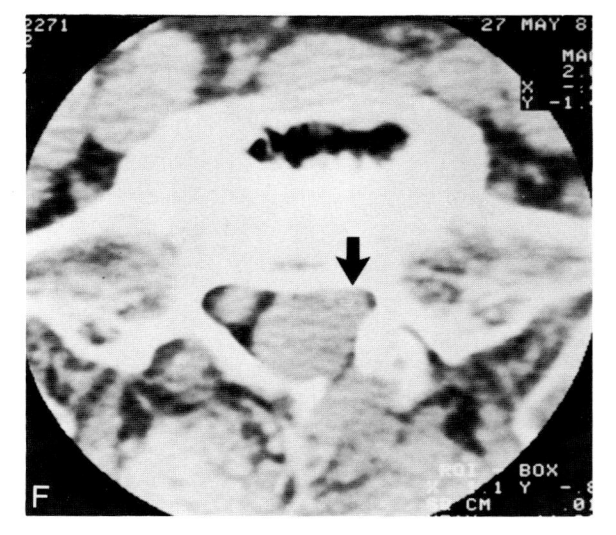

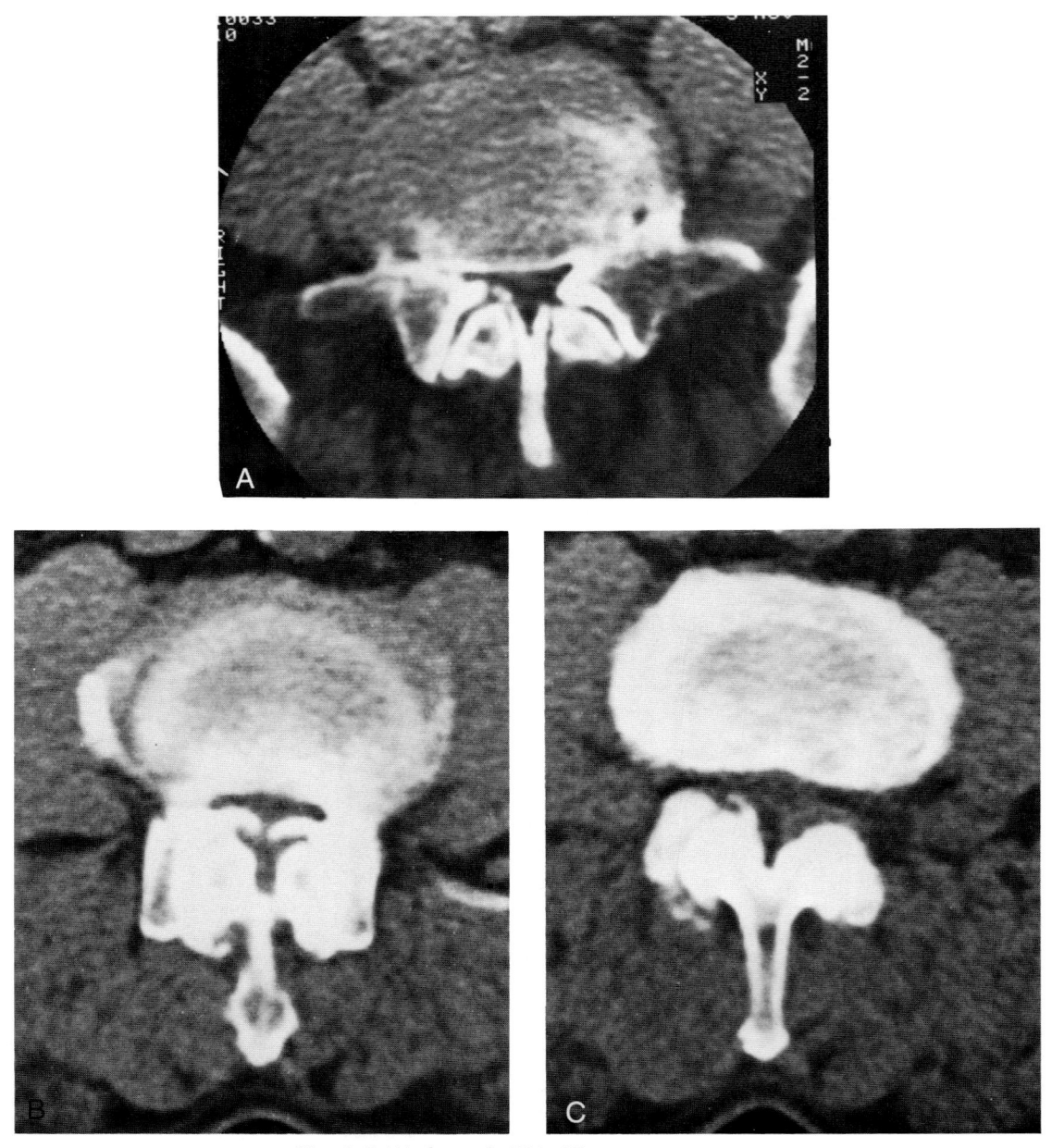

Fig. 9-5 (A) through (C). (*Figure continues*).

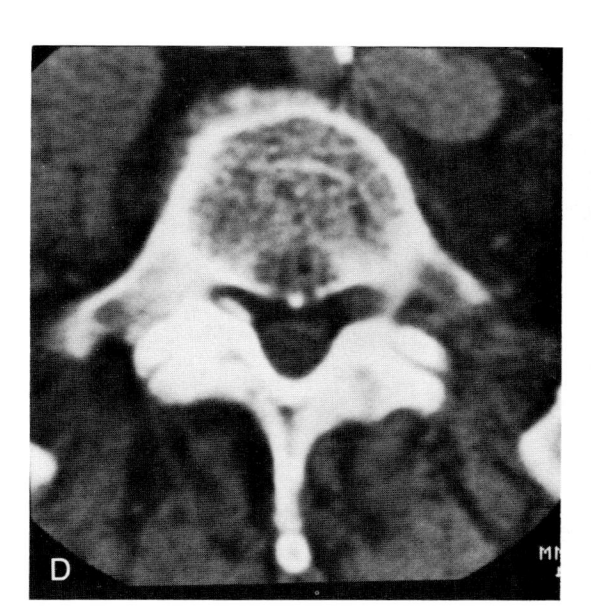

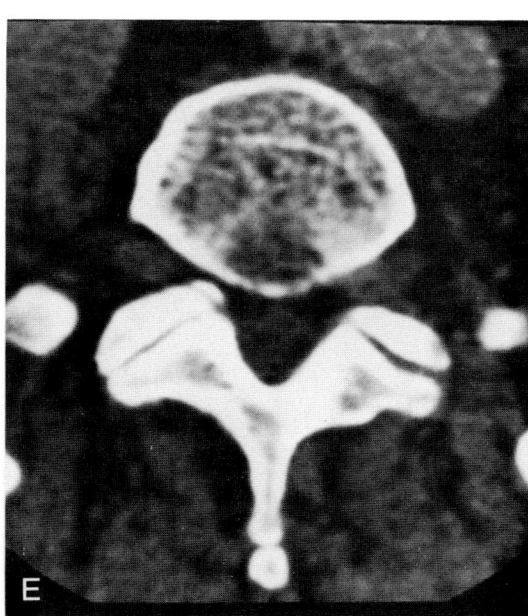

Fig. 9-5. (A) Central stenosis. CT scan at L5–S1. Enlargement of posterior facets on both sides has markedly narrowed the central canal. (B) Central stenosis. CT scan at L5–S1. Enlargement of posterior facets on both sides towards the midline has markedly narrowed the central canal. The presence of large osteophytes on the anterior surface of the superior facets has produced even further narrowing. (C) Unilateral central and lateral stenosis. Same patient as in (B). CT scan at L3–4. Enlargement of the posterior facets on the right has produced central and lateral stenosis. (D) Lateral stenosis. CT scan at the level of the pedicles of L4. The right lateral canal is slightly narrowed just above the point at which the L4 nerve exits. (E) Lateral stenosis. The same patient as in (D). CT scan 5 mm below the L4 pedicles. The right lateral canal is very narrow. The shadow of the L4 nerve can be seen lateral to the canal. This stenosis has entrapped the L4 nerve on the right. (F) Lateral stenosis. CT scan at L4–5. A large osteophyte is protruding medially from the left superior facet, the subarticular gutter is very narrow and the L5 nerve is entrapped between the superior facet and the back of the vertebral body.

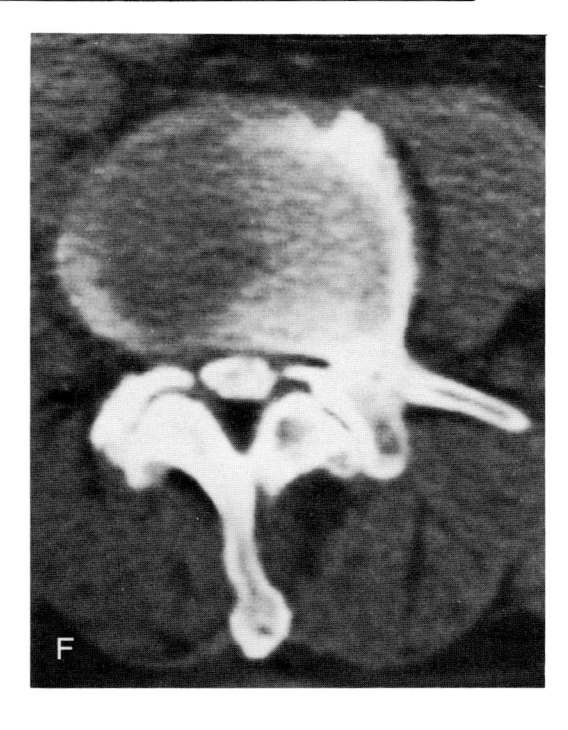

122 *Managing Low Back Pain • 9*

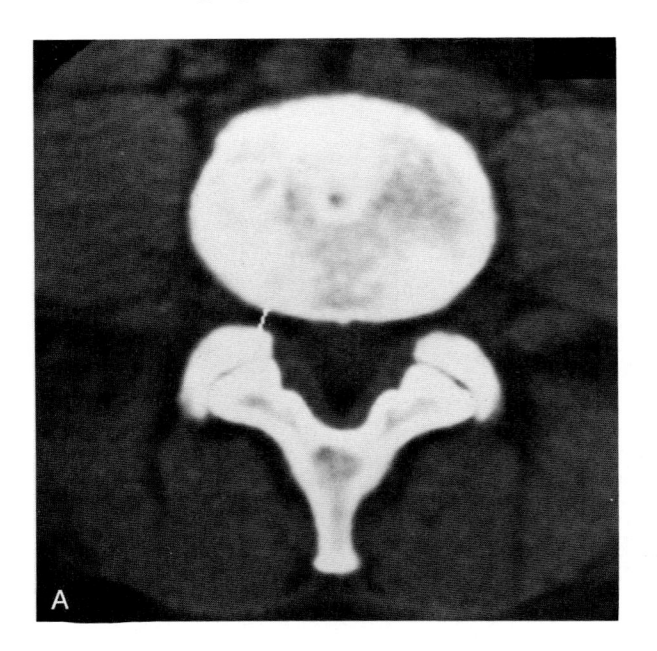

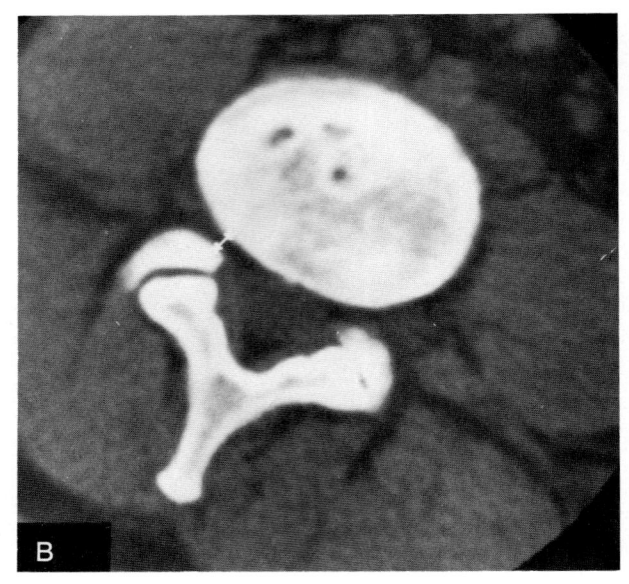

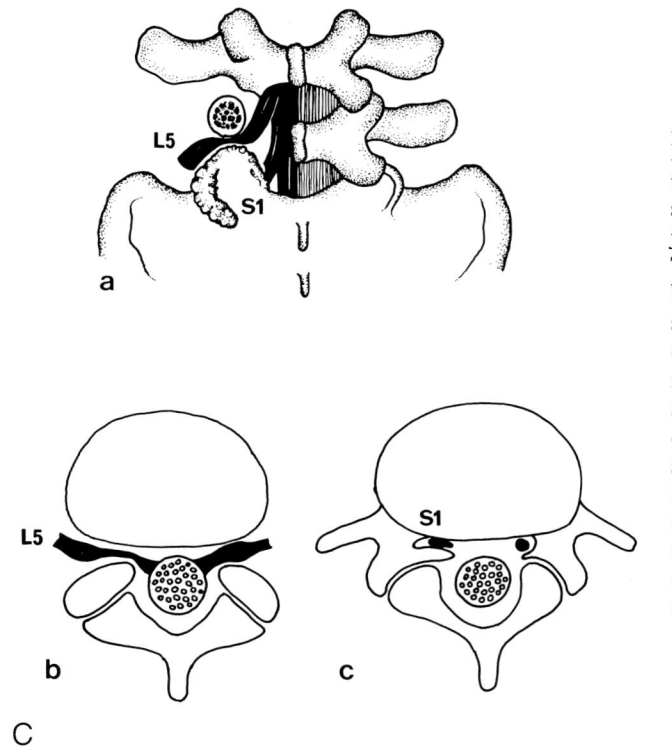

Fig. 9-6. (A) Dynamic lateral stenosis. CT scan at L4–5. Both lateral canals are slightly narrow. Note the diameter of the right canal (viewer's left). (B) The same patient as in (A). With rotation the posterior joint on the right (viewer's left) opens (Instability). The superior facet moves forward and the lateral canal becomes narrower than in (A). (C) Diagram to demonstrate how two nerves can be entrapped at one level (a) On the viewer's left at the L5–S1 level, the L5 nerve can be entrapped between the pedicle of L5 and the superior facet of the sacrum, and the S1 nerve can be entrapped by an osteophyte that narrows the subarticular gutter deep to the superior facet. (b) The L5 nerve can be entrapped between the superior facet of the sacrum and the pedicle of L5. (c) The S1 nerve can be entrapped between the superior facet of the sacrum and the back of the body of the sacrum or of L5.

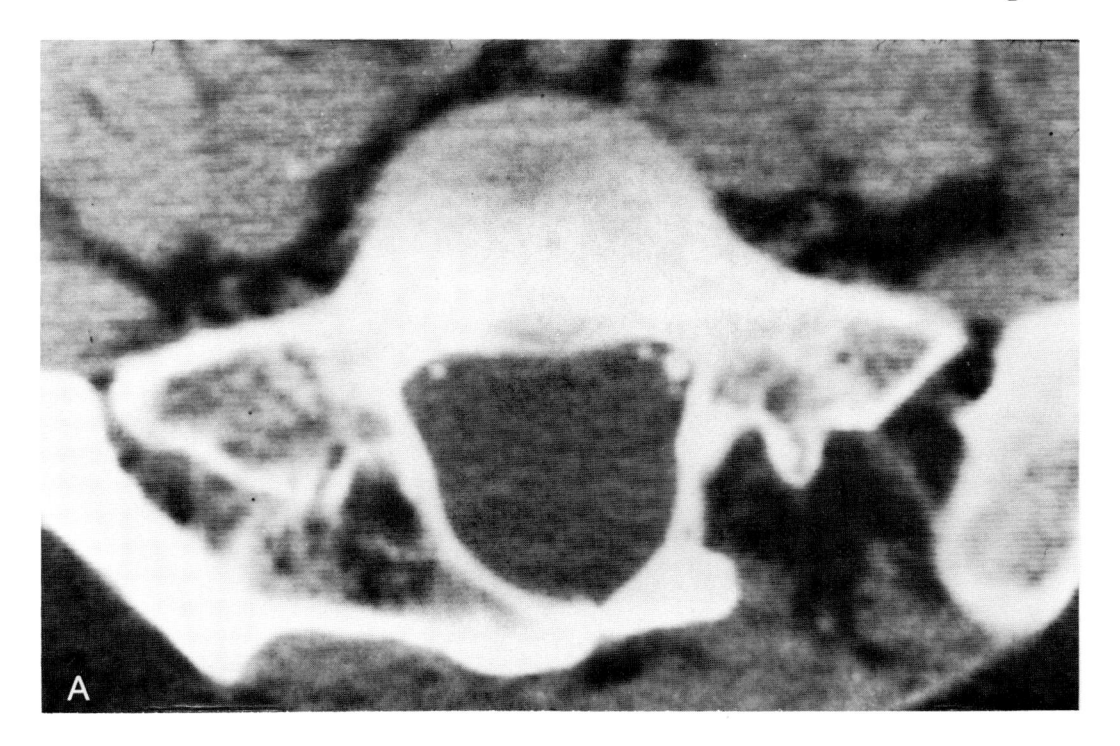

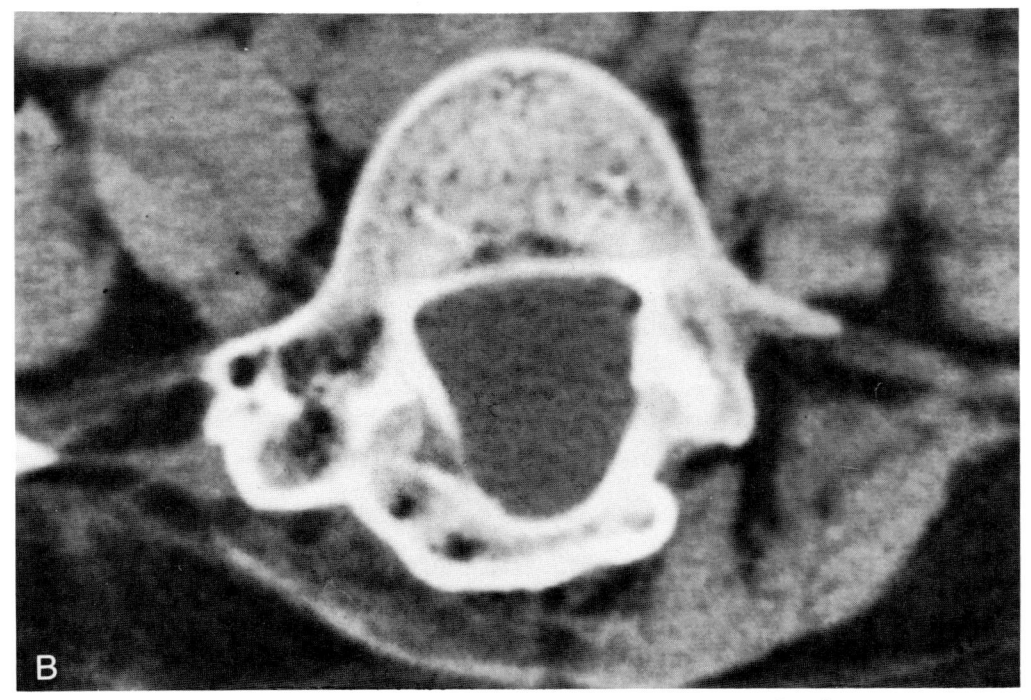

Fig. 9-7. (A) Successful fusion. CT scan at L5–S1. The facet joints are fused. An uninterrupted bar of bone is present posteriorly. (B) The same patient. At the L5 level the fusion is equally complete. (Figure continues).

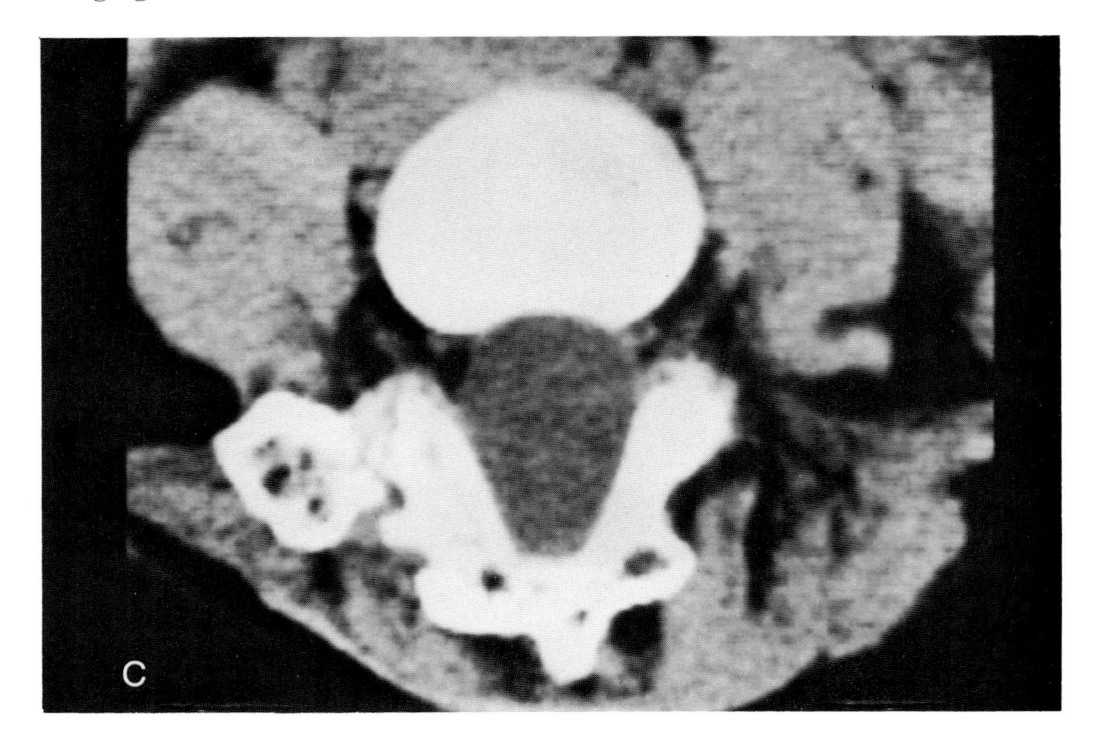

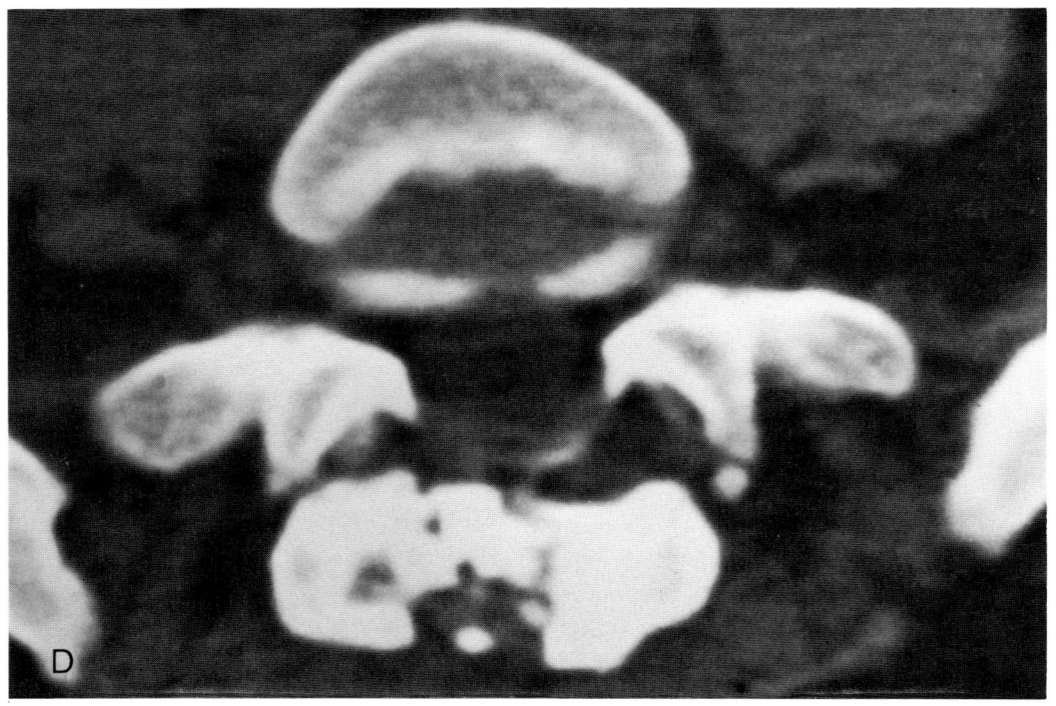

Fig. 9-7 (*Continued*). (C) The same patient. At the L4–5 level the fusion is equally solid. Fusion is complete from L4 to the sacrum. (D) Another patient. Failed fusion. CT scan at level of upper sacrum. The posterior fusion mass is fragmented (Figure continues).

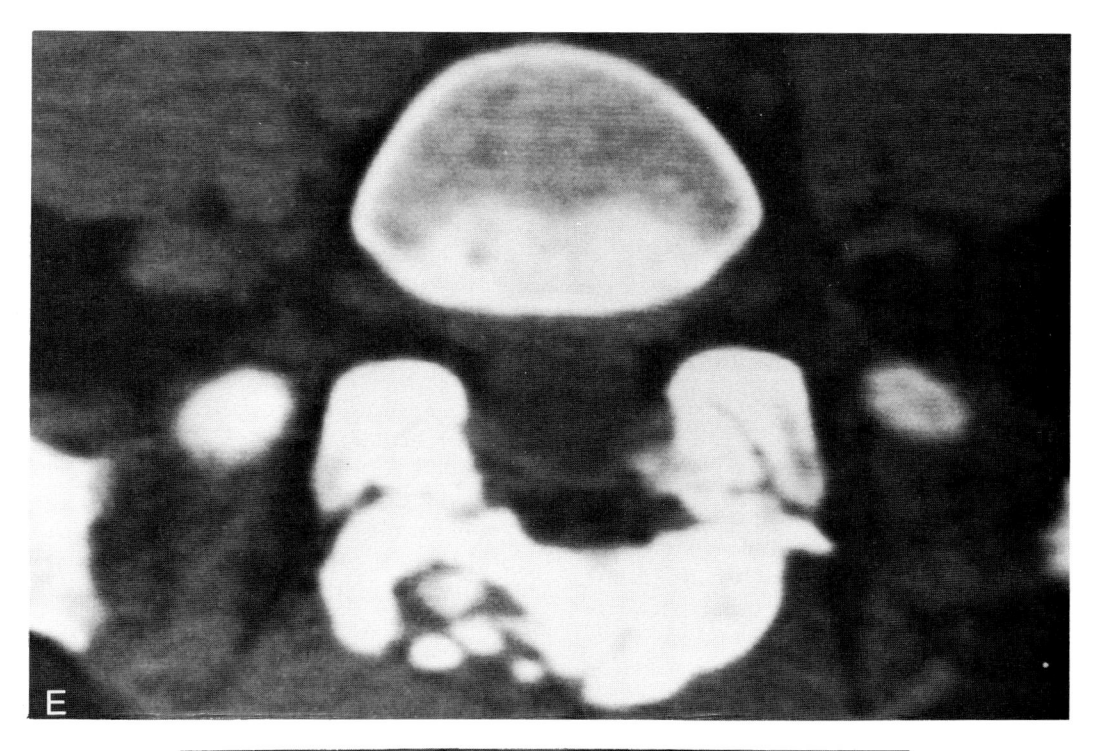

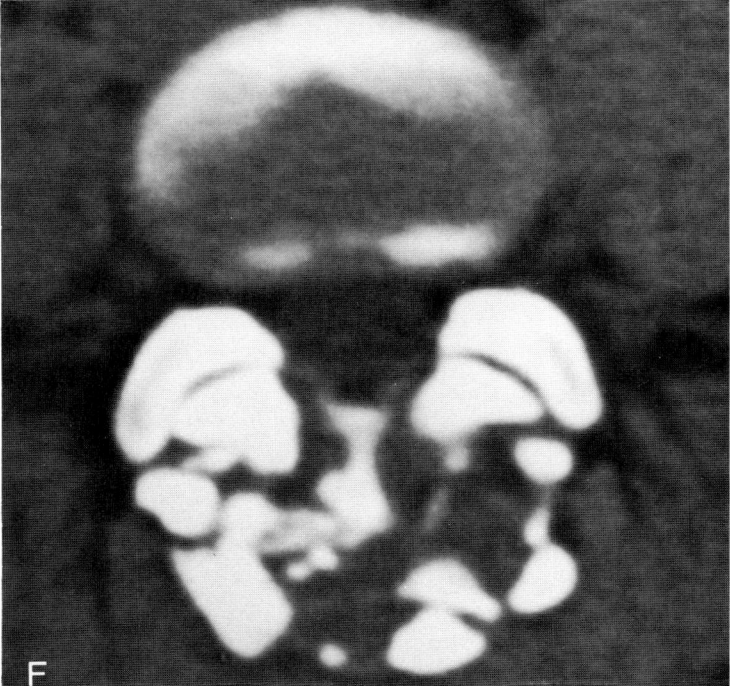

Fig. 9-7 (Continued). (E) The same patient. At the L5–S1 level the posterior joints are not fused. The posterior bar of bone is fragmented. (F) The same patient. At the L4–5 level the posterior joints are not fused. The posterior mass of bone is grossly fragmented.

Psychological Assessment

The value of psychological testing and of an interview with a psychologist interested in the psychological aspects of musculoskeletal lesions has been discussed in chapter 6. Before any decision is made to advise the patient to consider operative intervention, and in many other cases as well, it is essential that the physician and the psychologist sit down together to discuss the patient's problem in the framework of his or her personality. In some patients the problem is mainly a surgical one; in others mainly a psychological one, and in others it is mixed in nature. In the last group the risks involved in obtaining a good result must be carefully weighed. Often, even when the problem is mainly surgical, knowledge and understanding of the patient's personality and of minor psychological problems helps the surgeon to obtain a better result. Patients with a difficult personality and with major psychological problems often have a serious lesion that requires treatment and they should not be barred from this, provided that future expectations are carefully assessed and the patient informed of them. Many patients who have suffered back and leg pain for several years, especially those who have had several previous operations, are naturally depressed and have suffered a change in personality.

It is surprising how often the opinion of the surgeon and the considered assessment of the psychologist agree. When, on rare occasions, the latter advises strongly against further operative intervention, the wise surgeon heeds this advice.

SYNTHESIS OF CLINICAL EXAMINATION AND DIAGNOSTIC TESTS

The final step in the assessment is to synthesize all that has been done. The reader is again referred to Figure 5-1 in which the various aspects of the problem are set out in tabular form. Some examples serve to make this clear. This assessment gives a concise indication of the treatment required.

Matching the Phase and the Lesion. The patient in Phase I with posterior facet dysfunction is likely to respond to a course of manipulations or a facet injection. The patient in the early stage of Phase II may respond to rest and immobilization. Later in this phase fusion may be required to treat joint instability. In addition, decompression and fusion may be indicated when instability is complicated by a disk herniation or lateral stenosis. The patient in Phase III does not require fusion but may need a decompression for central and/or lateral stenosis.

The Type of Lesion. It is important to define the type of lesion accurately and fully. For example, the symptoms in a patient with central stenosis may be caused largely by interference with the blood supply to the cauda equina and spinal nerves; a decompression should be large enough to relieve this. The patient with several previous operations may be suffering from irritation and stimulation of the sympathetic nervous system. Further operative intervention may make the patient worse. What is required is an epidural steroid injection, a caudal block, or selective nerve block with bupivacaine.

Differential Diagnosis

It is clearly important to consider other conditions that mimic degenerative lesions. We recall the patient with symptoms and signs of an L5–S1 disk herniation who in fact had an abscess in the L5–S1 disk space caused by vertebral osteomyelitis. It may be difficult to differentiate neurogenic and vascular claudication. A neuropathy due to diabetes may mimic a disk herniation or spinal stenosis.

Psychological Assessment

Enough has been said in chapter 6 for us to appreciate the importance of such evaluation before deciding to carry out any operative procedure and in other cases as well.

REFERENCES

1. Burton CV, Heithoff KB, Kirkaldy-Willis WH, Ray CD: Computed tomographic scanning and the lumbar spine. Spine 4: 356, 1979

2. Kirkaldy-Willis WH: Five common back disorders: how to diagnose and treat them. Geriatrics 33: 32, 1978
3. Kirkaldy-Willis WH, Hill RI: A more precise diagnosis for low back pain. Spine 4: 102, 1979
4. Kirkaldy-Willis WH, Heithoff KB, Bowen CVA, Shannon R: Pathological anatomy of lumbar spondylosis correlated with the CT scan, Radiographic Evaluation of the Spine. Edited by Post MJD. New York, Masson, 1980
5. Kirkaldy-Willis WH, Farfan HF: Instability of the lumbar spine. Clin Orthop, 165: 110, 1982
6. Mooney V, Robertson J: The facet syndrome. Clin Orthop 115: 149, 1976
7. Tajima T, Furukawa K, Kuramochi E: Selective lumbosacral radiculography and block. Spine 5: 69, 1980

10 Differential Diagnosis of Low Back Pain

J. H. Wedge and S. Tchang

INTRODUCTION

Many different diseases can present as low back pain. The purpose of this chapter is not to classify the numerous different causes of back pain but rather to describe a method of approaching the problem of differential diagnosis. The reader is referred to other sources for an exhaustive encyclopedic classification of the etiology of low back pain.

We find Macnab's classification[1] of back pain simple, concise, and useful. He lists the causes as follows:
1. Viscerogenic
2. Neurogenic
3. Vasculogenic
4. Psychogenic
5. Spondylogenic

As soon as the physician thinks of back pain in this way, the likelihood of mistaking a more serious cause for degenerative disease is reduced. There are a small number of causes of back pain that often lead to diagnostic problems. Failure to do a thorough examination or to order the appropriate investigations at the outset is the usual error. A thorough abdominal examination may direct attention away from the spine to the source of viscerogenic pain, an elevated ESR to an infection, and a bone scan to a tumor.

We will emphasize those conditions that are commonly missed. It is extremely valuable always to remember the lesions listed in Table 10-1.

VISCEROGENIC BACK PAIN

In practice, visceral pain is not very often confused with pain originating in the spine. Usually, sufficient specific symptoms and signs are present to localize the problem correctly. For example, carcinoma of the pancreas can cause severe and persistent back pain. However, this lesion causes other problems that turn attention away from the spine. Hollow viscus perforation or colic seldom closely mimics "typical back pain," nor do gynecologic conditions. Low back pain of mechanical spondylotic origin is normally relieved by rest, whereas lesions in solid or hollow viscera are not so relieved.

NEUROGENIC BACK PAIN

Serious delay in diagnosis can result from failure to appreciate the fact that neoplasms of the cord and cauda equina and nerve roots and inflammatory lesions can mimic spondylogenic pain. Neurofibromata and neurilemmomata cause erosion of bone, often at the intervertebral foramina (Fig. 10-1). Spinal cord and cauda equina tumors give characteristic appearances on myelography (Fig. 10-2). Central and lateral spinal stenosis (see chapter 8 for symptoms and signs) can be diagnosed by myelography and CT scanning.

Diabetic neuropathy can cause nerve root irritation.[2] A clinical picture that is indistingusha-

Table 10-1. Important and Often Missed Causes of Back Pain

Vasculogenic
    Abdominal aortic aneurysm
    Peripheral vascular disease
Neurogenic
    Nerve Root Tumors
        Neurofibroma
        Neurilemmomata
    Spinal cord tumors
    Diabetic neuropathy
Spondylogenic
    Multiple myeloma
    Secondary malignancy
    Osteoid osteoma
    Pathologic fracture (osteoporosis)
    Vertebral osteomyelitis
    Ankylosing spondylitis

ble from sciatica can result and this similarity may lead to long and serious delays in diagnosis. One often sees patients with symptoms unrelieved by laminectomy in whom the diagnosis of diabetes has been missed or ignored simply because this condition was not suspected and a fasting blood sugar was not done.

VASCULOGENIC BACK PAIN

Abdominal aortic aneurysm can produce nagging, chronic back pain. Careful examination of the abdomen including auscultation may reveal the source of the symptoms. The lateral radio-

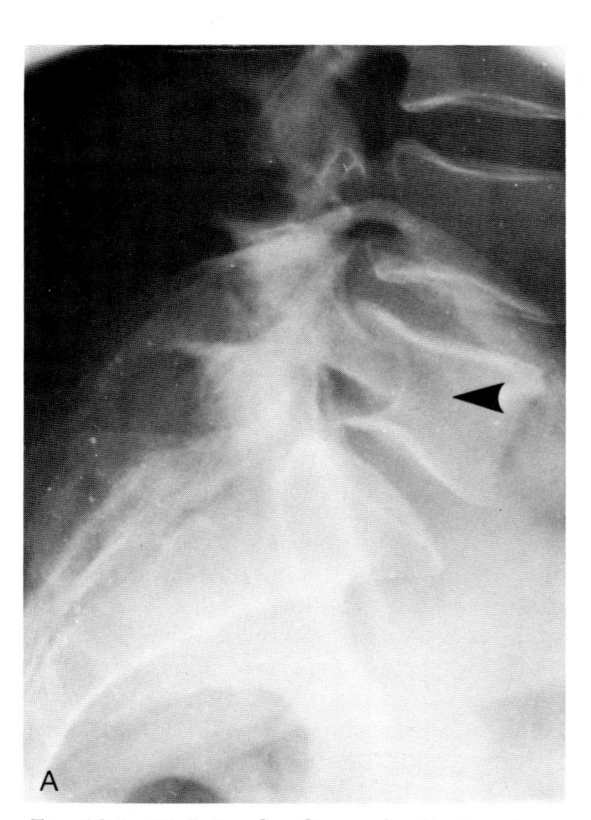

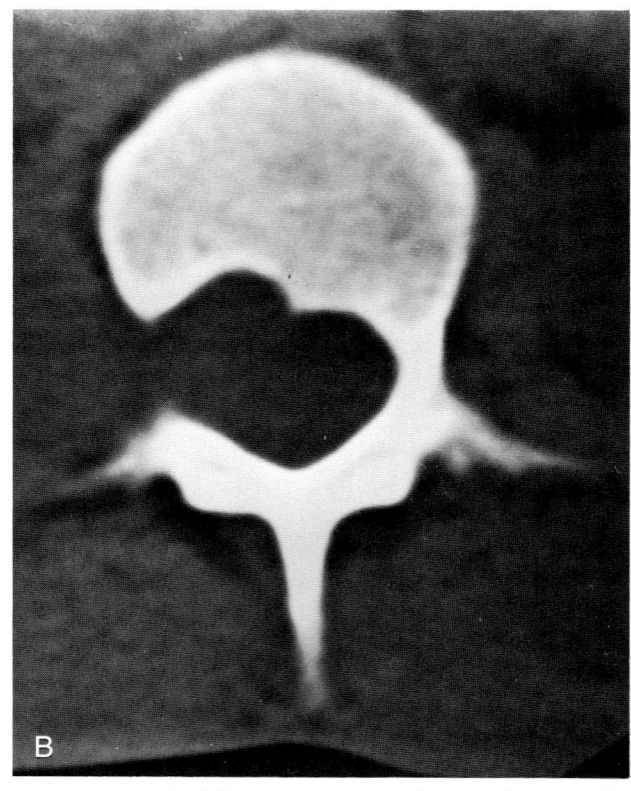

Fig. 10-1. (A) Lateral radiograph of spine shows enlarged intervertebral foramen typical of neurofibroma (B) In another patient CT Scan reveals neurofibroma that enlarges the foramen and erodes the posterior aspect of the vertebral body.

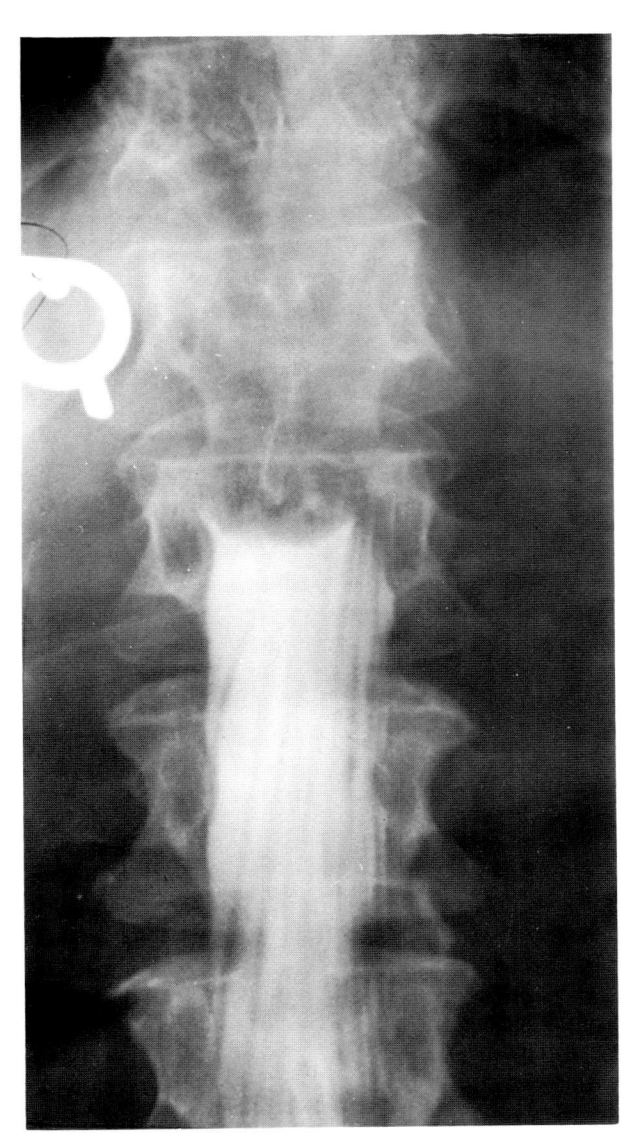

Fig. 10-2. Typical myelogram (water-soluble contrast) of an intrathecal tumor, in this instance a meningioma.

graph of the lumbar spine may show erosion of the anterior aspect of the vertebral bodies or calcification of an enlarged aorta (Fig. 10-3).

Peripheral vascular disease with claudication can be confused with spinal stenosis. The major difference in the clinical features is the response of the pain to rest. While pain from both vascular and neurogenic claudication is relieved by rest, neurogenic pain may not be induced as quickly by exercise done with the spine held in flexion (as in bicycling). Vasculogenic pain will be induced more quickly regardless of the position of the spine. Pain from spinal stenosis may actually be temporarily reduced by walking, but not that originating from vascular disease. The pain from stenosis is not usually relieved as promptly by rest as is pain of vascular origin.

PSYCHOGENIC BACK PAIN

Back pain is seldom ever purely psychogenic in origin. It is unwise to assume that the complaint of low back pain is made solely to gain attention or receive compensation, though this does happen occasionally. Outright malingering is rarely seen. This very complex issue is discussed in chapter 6.

SPONDYLOGENIC BACK PAIN

The symptoms produced by bone lesions are relatively limited in nature and quality: the conditions producing these symptoms are numerous. However, subtle variations in the symptoms together with other clinical findings lead to suspicion of the correct diagnosis. The age of the patient, the character of the pain, weight loss, fever, deformity, and bone tenderness are most helpful in making the correct diagnosis.

Multiple myeloma is the most common malignant primary bone tumor and early in its course can easily be overlooked as the cause of back pain. The complaints may be nonspecific, but the astute physician senses the general lack of well-being of the patient. Abnormalities on serum-protein electrophoresis studies and the presence of Bence Jones proteinuria usually clinch the diagnosis. However, at times both findings may be absent. Further difficulty may be encountered because the early radiographic picture is that of diffuse osteoporosis (Figs. 10-4, 10-5). The typical appearance of multiple "punched out" lesions is often absent (Fig. 10-6). Sternal puncture to obtain bone marrow for histology may be necessary.

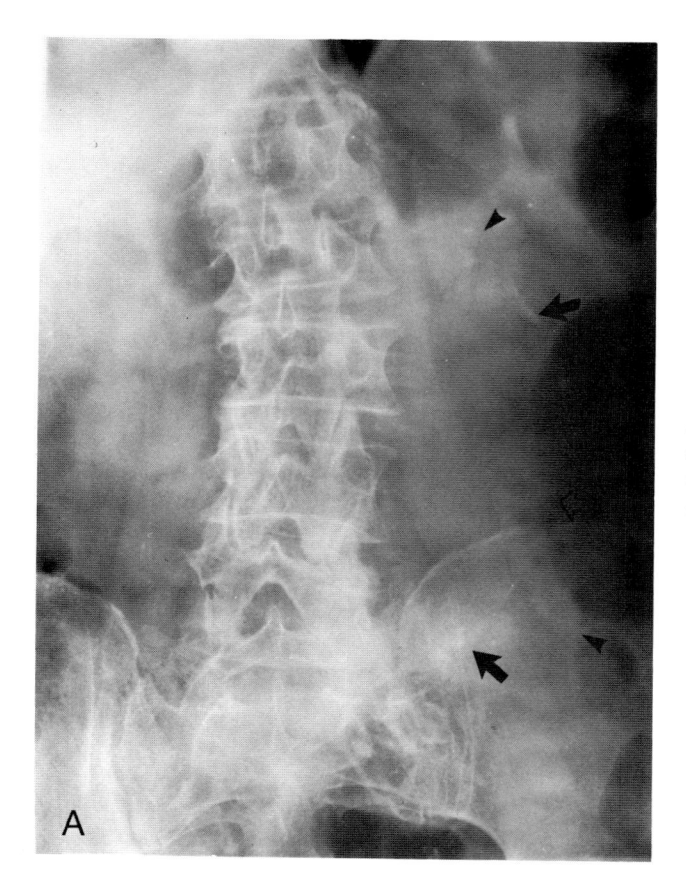

Fig. 10-3. (A) AP radiograph of spine in a patient with a large abdominal aortic aneurysm. Note calcification outlining the aneurysm (arrows). (B) In another patient CT scan shows an aneurysm eroding anterior aspect of lumbar vertebral body.

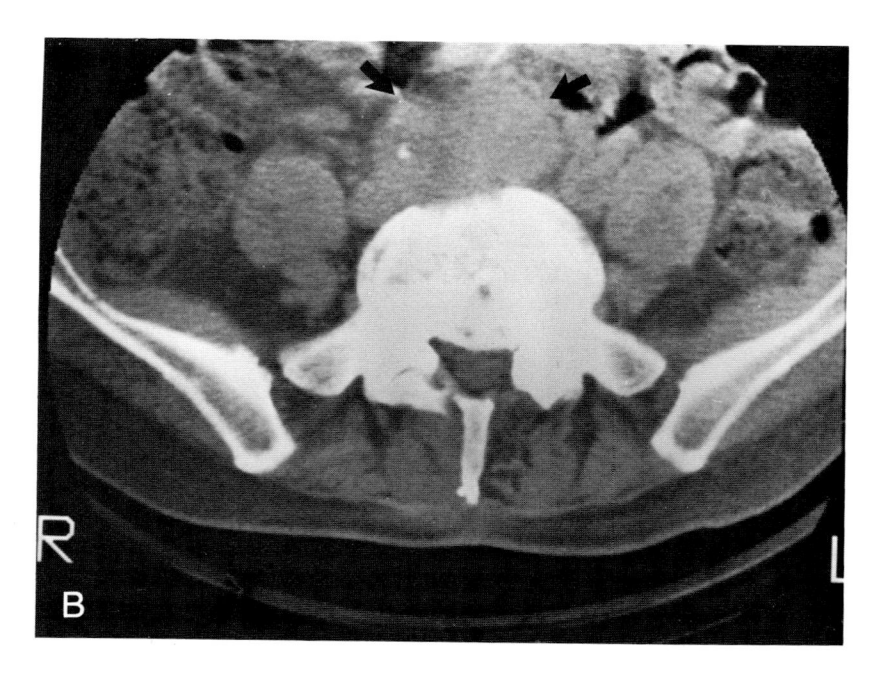

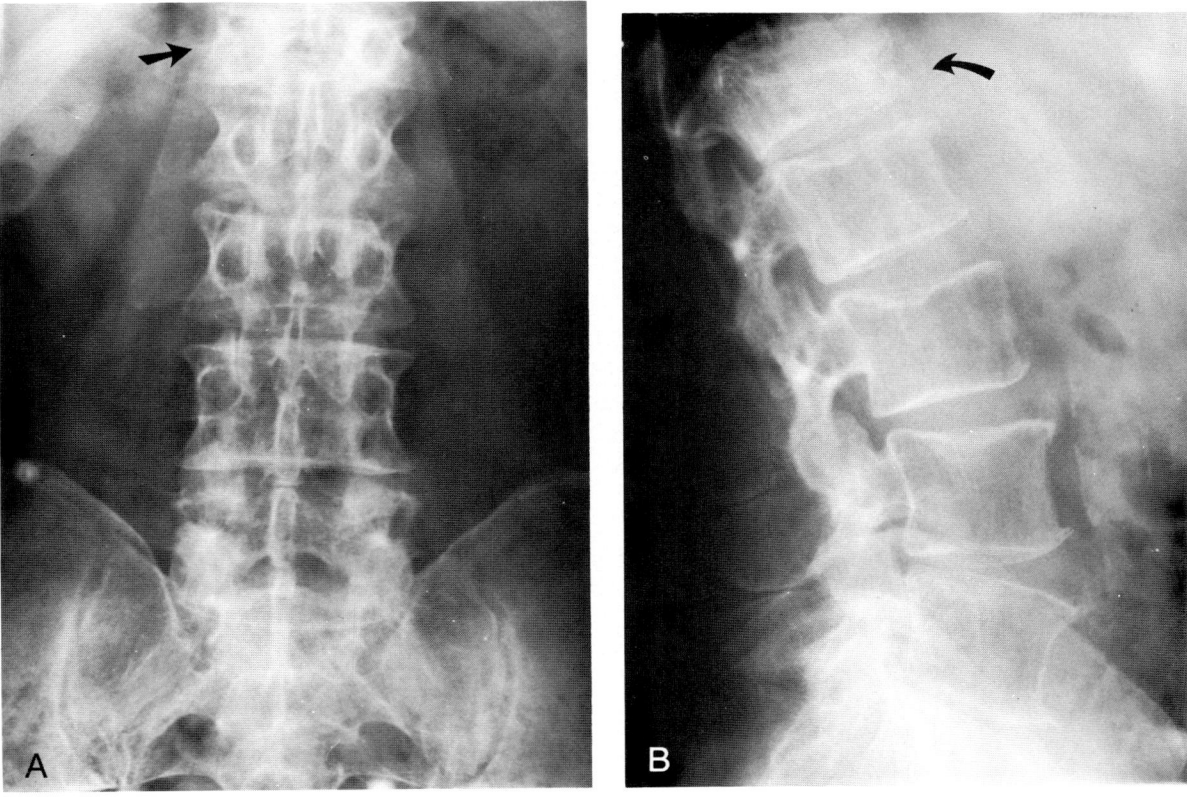

Fig. 10-4. AP (A) and lateral (B) radiographs showing diffuse osteopenia and fracture of L1 in multiple myeloma. The typical appearance of multiple punched-out lesions is often absent.

Secondaries from breast, thyroid, lung, kidney, and prostate can present as back pain. The distinguishing feature is the unrelenting, intense, and progressive nature of the pain. The patient looks anxious, fatigued, and often desperate for relief. Back pain due to degenerative disease is seldom if ever unrelenting and, as stated previously, usually responds to bed rest. Removal of a breast primary may be so far remote from the present that the patient does not volunteer the essential information. It is wise to assume that low back pain following a mastectomy is due to secondaries until proof to the contrary is obtained. Once such metastases are suspected, appropriate investigations lead to the correct diagnosis (Figs. 10-7, 10-8). Often a needle biopsy of the spine under fluoroscopic control is the most direct route to the diagnosis (Fig. 10-9). However, it is important to remember that neoplasms that metastasize to bone may lose their characteristic microscopic appearance. Often the pathologist can be confident that malignant tissue is present but may not be able to diagnose the tissue of origin.

Osteoid osteoma or osteoblastoma of the spine can also present a diagnostic problem. The characteristic history of night pain relieved by mild analgesics may be missing. Hamstring spasm with marked limitation of straight leg raising is often found with osteoid osteomata of the lumbar spine but can lead the physician further away from the correct diagnosis. Persistent back pain in a young adult in the absence of radiographic findings is an indication for a radioisotope bone scan (Fig. 10-10). Tomography of the area of increased isotopic uptake will usually localize the lesion to an articular process, lamina, or pedicle. The CT scan

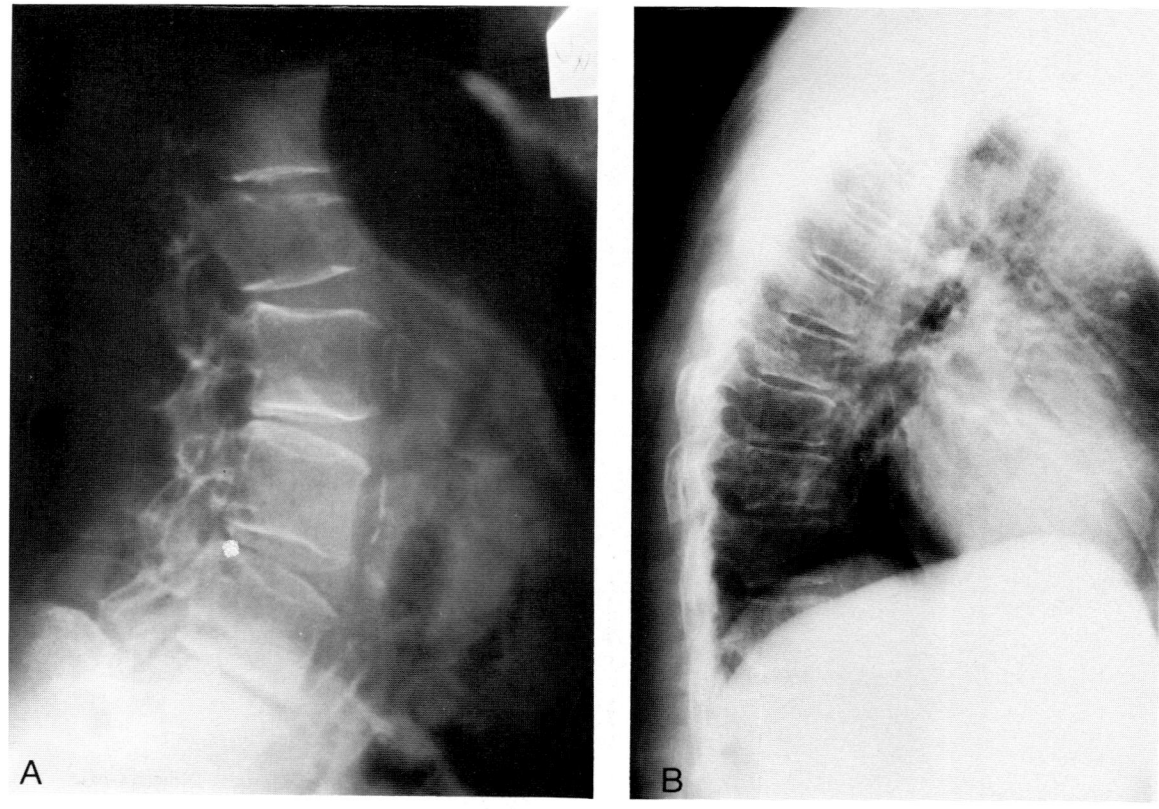

Fig. 10-5. Another patient with diffuse osteopenia and a fracture of L2.

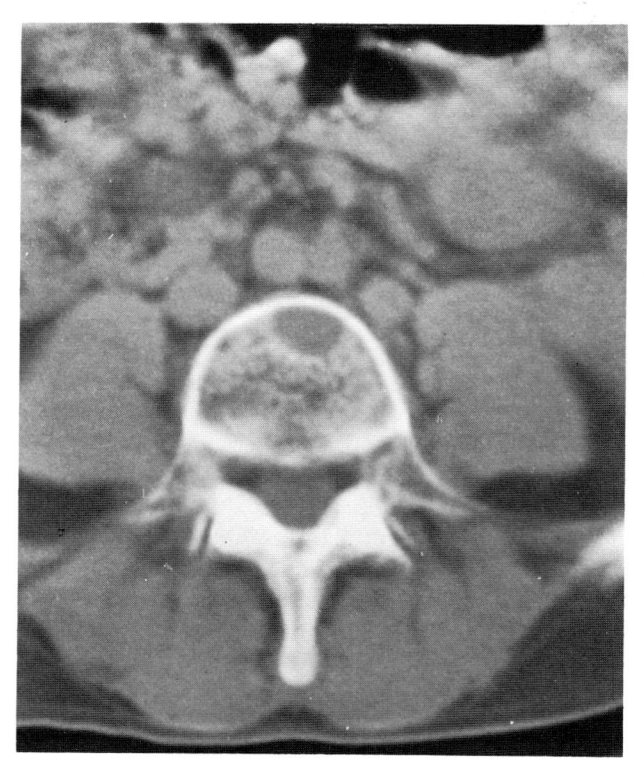

Fig. 10-6. CT scan showing typical lesion of multiple myeloma in the anterior aspect of a vertebral body.

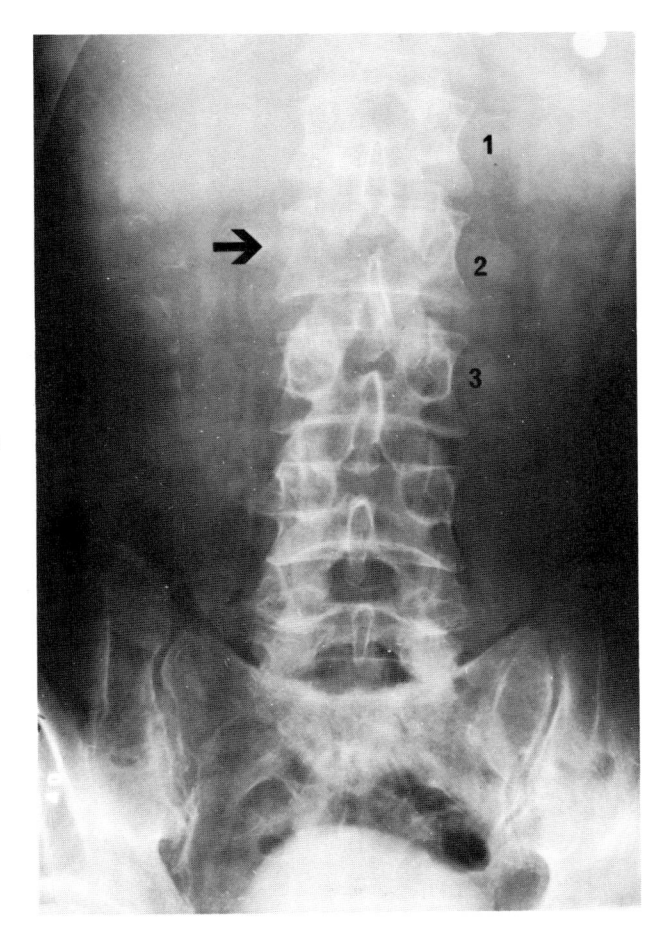

Fig. 10-7. Secondary to the spine from carcinoma of the colon. Note destroyed pedicle of L2 (arrow).

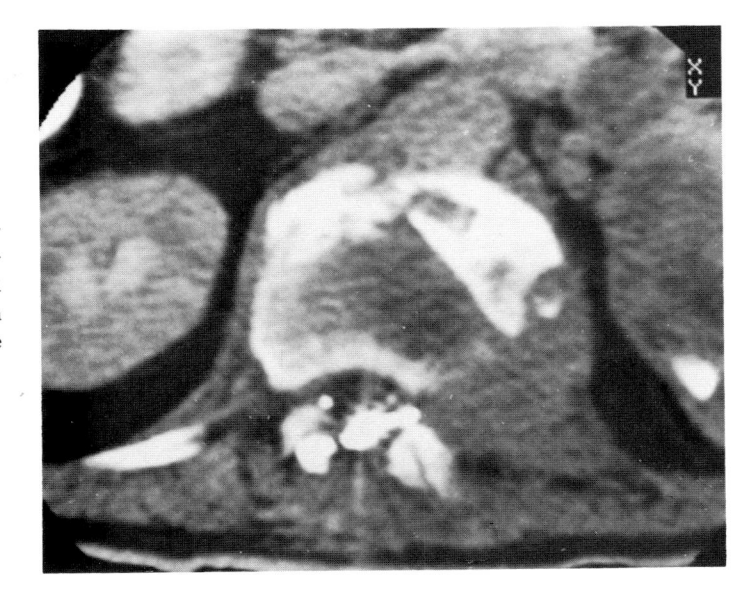

Fig. 10-8. CT scan of secondary from renal carcinoma. Often the CT scan of lumbar secondaries reveals the primary tumor in the abdomen on the same cut. The tumor of the kidney, which is enlarged, can be seen on the left of the figure (viewer's right).

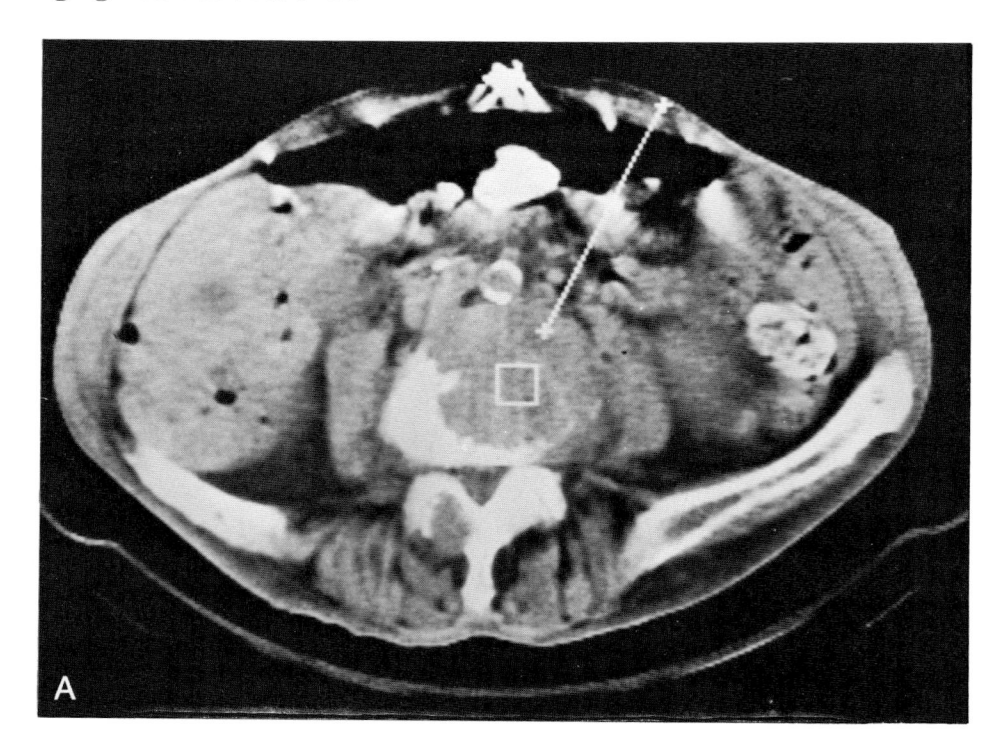

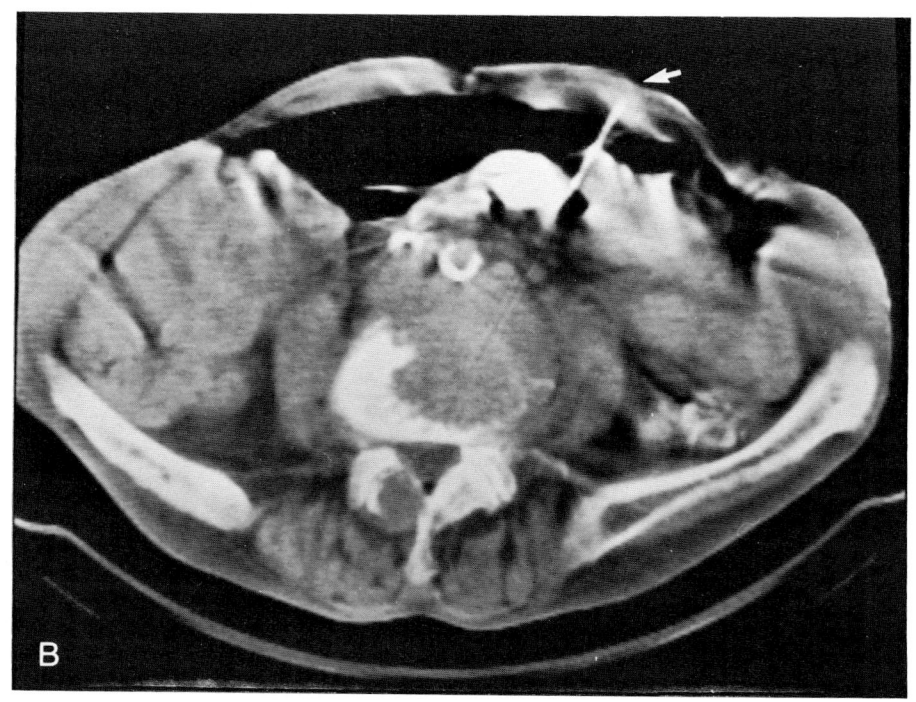

Fig. 10-9. The CT scanner is valuable in selecting the site for introduction of a biopsy needle. A. Secondary in the vertebral body and the safe route from the exterior for the needle are shown. B. Biopsy needle is introduced under CT control.

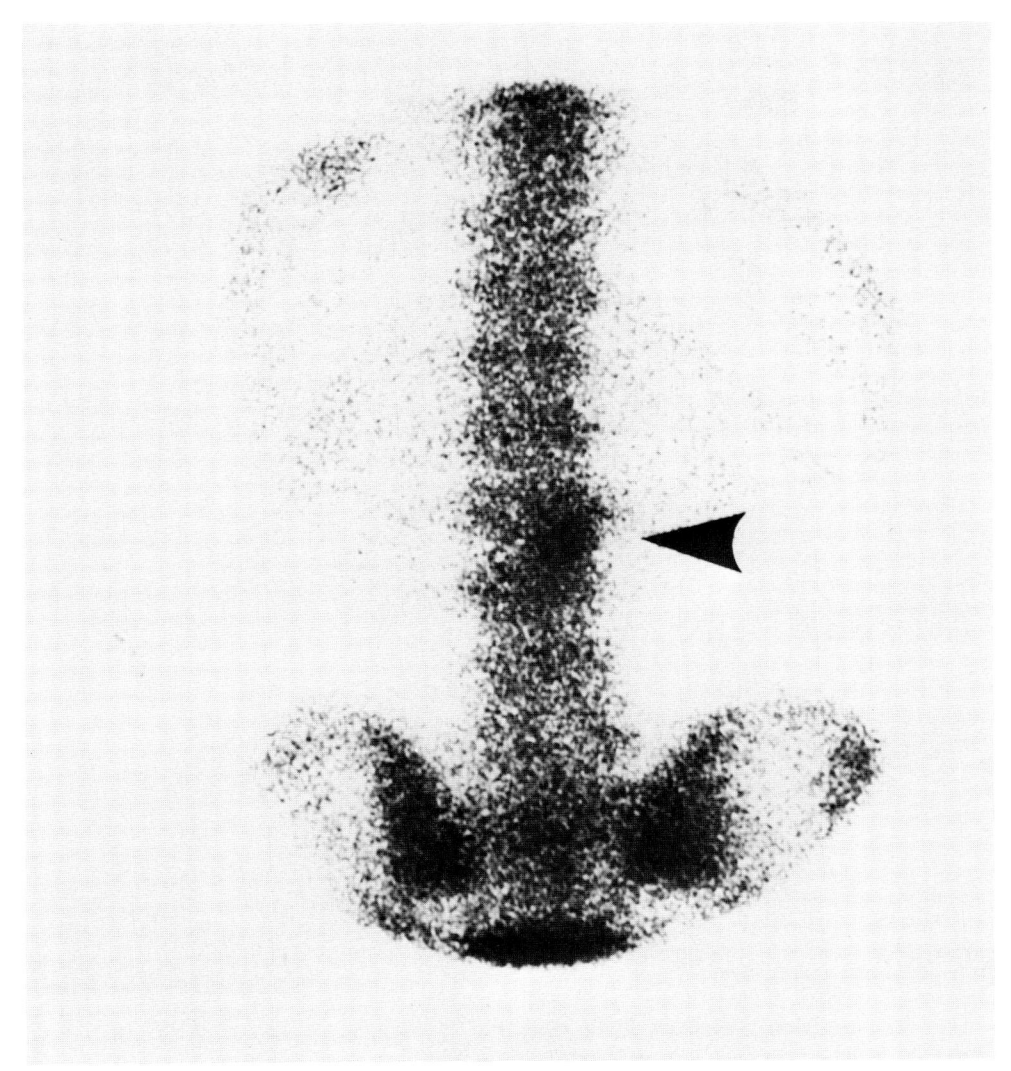

Fig. 10-10. Radioisotope bone scan of an osteoid osteoma in lamina of L2 (arrow).

is extremely valuable in localizing the lesion (Figs. 10-11, 10-12).

Osteoporosis can result in compression fractures. Acute pain superimposed on chronic discomfort, often in the absence of a history of trauma, may be the presenting symptom. The patient may recall only a "snap" associated with mild back pain that occurred when she simply bent to pick up a small object. More intense pain may not develop for hours or until the next day. A fracture may not be seen on the initial radiographs. Usually, however, osteoporosis and biconcave vertebral bodies as well as a recent fracture are seen on the radiograph (Fig. 10-13). It is important to think of the possibility of compression fracture in the osteoporotic spine so that the patient is not subjected to the cost and inconvenience of extensive investigations.

Vertebral osteomyelitis due either to Mycobacterium tuberculosis or pyogenic organisms is perhaps the most frequently missed diagnosis. It is particularly important to remember infection as

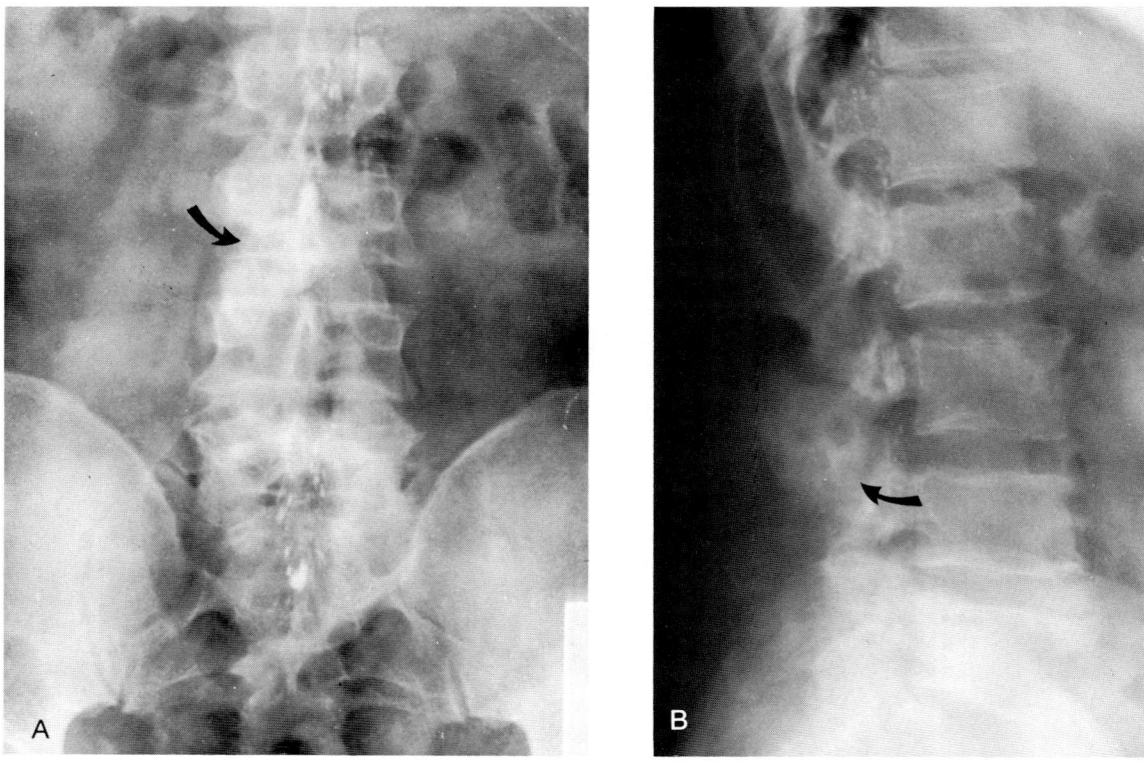

Fig. 10-11. AP (A) and lateral (B) radiographs of an osteoblastoma in the inferior articular process of L3.

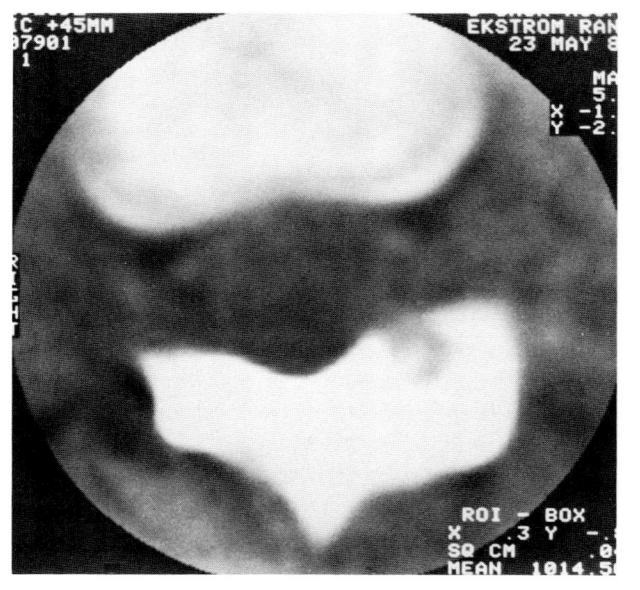

Fig. 10-12. CT scan of osteoid osteoma showing radiolucent nidus and surrounding sclerotic bone.

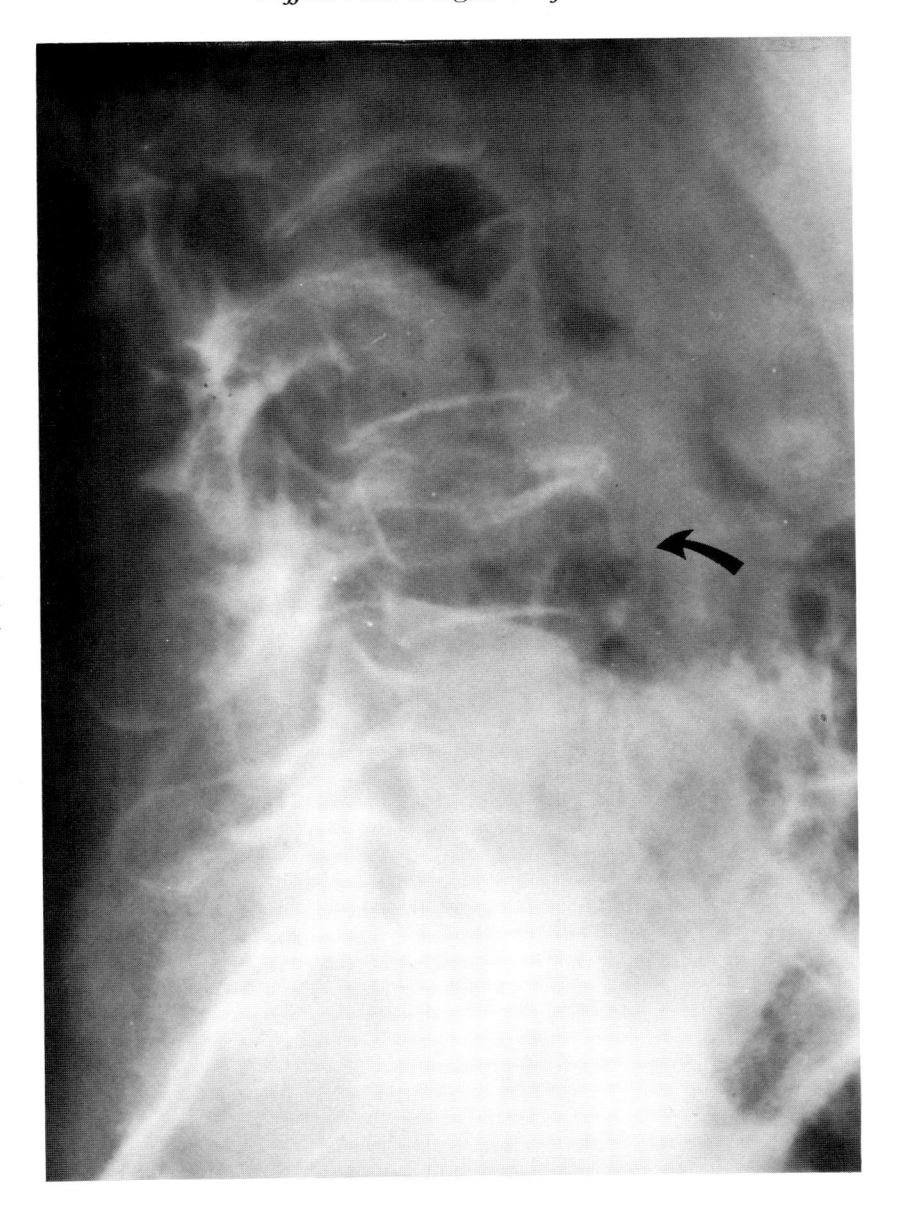

Fig. 10-13. Severe osteopenia and fracture of L3 in a 54-year-old woman who had been on corticosteroid therapy for many years.

a cause of low back pain in diabetics, drug addicts, alcoholics, patients on corticosteroid drugs, those who have had recent urethral instrumentation, those with disseminated malignancy, and otherwise dibilitated patients. No rise in body temperature may be present and the white blood cell count may be normal. In a recent series of cases of osteomyelitis diagnosis was delayed more than 3 months from the appearance of initial symptoms in 50% of patients.[3] The most constant clinical finding is marked tenderness over the spinous process of the involved vertebra and the erythrocyte sedimentation rate is almost invariably elevated. Early in the course slight disk-space narrowing

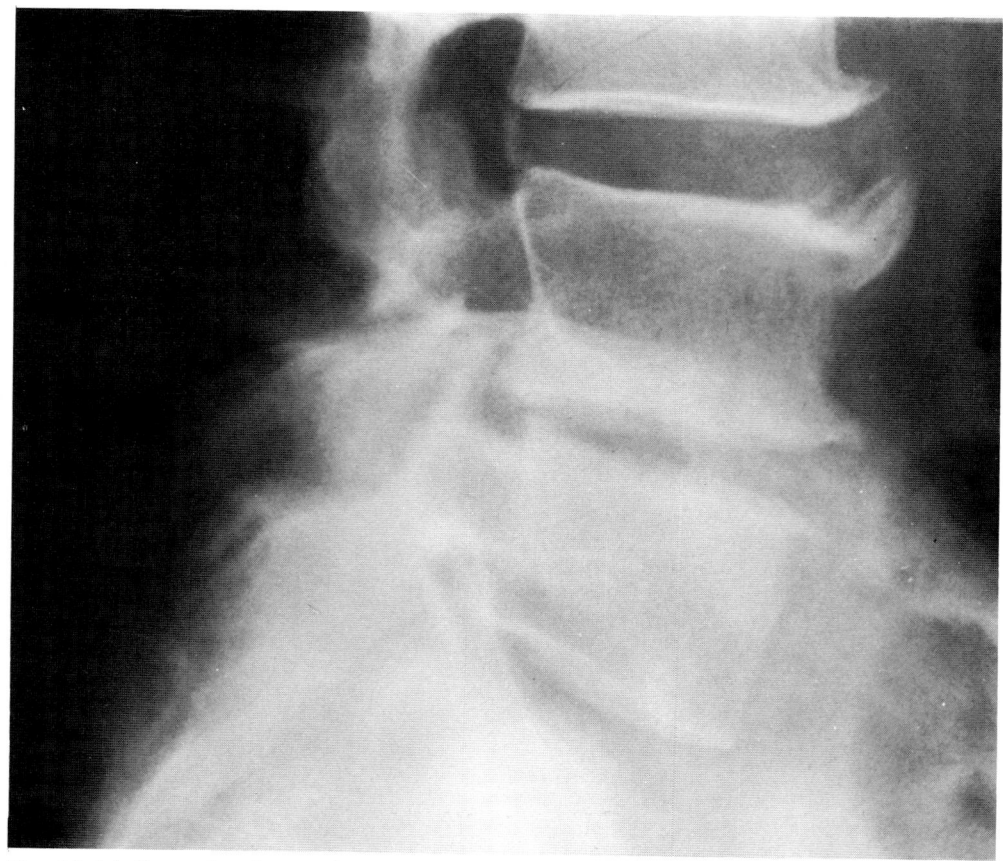

Fig. 10-14. Lateral radiograph showing early osteomyelitis of the inferior aspect of L4 with L4–5 disk-space narrowing. Initially attention was diverted to the obvious degenerative changes at L3–4, which were thought to be the source of the symptoms.

and minimal adjacent vertebral body erosion may be the only radiographic findings (Figs. 10-14, 10-15).

Ankylosing spondylitis may be another diagnostic enigma. Night pain and morning stiffness may be the major complaints, but asymmetric sacroiliac involvement with radiation into the buttock and thigh is not unusual. In fact, it is not unknown for these patients to come to laminectomy before the correct diagnosis is made. Early in the course of the disease, no obvious radiographic changes in the spine or sacroiliac joints may be present (Figs. 10-16, 10-17). An elevated sedimentation rate, a positive HLA-B27 antigen test, and increased uptake on a radioisotope bone scan strongly suggest the diagnosis.

SUMMARY

Table 10-1 lists the conditions that are frequently confused with low back pain caused by

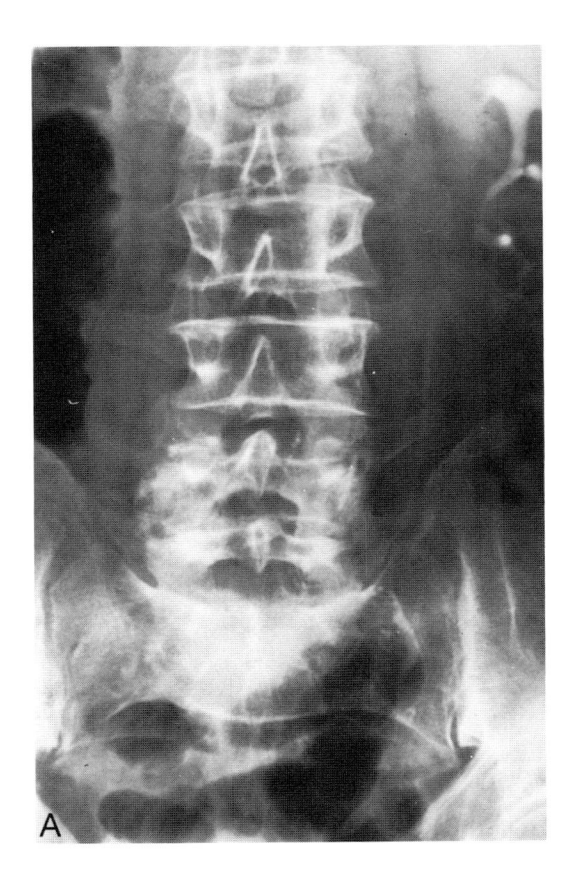

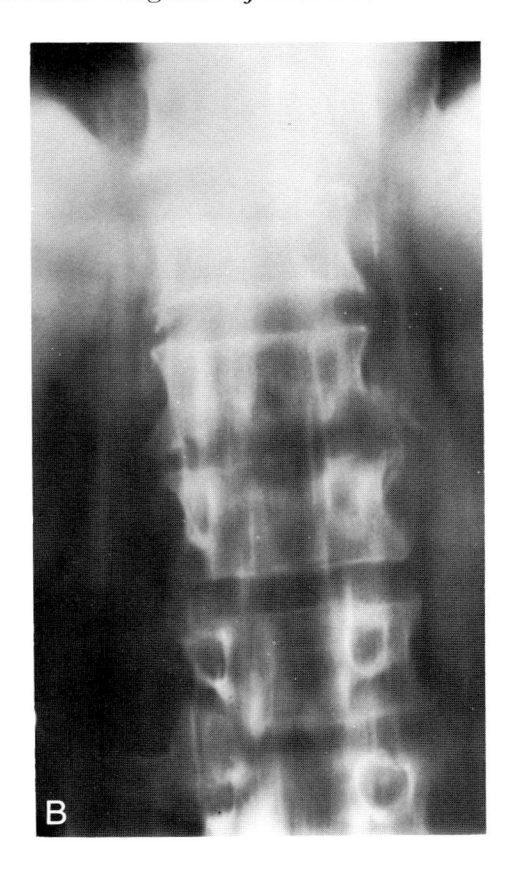

Fig. 10-15. (A) Vertebral infection at L1–L2. This AP radiograph taken 1 week after onset of symptoms does not direct attention to the site of the infection. AP (B) and lateral (C) tomograms taken 6 weeks later show typical appearance of pyogenic infection of the spine.

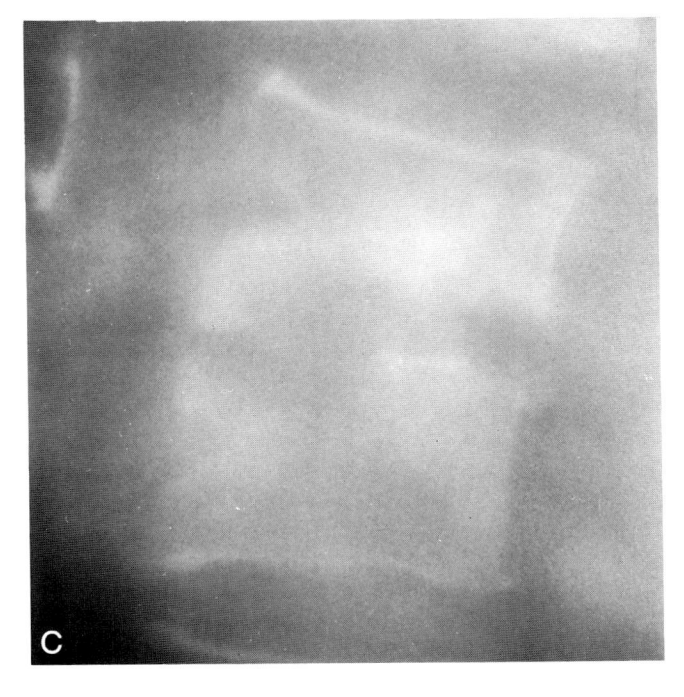

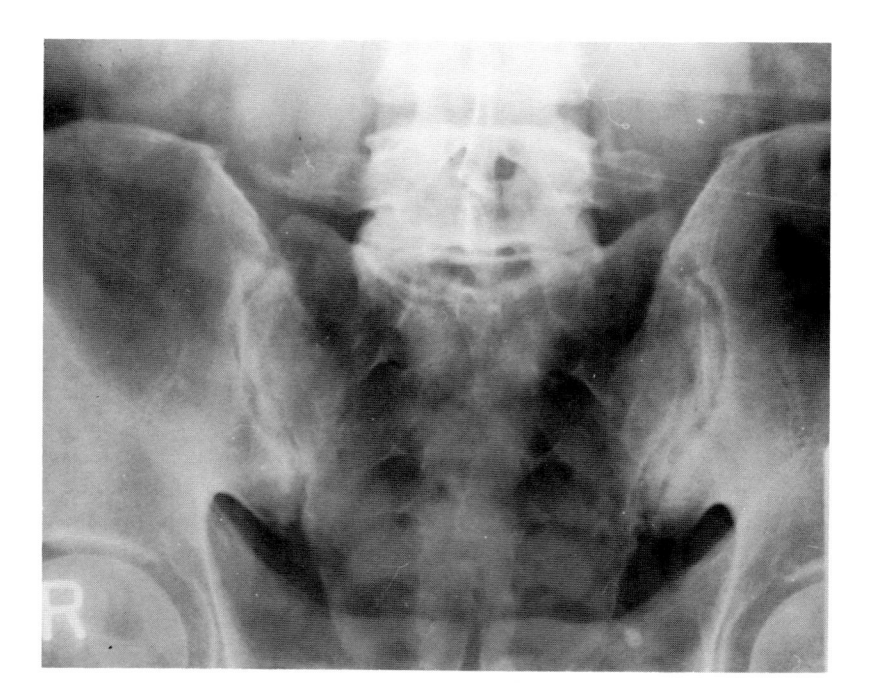

Fig. 10-16. Early ankylosing spondylitis. The sacroiliac joints can be clearly visualized, but note the para-articular sclerosis.

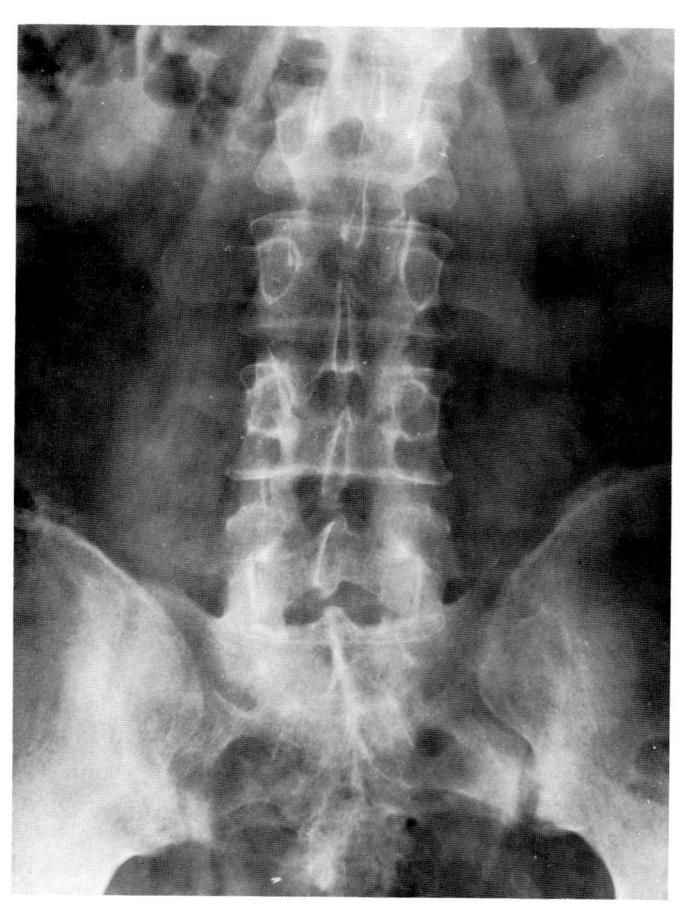

Fig. 10-17. Moderately advanced ankylosing spondylitis. Note obliteration of right sacroiliac joint (viewer's left).

degenerative lesions in the lumbar spine. The wise physician has this list in mind when examining any patient who presents with the symptoms and signs of low back pain. When the problem is approached in this way, particularly if the patient does not respond rapidly to simple conservative measures of treatment, failure to arrive at the correct diagnosis will be a rare occurrence.

REFERENCES

1. MacNab I: Backache. Baltimore, Williams & Wilkins, 1977
2. Tile M: Diabetic Neuropathy in Orthopaedic Practice. J Bone Joint Surg [55B:] 662, 1973
3. Wedge JH, Oryschak AF, Robertson DE, Kirkaldy-Willis WH: Atypical manifestations of spinal infections. Clin Orthop 123: 155, 1977

Part III Treatment

11 A Comprehensive Outline of Treatment

W. H. Kirkaldy-Willis

In this chapter we shall consider the treatment of each specific clinical lesion seen during the three phases—Dysfunction, the Unstable Phase, and Stabilization—of the degenerative process. Detailed descriptions of treatment modalities, including operative techniques, will be dealt with in subsequent chapters.

SURVEY OF MANAGEMENT OF LOW BACK PAIN

An overall view is set out in Table 11-1. Of course, so brief a summary is no more than a guide for the reader. It cannot be applied rigidly in every case. There are many exceptions.

Planning treatment as advocated by the writer is rather complex because of the need to consider two aspects in each instance: the phase and the type of clinical lesion. If readers bear this in mind, they should not experience much difficulty in following the rationale suggested below. Conservative measures are considered first because they apply to all patients with low back pain. Consideration of the clinical lesions seen in Dysfunction (Phase I) comes next. Dysfunction of the intervertebral joints affects both the facet joints and the disk, but the joint symptoms predominate. A discussion of the treatment of Instability (Phase II) and Stabilization (Phase III) follows because all subsequent lesions may present in either of these phases. Then Herniation of the Nucleus Pulposus is considered because it may occur in any of the three phases, though it is seen most commonly at the end of Phase I or the beginning of Phase II. The other clinical lesions that are discussed subsequently are encountered in both Phases II and III.

CONSERVATIVE TREATMENT

The term conservative treatment is frequently used to describe the measures discussed just below. However, it is not altogether accurate because more aggressive methods sometimes prove more conservative in the sense of conserving, that is of restoring, normal function quickly. The term "nonoperative measures" has also been used.

Spine Education Program

Every patient should attend a class in spine education as early as possible (see chapter 12 for discussion). Instruction is given by a physiotherapist and an occupational therapist. The structure and function of the lumbar spine are taught in simple terms. The different types of lesion and the way in which these can cause pain are discussed. Instruction is given in low back care, especially as related to the activities of daily living. The class is taught correct posture and pelvic tilting and

Table 11-1. Overall View of Scheme of Treatment

Phase	Lesion	Treatment
Dysfunction	Facet joints	Manipulation, injection
	Sacroiliac joint	Manipulation, injection
	Quad. lumb.	Stretching, injection
	Piriformis	— Injection
	Disk herniation	Decompression —
Unstable phase	Disk herniation	Decompression, fusion
	Instab. alone	— Fusion
	Lateral stenosis	Decompression, fusion
	Central stenosis	Decompression, fusion
	Degen. olisthesis	Decompression, fusion
	Isthm. olisthesis	Decompression, fusion
Stabilization	Disk herniation	Decompression —
	Lateral stenosis	Decompression —
	Central stenosis	Decompression —
	Degen. olisthesis	Decompression —
	Isthm. olisthesis	Decompression —

exercises to be done twice daily to strengthen muscles, especially the abdominal muscles that provide most strength to the back. Weight reduction is often advocated, and the patient may be sent to consult a dietician about this. Individual instruction should be given to each patient at the end of the class, explaining in more detail the nature of the patient's lesion and the way in which the patient can become his or her own doctor to deal with it. A second period of instruction to reinforce what has been taught during the first session is highly desirable.

Manipulation

As discussed in chapter 13, manipulation is greatly beneficial to many patients in Phase I.

More Intensive Therapy

Many patients benefit greatly from one attendence at the Spine Education Programme. Some require further help. For these an intensive course of physiotherapy and occupational therapy is given for several hours a day for 2 to 3 weeks. It is convenient to lodge patients attending from a distance in a hostel adjacent to the hospital. A light elastic garment is often provided for the patient to wear whenever not in bed. It provides support to the back and helps the patient to pull in the abdominal muscles. It permits almost full movement of the spine, and thus does not contribute to muscle atrophy (Chapter 14).

DYSFUNCTION: THE POSTERIOR FACET SYNDROME

As discussed previously, this syndrome is caused by rotational strain to both facet joints and annulus fibrosus. Dysfunction of the facet joints produces most of the symptoms, and treatment is mainly directed there (Table 11-2).

For the acute lesion with severe incapacitating pain, treatment with suitable analgesics and a few days of bedrest is indicated. The value of muscle relaxants and of anti-inflammatory drugs is doubtful.

For less acute and for recurring and chronic lesions the conservative treatment described above is prescribed. At this point the physician has a choice between two apparently different forms of treatment.

Manipulation

Undertaken by a practitioner well versed in the art and given daily for 7 to 10 days, manipulation relieves many patients of their symptoms. Few physicians or surgeons have acquired the necessary skill. The physician needs to choose a practitioner whose skill he knows and whose judgement

Table 11-2. Plan of Treatment: Phase I: Dysfunction

	Treatment			
Lesion	Conservative	Manipulation	Injection	Operation
Facet joints	Yes	Facets	Facet and muscle	—
Sacroiliac joint	Yes	Sacroiliac and muscle	Joint and muscle	—
Quadratus lumborum	Yes	Stretch muscle	Muscle	—
Piriformis syndrome	Yes	—	Muscle	—
Disk herniation	Yes	Rarely	Epidural steroids	Sometimes

he trusts. The way in which this modality works has long been the subject of controversy. The most reasonable explanation is that manipulation produces a three-fold effect: (1) a direct mechanical effect on the facet joints, which may reduce a subluxation of 1 to 2 mm; (2) stretching of hypertonic posterior segmental spinal muscles by the thrust applied by the manipulator with abolition of pain coming from the muscles, ligaments, and tendons because of stretching; (3) increased neural output produced by mechanoreceptor stimulation that may modulate pain perception through the gate control mechanism.

Facet Injection

The technique will be described in detail in a later chapter.[1] After the skin is anesthesized, a lumbar puncture needle is passed, under fluoroscopic control, to the posterior joint considered to be mainly affected. A 1-ml dose of 0.25% bupivacaine (Marcaine) is injected into the joint. As the needle is withdrawn, 3 to 4 ml are injected into the muscle overlying the joint. The patient then stands and puts the back through a full range of movement. In many cases injection at one level, usually L4–5, relieves the patient of his pain. If the pain is relieved, no further injection is given, but in some cases it is necessary to repeat the procedure at a second or third level. Facet injections nearly always relieve the patient of pain for several hours. In approximately 50% of cases the patient is free of pain for weeks or months. In some cases relief is permanent. The explanation that best explains the success of injection is (1) that the nerve supply to the joint and capsule is temporarily anesthetized, permitting a minor subluxation to be reduced; (2) that hypertonic contracted ischemic muscle is relaxed when pain coming from it is abolished; (3) that relaxation of the muscle overlying the joint allows the subluxed articular surfaces to move back into correct alignment; (4) that sustained neural activity that summates to produce pain is interrupted and the vicious circle of pain is broken.

Each of the two modalities brings relief to many patients. No guideline can be given as to which should be tried first. If one fails, the other should be given a trial. Sometimes facet injection followed by manipulation gives good results. In each case the treatment is followed by adherance to the conservative measures outlined above. In recalcitrant cases, where both manipulation and injection have failed, the application of a "light cast" body jacket to immobilize the spine for 4 to 6 weeks may be very effective. This assists resolution of the inflammatory synovitis in the joint and healing of tears in the capsule and annulus (Fig. 11-1).

Denervation of posterior joints is occasionally indicated when all other methods have failed to give relief of pain.

DYSFUNCTION: THE SACROILIAC SYNDROME

The presentation is rarely acute and nearly always subacute or chronic. We have seen (chapter 8) that the symptom complex is well-defined even though the exact pathological nature of the lesion is obscure. The response to treatment is as well-

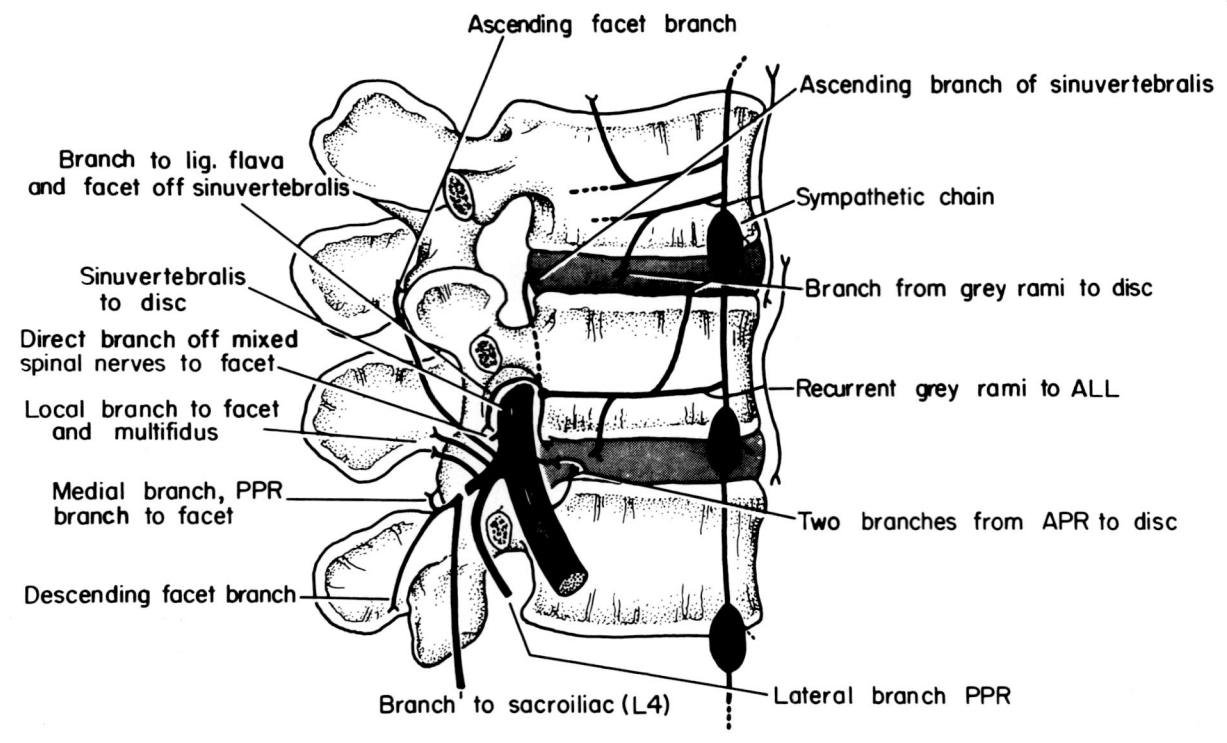

Fig. 11-1. Innervation of the posterior joints. Each posterior joint is innervated by branches of the posterior primary rami from three levels. At each level a small nerve passes directly from the main nerve to the posterior joint. (Figure courtesy of Dr. Stanley Paris).

defined as the clinical syndrome. Conservative measures are prescribed as listed above. Definitive treatment is started as soon as the diagnosis is made.

Manipulation

The patient nearly always has reduced movement of the sacroiliac joint as well as pain. Manipulation for 3 to 4 days often relieves the pain and restores the joint movement. Sometimes daily manipulation for 10 days is required. Three types of adjustment are employed: a superior, a direct, and an inferior sacroiliac manipulation. This modality is by far the most certain way of relieving the patient's pain.

Injection

When manipulation fails, injection of 3 to 4 ml of 0.25% bupivacaine into the overlying muscle, the posterior ligaments, and, if possible, the joint sometimes produces marked relief of pain. It is difficult to be certain that the local anesthetic has penetrated into the joint.

The mechanism by which manipulation relieves pain is probably that it reduces hypertonicity (spasm) in the posterior muscles that maintain the point in a state of fixation; the treatment may also result in restoring movement by shifting the ilium 1 to 2 mm on the sacrum. It is reasonable to assume that injection acts by relieving muscular hypertonicity.

DYSFUNCTION: THE QUADRATUS LUMBORUM SYNDROME

The pain and tenderness over one segment of this muscle result from local injury followed by hypertonicity and ischemia.

Passive stretching of the muscle followed by active exercises to stretch the muscle sometimes relieves the pain.

Injecting 2 to 3 ml of 0.25% bupivacaine into the painful area in the muscle is usually effective when stretching and exercises have failed. An exercise program should follow.

DYSFUNCTION: THE PIRIFORMIS SYNDROME

Injection

The treatment is to inject 2 to 3 ml of 0.25% bupivacaine into the muscle medial to the spine of the ischium. The injection is made from the buttock with a finger in the rectum or vagina. Details are given in Chapter 16. Almost instantaneous relief of pain is obtained.

THE UNSTABLE PHASE AND STABILIZATION

The Unstable Phase

The clinical diagnosis depends on both the presence of low back pain and radiological evidence of increased abnormal movement. Instability may occur alone. In that case only the instability should be treated. Alternatively, it may accompany a disk herniation, spinal stenosis, and other clinical lesions. In this case treatment of the clinical lesion should be followed by treatment of the instability. Patients with mild instability may respond to the conservative measures outlined above. The application of a "light cast" body jacket may be helpful. Apart from this there are two main methods of treatment of instability: denervation and fusion (Table 11-3).

Denervation of Posterior Joints

The rationale of this procedure is to reduce the number of impulses from pain fibers (S) arising in the posterior joints and thus to prevent summation of impulses from posterior joints and disk and so to inhibit pain. Denervation may be carried out percutaneously by creating a thermal lesion that destroys part of the innervation of the posterior joint or by open operation when a more thorough denervation can be performed. It is indicated, occasionally when other modalities fail to relieve pain in Dysfunction and, more often, early in the Unstable Phase in an attempt to obviate the necessity for spinal fusion.[2]

Table 11-3. Plan of Treatment: Phase II: Unstable Phase

Lesion	Conservative	Decompression	Fusion
Disk herniation Instab. mild	Yes	Yes	No
Disk herniation Instab. marked	Yes	Yes	Yes
Instability alone Mild	Yes	Cast Immobilization	Denervation
Instability alone Marked	No	No	Yes
Lateral stenosis Instab. mild	Yes	Yes	No
Lateral stenosis Instab. marked	No	Yes	Yes
Central stenosis Instab. mild	Yes	Yes	No
Central stenosis Instab. marked	No	Yes	Yes
Degen. olisthesis	Yes	Yes	Yes
Isthmic olisthesis	Yes	Yes	Yes

Table 11-4. Plan of Treatment: Phase III: Stabilization

Lesion	Treatment		
	Conservative	Decompression	Fusion
Disk herniation	Yes	Yes	No
Lateral stenosis	Yes	Yes	No
Central stenosis	Yes	Yes	No
Combined stenosis	Yes	Yes	No
Degenerative spondylolisthesis	Yes	Yes	No
Isthmic spondylolisthesis	Yes	Yes	No

Spinal Fusion

In the past there has been much confusion over the role of fusion in treating low back pain. This confusion continues at the present time. Some surgeons advocate fusion of one or two levels when a period of bed rest and wearing a rigid corset or brace or immobilization in a "light-cast" jacket have failed to relieve the patient's pain. Others reserve fusion for patients who have had prolonged conservative treatment followed by one or more operations for decompression and still have low back pain; in effect they say, "This patient has had every other form of treatment with no relief of pain; a small percentage of patients benefit from fusion; therefore fusion is indicated." Still others choose anterior or posterior interbody fusion for the same reason when a posterior or posterolateral fusion has failed to relieve pain. In the opinion of the writer these approaches are not logical.

The only logical reasons and indications for spinal fusion are, first, that other modalities have been tried and failed, second, that from a psychological viewpoint the operation is reasonable, and, third, that the instability is present at one or at two levels. The definition of instability (the Unstable Phase) is pain with increased abnormal movement (as discussed and illustrated by stress radiographs and CT images in chapter 7). There appears to be no adequate reason for fusion other than radiological demonstration of increased abnormal movement.

At present no consensus as to when posterior and when interbody fusion is the best form of treatment exists. Fusion relieves pain by abolishing movement.[3]

Stabilization

As seen in chapter 7, this final phase in the degenerative process can be diagnosed with accuracy by stress radiographs. When this phase is nearly reached, the surgeon can with confidence assure the patient that soon the low back pain will abate. When stabilization has been reached, fusion is seldom if ever indicated though decompression may be required to treat central or lateral spinal stenosis (Table 11-4).

HERNIATION OF THE NUCLEUS PULPOSUS

The pathology, pathogenesis, and clinical picture have been described in previous chapters. To recapitulate briefly, two mechanisms are involved. First, recurrent rotational trauma produces lesions in the facet joints and the annulus fibrosus. In this type circumferential tears coalesce to form radial tears. The posterior annulus thins out at one point. Further minor rotational trauma allows the annulus to bulge locally at that point (a disk protrusion) or to rupture completely (a disk extrusion). Second, a fall onto the buttocks with the lumbar spine in flexion may produce a sudden rupture of the posterior annulus with protrusion or extrusion of the nucleus pulposus.

The Three-Joint Complex

Nearly every case of disk herniation is accompanied by pathology in the facet joints. For this reason the wise physician, confronted by a patient with a disk herniation, considers the possibility that this lesion is complicated by facet lesions that may produce pain or instability and by facet subluxation that may result in lateral canal stenosis.

The Phase

Most commonly the herniation occurs at the end of Phase I or early in Phase II. More rarely, it takes place during Phase III, complicating spinal stenosis or degenerative spondylolisthesis.

Expectant Treatment

Resolution of a first disk herniation takes place in approximately 75% of patients over a period of 3 months. With recurrent herniation the chance of spontaneous relief of symptoms is reduced. During the acute stage the patient is hospitalized and put on bed rest with bathroom privileges. Adequate analgesics relieve the pain, and this helps the hypertonicity and spasm in muscle to subside. Gravity lumbar reduction (see chapter 15) is of considerable assistance to some patients. The amount of straight leg raising obtained without pain is a useful indication of recovery. At the onset often the leg can be raised no more than 20°. Over 1, 2, or 3 weeks the amount of straight leg raising slowly increases to 30°, 40°, 50°, and 60°. It is unusual to keep the patient in bed for more than 3 weeks. By this time in most cases the acute symptoms have subsided. In a few cases the pain is still severe and the patient is aware that other measures should be begun.

Chemonucleolysis

In several Canadian centers chemonucleolysis is the treatment of choice when expectant measures have failed. In this center it is reserved for patients below the age of 40 with minimal loss of motor power. We manage a large percentage of cases with expectant measures and thus fewer cases by chemonucleolysis. Undoubtedly this latter therapy has a place in treating disk herniations. An immediate complication is anaphylactic shock and a late complication the development of lateral stenosis from loss of disk height and subluxation of posterior facets. Both complications are uncommon. It is essential to order a CT Scan before embarking on chemonucleolysis in order to rule out the possibility that lateral stenosis is present along with the herniation.

Fraser, of the Flinders Medical Center, Adelaide, South Australia, reported on a double-blind study on the use of Chymopapain at the Toronto meeting of the International Society for the Study of the Lumbar Spine in June 1982. This author recommends the use of Chymopapain for the treatment of Sciatica due to proven intervertebral disk prolapse when conservative measures have failed before diskotomy is considered.

Microsurgery on the Disk

The rightful place of this type of surgery is not yet firmly established. It is reasonable to suppose that the procedure has a role provided that neither central or lateral stenosis, as shown by CT Scan, nor marked instability, as shown by stress radiographs, is present.

Diskotomy

As mentioned above it is essential to assess accurately not only the level of the disk herniation but also the presence or absence of instability and of lateral stenosis.

The uncomplicated herniation is approached by either a uni- or a bilateral minimal partial laminectomy after the level is accurately identified, if necessary by radiography at the time of surgery. The use of magnifying glasses, a headlight, and bipolar cautery minimize the danger of injury to nerves and blood vessels. The operative field should be bloodless throughout the procedure. After retraction of the dura and gentle retraction of the nerve, the disk herniation comes into view. The nerve is retracted medially or laterally as required; the annulus is incised; and the protruded or extruded nuclear material is removed using pituitary forceps. In the case of an extrusion, incising the annulus may not be necessary. It is important to make certain that no loose fragments of material are left within the disk or in the central or lateral spinal canals. Further confirmation of the size of the lateral canals is obtained by measuring them with gauges ranging from 2 to 5 mm in diameter.

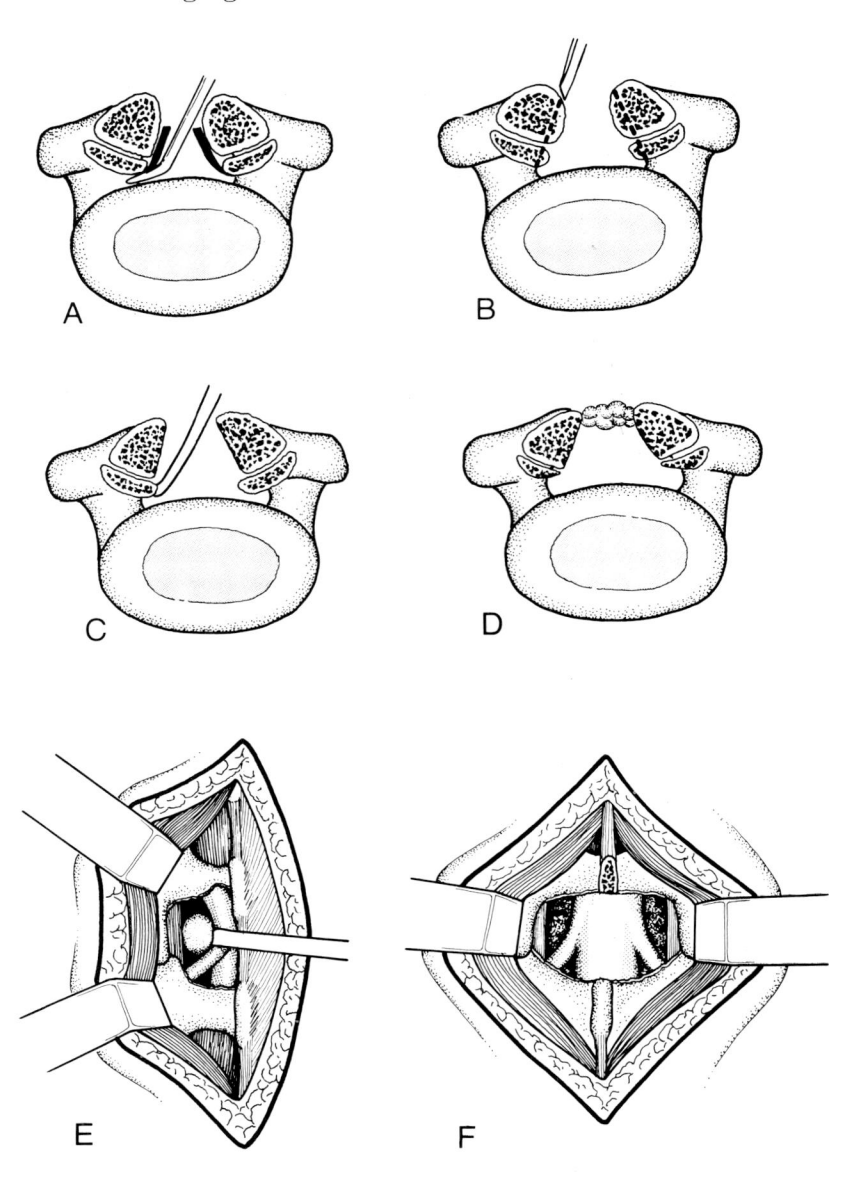

Fig. 11-2. Cross-sectional; illustration of the four steps in an operation to treat one-level or multilevel central and lateral stenosis. (A) A laminectomy has been performed and a gauge is inserted into the lateral canal to determine its size. (B) Removal of the medial third of the inferior articular process with an osteotome. (C) Removal of the medial and anterior parts of the superior articular process using the Quintron sonic tool. (D) The lateral canals have been enlarged and a free fat graft is placed posterior to the dura. (E) Posterior view of a unilateral approach for diskotomy. (F) Posterior view of a bilateral minimal partial laminectomy for one level central and lateral stenosis.

In treating a herniation with lateral stenosis, it is necessary to enlarge the lateral canals to 6 mm at this point, using the Quintron sonic tool, Kerrison forceps, or osteotome and mallet.

When the herniation is complicated by marked instability as demonstrated by stress radiographs, it is wise to perform a one-level spinal fusion. At the end of the operation a free fat graft is placed posterior to the dura to prevent adhesions (Fig. 11-2).

The after care is the same whatever the nature of the treatment because a concomitant lesion in the facet joints is virtually always present. The patient receives instruction in low back care and exercises. An elastic support should be worn for 2 to 3 months. The patient should rest at home for 1 month and avoid bending, lifting, twisting, and all heavy work for a further 2 months. It is wise to warn the patient that a disk does not become herniated unless the affected level has been weakened by recurrent injury. This implies that some extra care throughout life is necessary to avoid becoming overweight, to do exercises daily, and to follow the instructions given in the Spine Education Program.

ONE-LEVEL CENTRAL AND LATERAL STENOSIS

In the early stage, one-level central and lateral stenosis, diagnosed and assessed accurately by the CT Scan, may sometimes be managed by the type of conservative measures outlined above. These are specially indicated when an operation is hazardous because the patient's general condition is poor.[4-7]

Operation

When conservative measures fail, the level of the stenosis is approached through a one-level bilateral minimal partial laminectomy, as described for operation on a disk herniation. After the central portion of the ligamentum flavum is excised on both sides, it may be necessary to remove bone from both the lower edge of the upper lamina and the upper edge of the lower lamina. The inferior articular processes are identified and on each side the medial third of the process is removed using a 1-cm-wide osteotome and mallet until the cartilage of the superior articular process is reached. In doing this, care must be taken not to fracture the base of the inferior process. The medial third of the superior articular process is then removed using the Quintron sonic tool, Kerrison forceps, or osteotome and mallet. Central stenosis is usually relieved by excising the medial third of the inferior and the medial edge of the superior process. In treating lateral stenosis, it is usually necessary to remove more of the superior process until the lateral canal between the anterior surface of the superior process and the back of the vertebral body and disk is at least 6 mm in diameter. Confirmation of canal size is obtained as described above. Two nerves may be entrapped laterally at any one level. For example at the L4–5 level the L4 nerve may be entrapped just below the pedicle of L4 between the displaced superior process of L5 and the body of L4; the L5 nerve may be entrapped in a narrow subarticular gutter between an enlarged superior articular process of L5 and the back of the L5 vertebral body or the l4–5 disk (see chapter 9, Fig. 9-7C). In addition, one nerve may be entrapped at either or both of two levels as shown in Figure 11–3. At the end of the procedure a free fat graft, taken subcutaneously, is placed between the dura and the posterior muscles to prevent adhesions.

Instability

When more than a minimal amount of abnormal increased movement is detected by stress radiograms and/or at the time of operation, a one-level

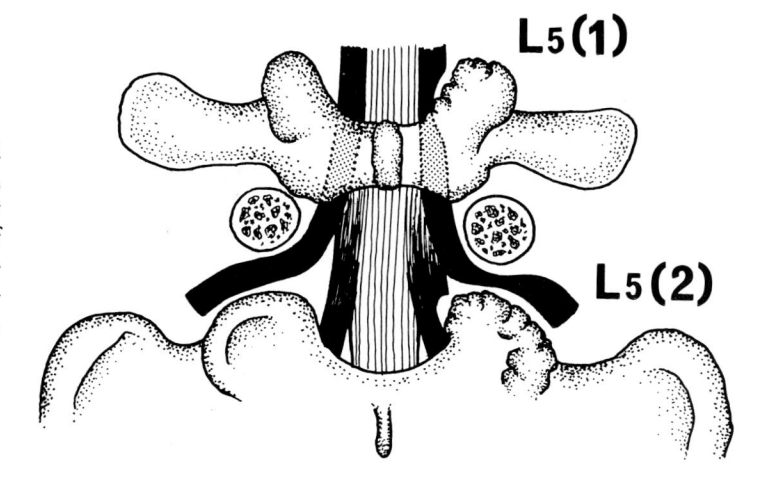

Fig. 11-3. The L5 nerve may be entrapped at one of two different sites: at the L4–5 level, by the medial edge of an enlarged L5 superior facet or between this facet and the back of the L5 vertebral body in the subarticular gutter; and at the L5–S1 level between the superior facet of the sacrum and the pedicle of L5.

fusion should be done at the same operation. Two methods are possible: a posterior facet and intertransverse fusion using iliac crest grafts or a posterior interbody fusion. Both of these will be described in detail in Chapter 16.[4,5,8]

CENTRAL AND LATERAL STENOSIS AT SEVERAL LEVELS

Conservative measures are again employed to treat early lesions but are less likely to be effective than in managing one-level stenosis.

Operation

Entry between the laminae is usually made at what is considered the upper or lower end of the stenotic segments. This method may be difficult and time consuming. It is often easier to expose the dura just above or just below the area of the lesion through a normal interlaminar space. Often the interlaminar space is much reduced in size. After the dura is exposed, the aperture is widened as described for treating one-level stenosis and the medial portions of inferior and superior facets are removed in the same way. From then on, the exposure can be lengthened with Kerrison forceps, with care taken not to injure the dura. It may be difficult to decide how long the laminectomy should be. To some extent this can be decided before the operation by studying the myelogram or CT scan and by correlating it with clinical findings. Three examples clarify this point. (1) The patient has clinical signs and symptoms of L5 nerve entrapment. The CT scan demonstrates central stenosis at the L3–4, L4–5 and L5–S1 levels. Decompression of the L5 nerve at the L5–S1 level may well be adequate. (2) The patient has symptoms and signs of entrapment of the L4 and L5 nerves. The CT scan demonstrates stenosis at L3–4, L4–5, and L5–S1. Decompression of the L4 and L5 nerves at the L4–5 and L5–S1 levels may well relieve the patient's symptoms. (3) The patient has bizarre symptoms and signs affecting almost the whole of both lower limbs. The CT findings are as described under (2). It is wise to decompress the whole length of the stenotic area.

The presence or absence of pulsation of the dura at operation is another useful guide. When pulsation is absent, the laminectomy should be extended proximally as far as the L2–3 level to restore pulsation. While the laminectomy should be as short as possible, a long laminectomy does not add to the risk of instability, provided that the lateral two-thirds of all the facet joints are preserved. At the end of the procedure, a free fat graft is placed posterior to the dura (Fig. 11-4).[6,7,9,10]

DEGENERATIVE SPONDYLOLISTHESIS

The condition presents either late in Phase II or early in Phase III. Assessment of the phase is most important in deciding what treatment is adequate. Erosion of the articular processes, usually at L4–5, allows the upper vertebra to move anteriorly on the lower as the disk yields. At the L4–5 level, for example, anterior displacement of the inferior process of L4 accompanied by marked erosion of

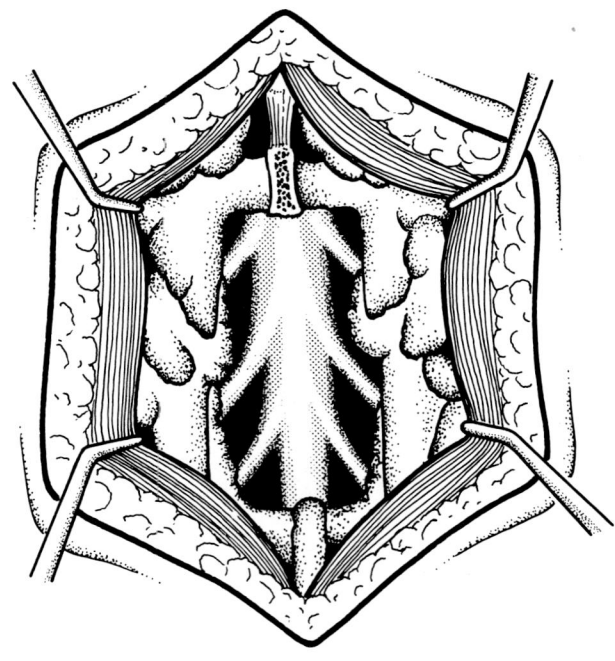

Fig. 11-4. Posterior view of a two-level decompression for central stenosis.

Fig. 11-5. Cross-sectional view illustrating the decompression for degenerative spondylolisthesis at L4–5: IAP, inferior articular process; SAP, eroded superior articular process. Anterior displacement of the inferior process has trapped the L5 nerves on both sides; the amount of the medial portion of the inferior articular processes to be removed is indicated by the dotted lines and shading.

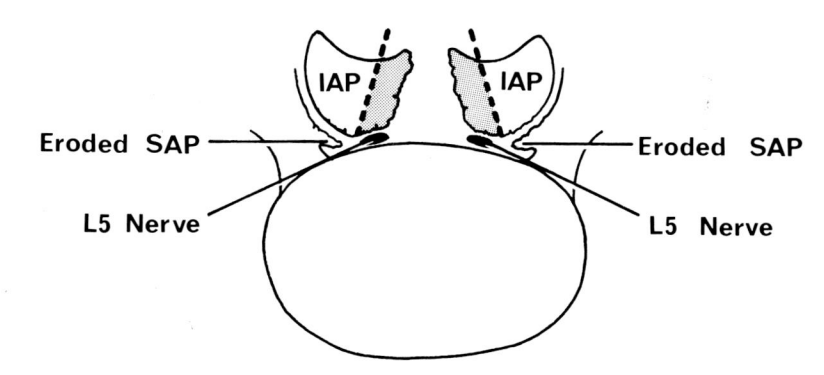

the superior process of L5 entraps the L5 nerve between the processes and the back of the vertebral body of L5.[11]

Conservative Measures

Such measures help some patients. However, it is likely that the patient must put up with back and leg discomfort and pain until the severity of this makes life miserable enough so that the patient requests an operation.

Operation

The approach and the size of the window, made by a bilateral minimal partial laminectomy, are as described for one-level central or lateral stenosis. The cephalocaudal dimension of the window needs to be slightly greater. Removing the medial part of the inferior articular process is more difficult because it is displaced far forward and because the superior process is eroded. The thin rim of the eroded superior process and the anterior portion of the inferior process are in contact with the nerve. This makes release of the trapped nerve time consuming and difficult.

When marked instability is present, undertaking a one-level fusion—usually a posterolateral fusion—is essential (Fig. 11-5).[11]

ISTHMIC SPONDYLOLISTHESIS

The presentation is most commonly at the L5–S1 level. Posterior joint pain is often at the level above the lesion, at L4–5. Leg pain is due to entrapment of the L5 nerve medial to the L5–S1 foramen. The nerve is compressed or put under tension by the upper part of the pars interarticularis, immediately above the defect.

Conservative Measures

Such therapy assists many patients. Pain arising in the posterior joints can be relieved by either manipulation or injection. In some patients the pain experienced arises in the sacroiliac joint. Often a sacroiliac syndrome arises as a complication of spondylolisthesis. The treatment for this has been discussed above.

Operation

The plan of treatment propounded by Wiltse[12] and Wiltse et al.[13,14] is a useful guide as to what type of operation should be done. In adolescents with back or leg pain, a fusion (from L5 to the sacrum for a slip at L5–S1 and from L4 to the sacrum for a slip at L4–5) is usually all that is required. In adults with back pain only, a fusion alone usually suffices. In adults with leg pain, decompression alone may be enough. (4) In adults with back and leg pain, the decompression should be followed with a fusion. (5) In patients with spondyloptosis both decompression and fusion should be performed.

Decompression

Removing the loose fragment alone is not enough. It is essential to expose the pars interarticularis just above the defect, identify the nerve and exact site of entrapment, and remove enough of the pars at this point to free the nerve (Fig. 11-6). The procedure can be done through a posterior midline incision or through two lateral incisions as described by Wiltse and his group.

Fusion

When fusion alone is to be done, the surgeon can choose either a posterolateral or an anterior-interbody fusion.

When fusion follows decompression, a posterolateral fusion can be undertaken at the same operation. Anterior interbody fusion requires a second operation. Posterior interbody fusion, which theoretically can be done at the same time as the decompression, in the writer's opinion is difficult because of the slip.[12-15]

A Word of Caution

Just as the back pain in spondylolisthesis may arise from a sacroiliac joint, pain after decompression or fusion may have the same origin. Awareness of this possibility and conservative treatment of this separate lesion may save the patient from a second decompression or fusion.

POST-FUSION STENOSIS

Two types are recognized: that due to degenerative changes in the joints just above the fusion—the most common type; and that caused by new bone formation beneath and anterior to the fusion.

Operation

One-level degenerative stenosis above the fusion is relieved by decompression through a bilateral minimal partial laminectomy. Stenosis beneath a fusion presents a more difficult problem. The dura should be exposed just above the top of the fusion and the central portion of the fusion mass removed in a caudal direction. This procedure is time consuming and difficult. Often the dura adheres to the anterior aspect of the fusion.

THE MULTI-OPERATED BACK

The first operation should be done with such meticulous attention to detail that it is the last. In practice it is often necessary to consider undertaking a second or third operation. In this situation the personality of the patient, the phase, and the exact site and nature of the lesion should be most carefully assessed.

The most commonly seen lesions, as recorded by Burton et al.,[8] are lateral spinal stenosis (58%), central spinal stenosis (7%), arachnoiditis (16%), recurrent disk herniation (12%), and epidural fi-

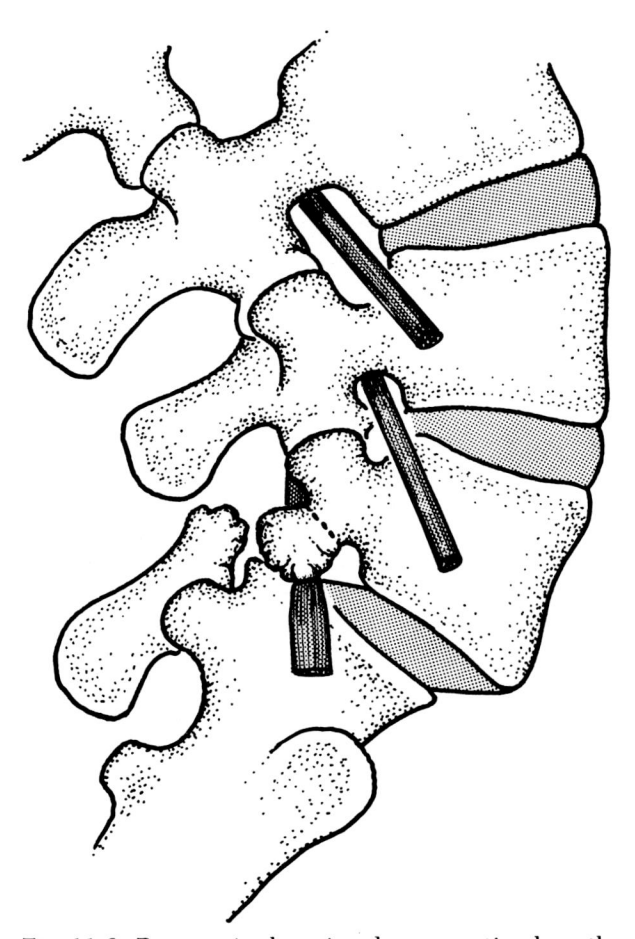

Fig. 11-6. Parasaggittal section demonstrating how the L5 nerve is entrapped by the pars interarticularis just above the defect in isthmic spondylolisthesis; the amount of bone to be removed is shown by the dotted line.

Fig. 11-7. Cross-sectional diagram of the four steps of an operation to decompress the nerves lateral to the dura and in the lateral canal when fibrosis in the multi-operated back is present. (A) A laminectomy has been performed. (B) On the left side the lateral expansion of the ligamentum flavum has been separated from the medial aspect of the inferior articular process and the medial third of this process has been removed. (C) The Sonic tool is inserted between the ligamentum flavum and the superior articular process to remove its medial and anterior portions. (D) The lateral canals have been enlarged and a free fat graft is placed posterior to the dura.

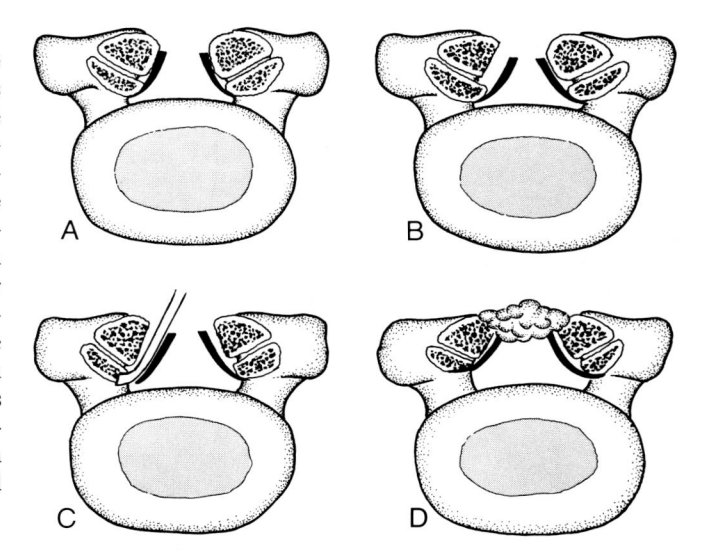

brosis (8%). Instability is more common than previously recorded.

Arachnoiditis and epidural adhesions sometimes benefit from epidural steroid injections or from a caudal block. In a few patients, found at reexploration to have marked intraspinal fibrosis, repeated epidural steroid administration following the operation has been beneficial.

Operation

The problems encountered are distortion of anatomy because of previous surgery, the presence of adhesions between the dura and the scar tissue posterior to it, and the presence of scar tissue surrounding spinal nerves. The risks encountered during operation are opening of the dura, damage to nerves, and damage to blood vessels leading to hemorrhage, postoperative fibrosis, and nerve ischemia. For these reasons, it is often wise to begin the decompression lateral to the lateral extensions of the ligamentum flavum. These are identified just medial to the inferior articular processes. The plane of cleavage between the ligamentum flavum and the articular processes is developed. The ligament is separated from the superior process anteriorly and laterally. The dura and overlying scar can then be retracted toward the midline, first on one side and then on the other. At this point it is easier to identify the site at which scar adheres to the dura and to excize the scar without opening the dura (Fig. 11-7).

SUMMARY

In this chapter the writer has attempted a brief overall survey of the therapeutic modalities for low back and leg pain. Each of these will be considered in more detail in later chapters in this section.

REFERENCES

1. Mooney V, Robertson J: The facet syndrome. Clin Orthop 115: 149, 1976
2. Edgar MA, Ghadially JA: Innervation of the lumbar spine. Clin Orthop 115: 35, 1976
3. Farfan HF, Kirkaldy-Willis WH: The present status of spinal fusion in the treatment of lumbar intervertebral joint disorders. Clin Orthop 158: 198, 1981
4. Crock HV: Isolated disk resorption. Clin Orthop 115: 109, 1976
5. Crock HV, Venner RM: Clinical Studies of isolated disk resorption in the lumbar spine. J Bone Joint Surg [Br] 4: 491, 1981
6. Getty CJM: Lumbar spinal stenosis. J Bone Joint Surg [Br] 62B: 481, 1980

7. Kirkaldy-Willis WH, Paine KWE, Cauchoix J, McIvor GWD: Lumbar spinal stenosis. Clin Orthop 99: 30, 1974
8. Burton CV, Kirkaldy-Willis WH, Yong-Hing K, Heithoff KB: Causes of failure of surgery of the lumbar spine. Clin Orthop 157, 191, 1981
9. Arnoldi CC: Intraosseous hypertension. Clin Orthop 115: 30, 1976
10. Dommisse GF: Arteries and veins of the lumbar nerve roots and cauda equina. Clin Orthop 115: 22, 1976
11. Cauchoix J, Benoist M, Chassaing V: Degenerative spondylolisthesis. Clin Orthop 115: 122, 1976
12. Wiltse LL: The Etiology of spondylolisthesis. J Bone Joint Surg 44A: 3539, 1962
13. Wiltse LL, Bateman JG, Hutchinson RH, Nelson WE: The paraspinal sacrospinalis—splitting approach to the lumbar spine. J Bone Joint Surg 50A, 5, 919, 1968
14. Wiltse LL, Widell EH, Jackson DW: Fatigue fracture: the basic lesion in isthmic spondylolisthesis. J Bone Joint Surg 57A: 17, 1975
15. Newman PH: Stenosis of the lumbar spine in spondylolisthesis. Clin Orthop 115: 116, 1976

12 Spine Education Program—Intensive Therapy—The Pain Clinic

W. H. Kirkaldy-Willis

SPINE EDUCATION

Introduction

Spine education for 8 to 10 patients at a time is invaluable in managing low back pain. All patients suffering from this condition should attend a spine education programme as early in their treatment as possible. It is as useful in helping the vast majority of patients with minor degrees of pathology as for patients recovering from major surgery. Many different kinds of programs have been set up in one city and another. Probably each patient needs two periods of instruction of 1½ to 2 hours each, followed 1 month later by an additional hour to reinforce what has been learned and test how much of the information given has been retained by the patient. The description given below is a composite from several different types of programs.

The instruction given should be as short and as simple as possible. It should be practical. The patient should participate as fully as possible.

The Setting

This should be as informal as possible, with mats or rugs on the floor and chairs, tables, or boxes arranged so that patients can relax lying on the floor with hips and knees flexed for at least part of the time spent in the class. An important part of the instruction is about rest and relaxation. The patient should be practicing this right from the start (Fig. 12-1).

The Objective

The most important objective is to teach the patient how to help him- or herself. This should be made clear right at the start and repeated two or three times. In our modern society we tend to want everything to be done for us. This attitude leads the patient to expect the physician or therapist to do all the work. For this reason we say,

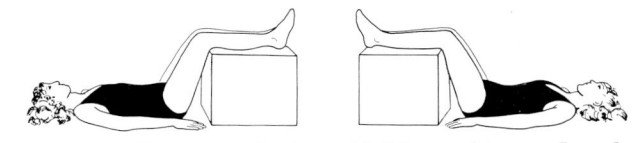

Fig. 12-1. Patients relaxing with hips and knees flexed.

"We understand your trouble. We cannot ourselves do more than a certain amount to help you. However, we can teach you to help and to cure yourself. You will have to work hard to do this. Learn to be good to your back and your back will be good to you." The rest of this chapter is concerned with ways in which the patient can be good to his or her back.

The Normal Lumbar Spine

It is necessary right at the start for the patient to have some knowledge of the way in which the

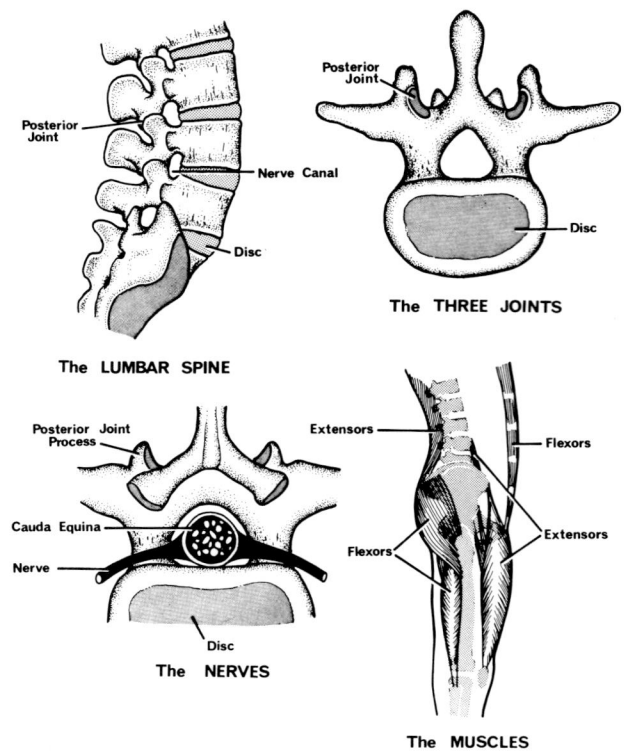

Fig. 12-2. The normal lumbar spine

normal lumbar spine functions. From top to bottom this region of the spine has five joints. Each joint has three parts, two small joints at the back and one larger joint in front—the disk. The movement of these three joints is controlled by muscles that bend the spine backward and forward, rotate (twist) it from side to side, and bend it to one side and another. A channel or tube runs down the center of the spine. This contains the nerves in a sheath (covering)—the dura. At each level a nerve passes from the sheath to left and right side. This passes along a smaller channel, leaves the spine, and joins other branches to form the nerves that supply the leg (Fig. 12-2).

Injury to the Lumbar Spine

The patient who knows something about the normal lumbar spine is better able to understand the reasons for low back and leg pain. Emphasis is placed on simple conditions that are by far the most common causes of pain. These are poor posture; twisting injuries that are usually minor ones, often repeated; and compression resulting from a fall onto the buttocks with the spine flexed (bent forward). The most common type of injury affects the two small posterior joints at one of the lower two levels and is called a posterior joint strain. Although this is not serious, it may cause severe pain and spasm (tightness) of the muscles that makes the pain worse. Other, less common conditions that result from these simple posterior joint strains should be mentioned briefly. These are a disk herniation, central stenosis (narrowing of the central tube), lateral stenosis (narrowing of the smaller tubes that contain individual nerves), and instability (weak joints at one level that allow more movement than normal). When the joints do not work normally, muscles also work abnormally. Sometimes they contract (tighten up) and increase the pain. Later on they become weak (flabby) and the spine loses its normal strength (Fig. 12-3). The diagnosis is written on each patient's requisition form. The leader of the class should be aware of all the diagnoses. Patients should be asked if they know what their own diagnosis is. If a patient is in doubt, it is helpful to explain what is wrong, pointing to the lesion on the diagram on the screen.

The Pain

As stated above, pain usually comes from irritation of nerves supplying the posterior joints. This condition may give leg as well as back pain. The common causes of leg pain are a disk herniation and central or lateral stenosis. Irritation of nerves supplying a joint produces electrical impulses that pass along the nerve to the spine and up to the brain, where they are recognized as pain.

The Gate. There are two kinds of nerves in the joint: those that are stimulated by movement,

Table 12-1. Factors That Decrease and Increase Pain

Factors That Decrease Pain
  Confidence
  Movement
  Rhythm
  Avoidance of painful activity
Factors That Increase Pain
  Fear
  Not understanding
  Holding back stiff
  Lack of knowledge of how to avoid pain

rhythm and activity and those stimulated by injury. The first kind shut the gate in the spine so that the patient does not feel pain. The second kind result in pain. When the "gate" is shut (by the first lot of nerves), the painful impulses cannot pass and so the patient feels less pain. It is useful to use the following analogy: Think of a gate on a farm between two fields. Cows (the good impulses that prevent pain) and sheep (the bad painful impulses) are waiting in one field by the gate. If the cows are passing through the gate to the second field, the sheep because they are smaller have a difficult job to go through; however, if the cows are making no attempt to go through the gate, it is easy for the sheep to do so.

The leader then tells the class how to stimulate the cows (the good impulses) to pass the gate. The following conditions stimulate the cows to go through the gate: (1) confidence that comes from understanding about one's back problem; (2) activity (movement), using the back as much as possible without causing pain; (3) rhythm, using the back as normally as possible; and (4) avoiding acts that aggravate back pain. The following conditions stimulate the sheep to pass through the gate: (1) fear, not knowing what is wrong or how serious it is; (2) holding the back stiffly so that it does not move or so that it moves in a jerky way; (3) not knowing how to avoid acts that increase the pain. In practice all this means that from the start rest and relaxation are important. As the back heals, it is extremely important for the patient to begin to use the muscles to move the back normally and with rhythm. Rhythm can be demonstrated by the leader doing a little "squiggly" movement from side to side. The point should be made that the patient is not likely to become pain free until he or she is moving the back almost normally again. Thus an early return to work

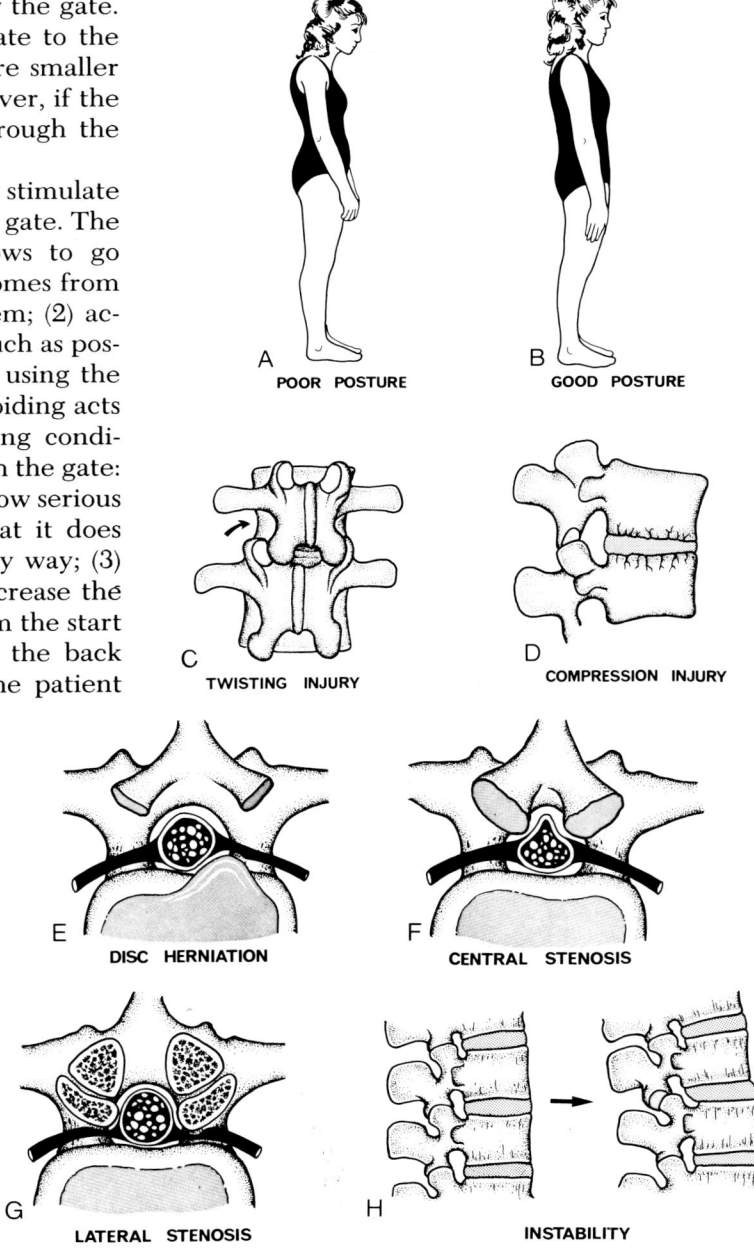

Fig. 12-3. The injured lumbar spine

164 *Managing Low Back Pain • 12*

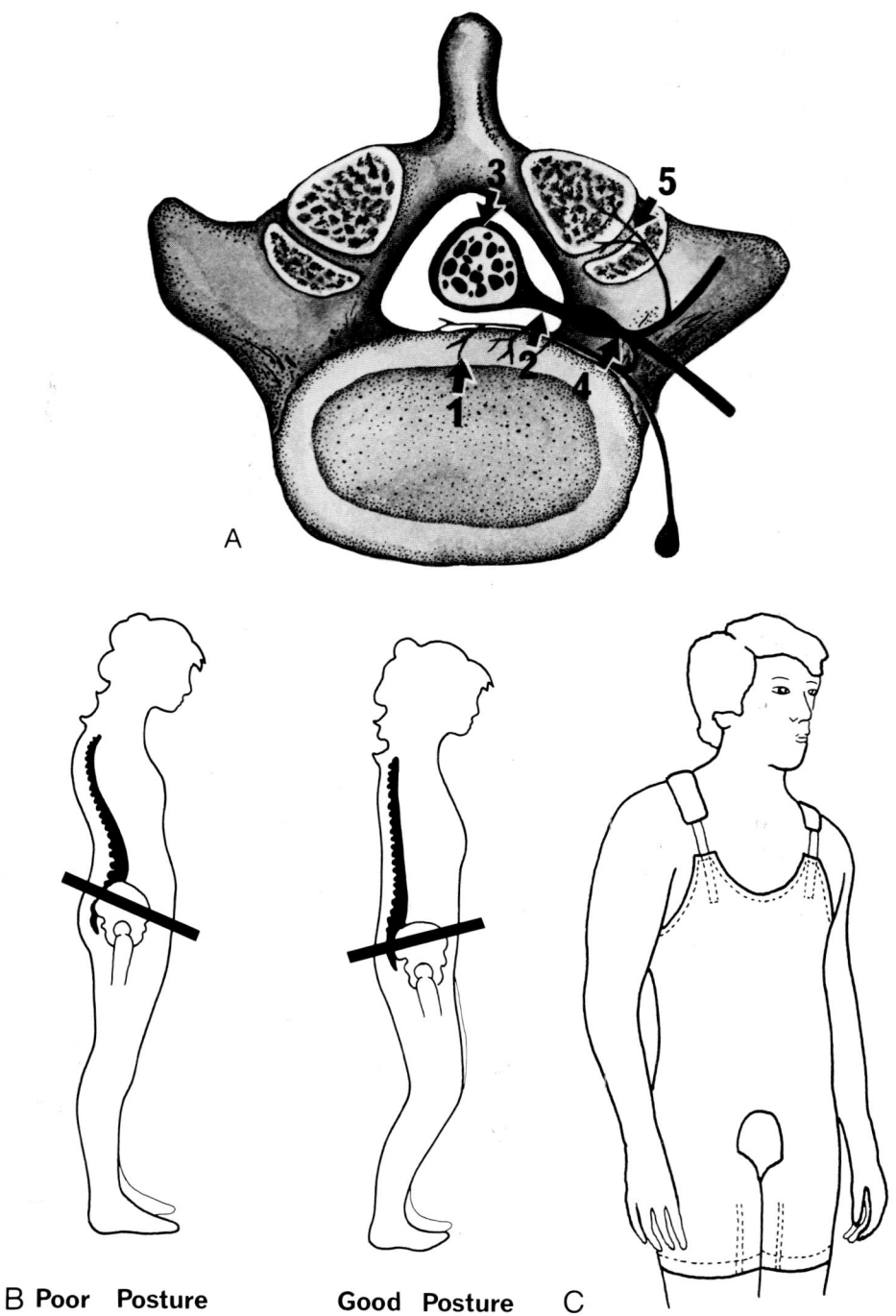

B **Poor Posture**   **Good Posture**   C

Fig. 12-4. (A) Common sites of nerve irritation. (1) Sinuvertebral nerve from central disk herniation, (2) main spinal nerve from more lateral disk herniation, (3) cauda equina from central stenosis, (4) main spinal nerve and ganglion from lateral canal stenosis, and (5) posterior joint nerves from degeneration of this joint. (B) Poor and good posture. (C) Elasticon support.

Table 12-2. Treatment of Back Pain

Rest and relaxation
A.I.M.
   *A*spirin
   *I*ce
   *M*ovement
Elastic support
Pelvic tilting
Reduction of obesity

(avoiding activities that cause pain) is a most important part of the treatment (Table 12-1).

Treating Back Strains

Most emphasis should be placed on treating back sprain, the most common and most easily treated condition. As the leader talks about this, the patients should be participating (doing the things the leader advises) as far as possible.

1. Rest and relaxation for several periods of time each day. (At this point the patients should be resting on their backs with hips and knees flexed.)
2. A.I.M. Aspirin, one or two tablets three to four times a day helps to relieve pain and counteracts inflammation. Ice, applied to the back several times a day, reduces muscle spasm (tightness). Movement stimulates the good nerves (the cows at the gate) and reduces pain.
3. Wearing a Camp elastic support or elastic body stocking helps pull in the tummy muscles and this relieves the pain.
4. Posture. Arching the back jams the posterior joints together and increases the pain. Pelvic tilting helps to avoid this by straightening the spine. This should be done with the patient in one of three positions: lying on the back on a couch with knees flexed 45°, in the same position with knees extended, and standing with the back to the wall and the knees slightly flexed. The patient should practice pelvic tilting for 5 to 10 minutes several times a day.

All of these activities should be demonstrated in each instance on at least one or two patients so that each patient participates in the programme as fully as possible. In many instances all the patients can take part together.

5. Obesity. At some point the importance of losing weight, of building up abdominal muscles to strengthen the back, and of avoiding stress to the back in order to obtain a rapid return to normal health should be stressed (Fig. 12-4, Table 12-2).

EXERCISE PROGRAM

(Courtesy of the Spine Education Center, Inc., Dallas, Texas)

General Rules

1. Do each exercise slowly.
2. Start with five repetitions and work up to 10.
3. Do the exercise for 10 minutes twice a day.
4. Omit painful exercises from the programme.
5. Do the exercises every day without fail.

Fig. 12-5A. Pelvic Tilting. Lie on your back with knees bent and feet touching the floor. Place your hand under your back and press against your hand with the small of your back. You will feel your stomach muscles tightening as you flatten your back against the floor. This corrects arching of the back.

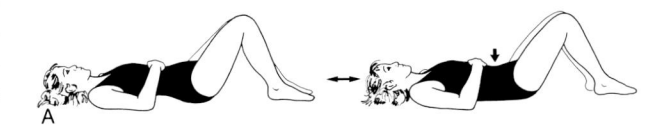

Fig. 12-5B. Modified Sit-ups. Begin as in A. Keep your hands by your side. Lift your head so your chin almost touches your chest. Lift your shoulders off the floor as you reach for your knees. Touch the top of your knees with your fingers, then lower your shoulders slowly to the floor. Keep your chin tucked in. Then lower your head slowly to the floor. Be sure you do not arch your back during any part of this exercise.

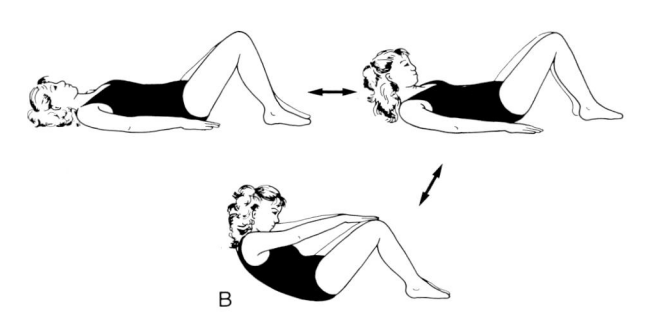

Fig. 12-5C. Double Knee-to-Chest or Low-Back Stretch. Begin as in A. Bring both knees to your chest, one at a time. Hug your knees tight enough to feel a mild stretch in your low back. Lower your legs slowly to the beginning position, one at a time. Be sure you do not arch your back during any part of this exercise.

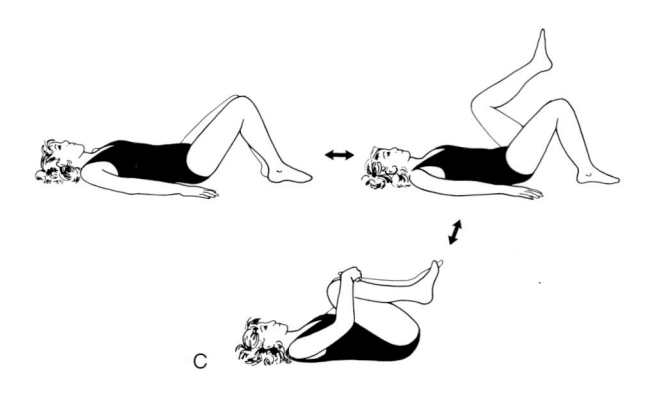

Fig. 12-5D. Sidelying Leg Raise. Lie on your side. Keep the top leg in line with your body. The bottom leg may be slightly bent. Raise the top leg straight up, slowly, and lower it to the beginning position. Do this with the other leg also.

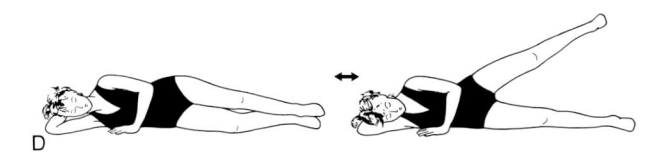

Fig. 12-5E. Mountain and Sag, Knee to Elbow. Start on hands and knees. Make a mountain out of your back, then let it slowly sag, like an old horse. Repeat 5 to 10 times. Bring your knee to your elbow, then straighten your leg behind you. Watch underneath and do not lose sight of your toes—you do not want to arch your back. Repeat with the other leg.

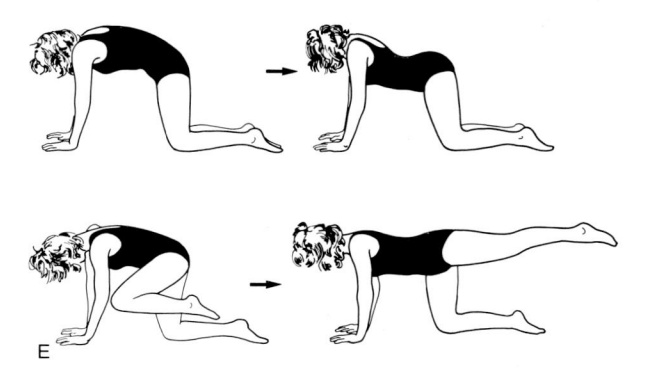

Fig. 12-5F,G,H. Hamstring Stretch. This can be done lying, standing, or sitting.

(F) Lying on your back, put your hands under your buttocks. Slowly, lift your legs over your head. *Do not* keep your legs straight when lifting them. Then, flap your feet.

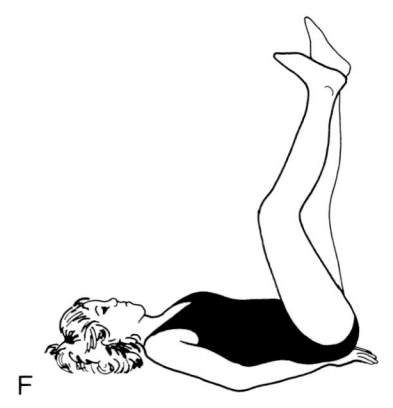

(G) Stand with one leg propped on a table or back of a chair. Bend the leg you are standing on until you feel a mild stretch under your thigh.

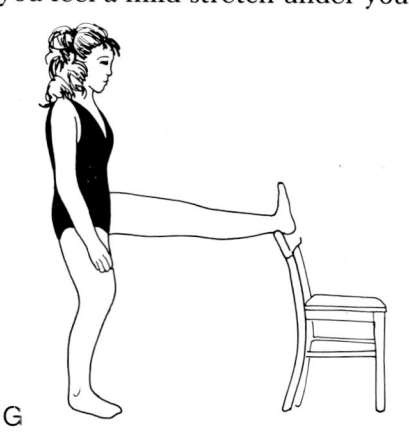

(H) Sit on the floor with one leg bent and the other almost straight. Lean toward the bent leg until you feel a mild stretch under the other thigh. Repeat with the other leg.

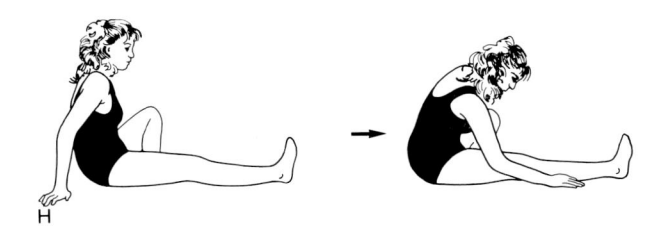

Swimming Exercises

Swimming in warm water is one of the best activities for patients with low back pain, but diving is inadvisable.
1. With back to the wall, bring knees to chest and rotate to the right and then to the left. Do all exercises 10 times.
2. Bring knees to chest. Straighten legs, but keep them at a right angle to your body. Spread legs apart, then bring them back together.
3. With legs out in front, (as in 2), open legs and then cross them like a pair of scissors.
4. Stand up with back to the wall, raise one leg straight in front, then pull back down. Repeat with other leg.
5. With back to wall, raise knee up to hip level, allowing knee to bend. Straighten and bend knee. Repeat with other leg.
6. Turn with side to wall. Kick outside leg up in front, then behind, then out to side and down. Repeat on other side.
7. Face wall and kick one leg out behind keeping leg straight. Repeat with other leg.
8. Facing bar, put both feet on bar. Bend and straighten knees.
9. With back to the wall, pretend you are riding a bicycle.
10. Back to wall, make a circle with one leg. Be sure foot touches surface of water as well as bottom of pool. Reverse direction. Repeat with other foot.

Summary

The instruction given so far together with the exercises demonstrated is as much as most patients can absorb in one session. During this first session it is good to have a ten minute coffee break before starting on the exercises.

During the second session attention is given to basic body mechanics (activities of daily living). In centers where patients attend from a long distance it may be best to hold the first session in the morning and the second session during the afternoon of the same day. Where patients live close to the Spine Education Center, it is ideal to hold the second session one week later than the first.

BASIC BODY MECHANICS

(Courtesy of the Spine Education Center, Inc., Dallas, Texas)

Fig. 12-6A. Standing. One foot forward, knees slightly bent; one foot up to change position.

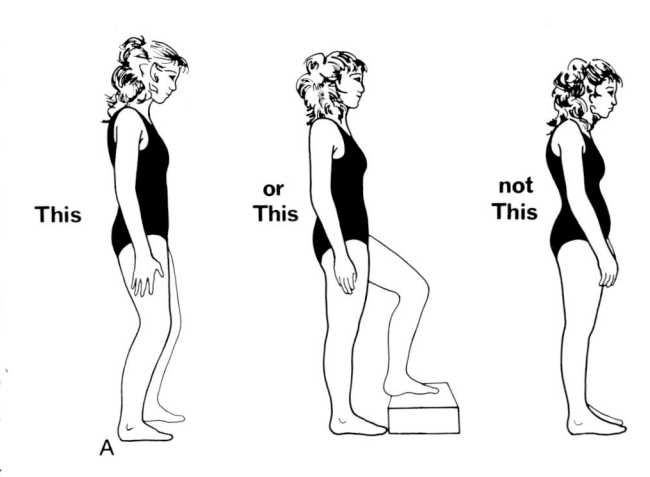

Fig. 12-6B. To Sit. Flex the lumbar spine; flex hips and knees; do not bend forward from the

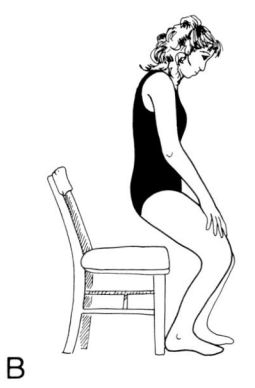

168 Managing Low Back Pain • 12

hips. Lower yourself to the chair; use your hands to help if necessary. **To Get Up.** Reverse the procedure.

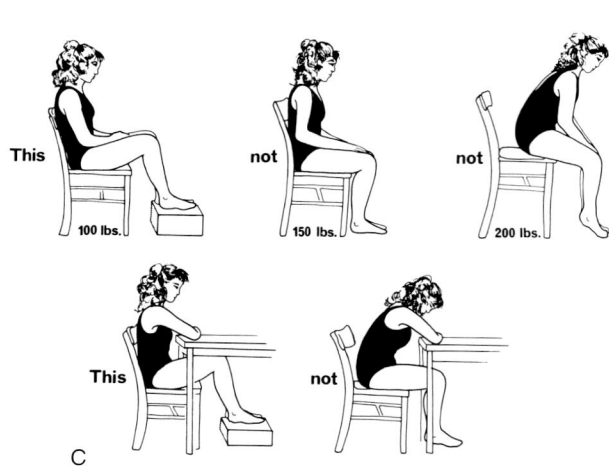

Fig. 12-6C. Sitting. Sit slightly reclined, knees higher than hips. Get close to work with chair, not with head.

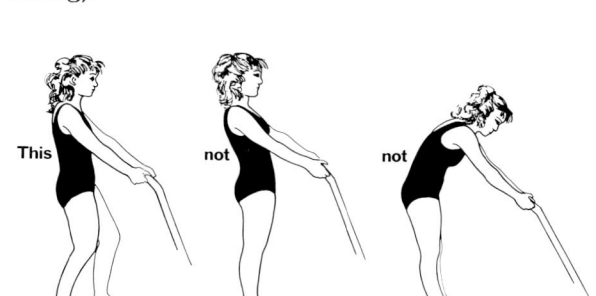

Fig. 12-6D. Reaching.

Fig. 12-6E. Brushing Teeth. Bend and rest knees. Open cabinet door, one foot up.

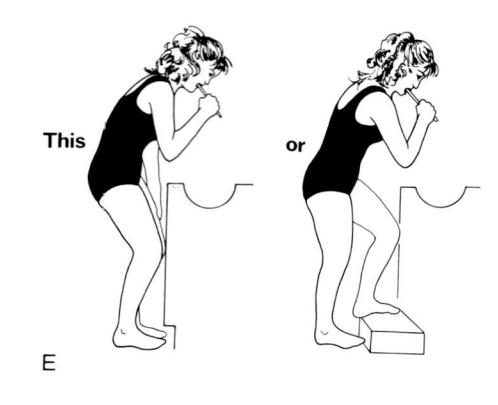

Fig. 12-6F. Weight Shift and Diagonal (Vacuuming).

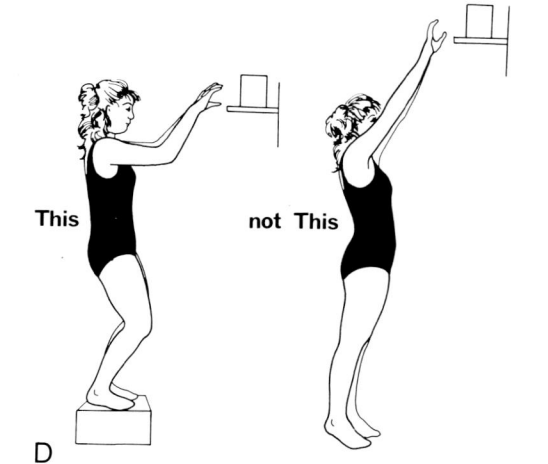

Fig. 12-6G. Push More Than Pull.

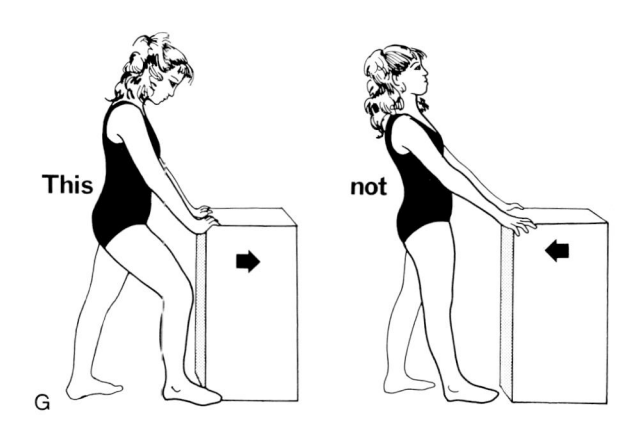

Spine Education Program—Intensive Therapy—The Pain Clinic   169

Fig. 12-6H. Lifting. For light objects, leg in air. Partial squat.

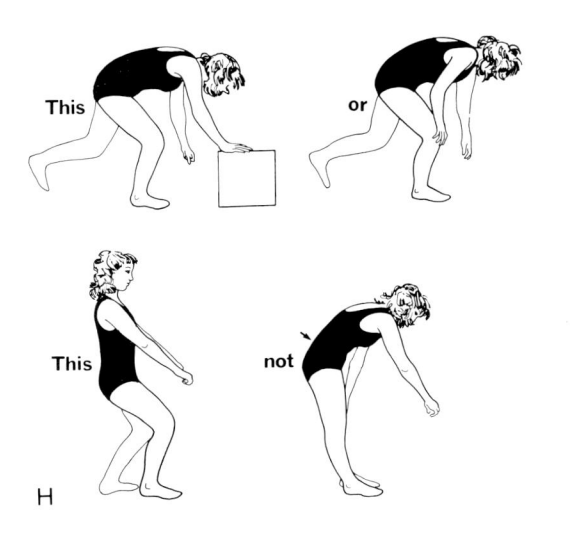

Fig. 12-6K. Shift Weight to Back Leg Before Walking.

Fig. 12-6I. More Lifting. Full squat with one foot forward.

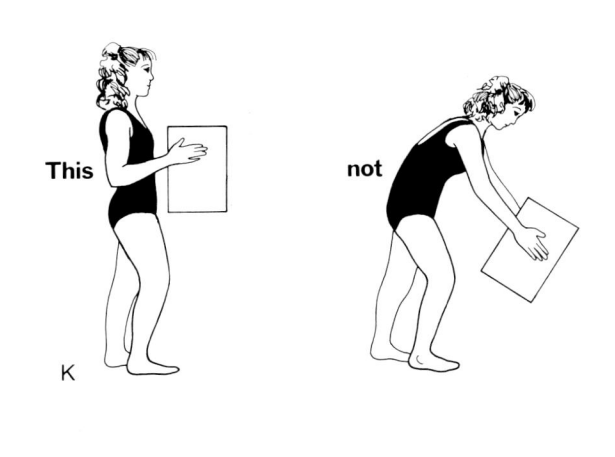

Fig. 12-6L. Recommended Sleeping Positions.

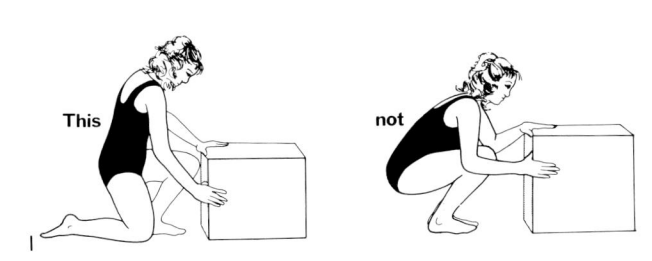

Fig. 12-6J. Keep Load Close.

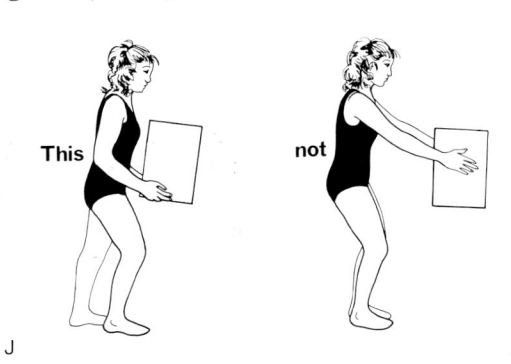

Fig. 12-6M. Getting in and out of Bed. If your right side is more painful get in on the right side of the bed. (1) Sit on edge of bed with knees bent. (2) Let your head and trunk down onto the bed to lie on the right side and bring your legs onto the bed. (3) Roll carefully onto back with knees bent. (4) Reverse the procedure to get out of bed.

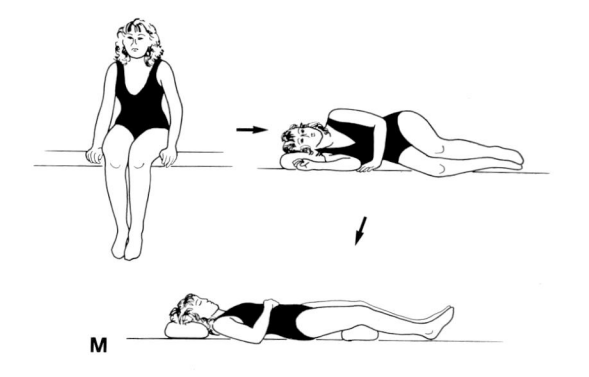

Fig. 12-6N. Getting into Car. Bend hips and knees with spine slightly flexed and lower yourself onto the seat facing the door. Use your hands on the door to help. Flex hips and knees further to bring your feet into the car. Using your hands, turn your whole body and legs as one unit to face forward in the car without twisting your low back. To get out of the car reverse the procedure.

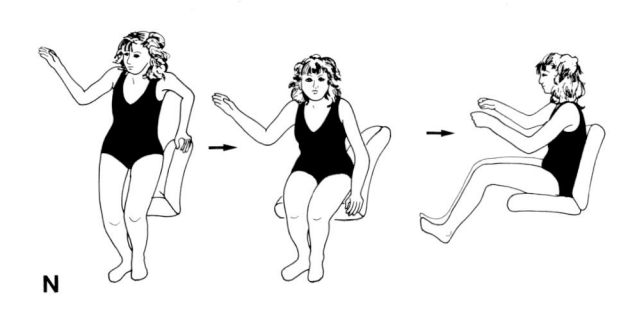

Fig. 12-6O. Sitting in Car.

Do not attempt to drive your car when you have severe back pain.

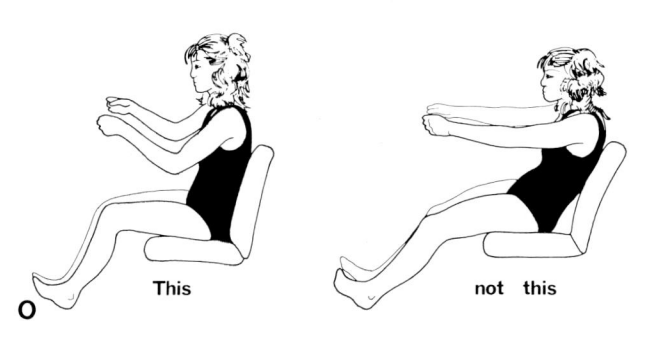

Fig. 12-6P. Use Bumper on Car.

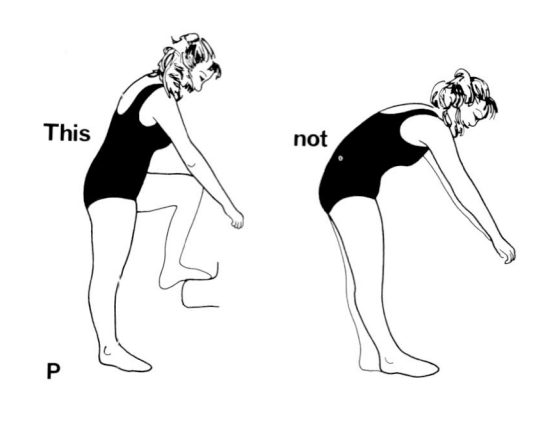

Do's and Don'ts

When Your Back is Painful

Sitting. Avoid sitting. If you must sit, (1) get up and move around every 20 minutes. (2) Use back and/or feet support. (3) Legs must not be straight out in front, as in sitting in bed, in the bathtub, or on the floor. (4) Use a small towel roll or magazine roll behind your low back. This will help straighten the curve in the low back. (5) When standing up, move to the edge of the chair; position one foot in front of the other; and use your legs to stand without leaning forward. Sitting with poor posture is certain to aggravate your back pain.

Driving. When your back is painful, try to avoid driving. As a passenger you can lie down on the back seat and bend your knees. When driving, bring the seat up close to the wheel so that your knees are slightly higher than your hips. Do not get so close to the wheel that you cannot turn it. Use a towel roll or magazine behind your low back.

Bending Forward. When your back is hurting,

try to avoid bending forward at the waist. Bending increases pressure on the disk. Kneeling to make beds and to reach low levels is a good alternative when your back is painful.

Lying. A good firm support is desirable. The floor is too firm, a saggy mattress is too soft. When getting out of bed, turn to one side, draw your knees up and drop your feet over the edge. At the same time, push yourself up with your arms and avoid bending forward at the waist.

Coughing and sneezing. When your back is painful, stand up, if you can, and bend your knees. If a wall is handy, brace yourself against it. If you are sitting and cannot stand, lean back in your chair. Always avoid leaning forward at the waist.

When You Are Feeling Better

Sitting. Sit with a back support cushion. You may also maintain the same position with your own muscles. While you sit, do the hump and sag exercise for the low back to work out sore spots. Get up and move around every 30 to 45 minutes. If you are driving long distances, stop every hour or two to walk around.

Recurrence

The next time you feel the warning signs of impending back pain:
1. Use the first aid techniques—ice–massage–stretching–aspirin (A.I.M.) to get rid of any muscle spasm.
2. Do the exercises that helped decrease the pain during the last episode.
3. If the first aid regimen every hour does not help significantly in the first 48 hours or if you experience a different back or leg pain from that experienced before, go and see your doctor and follow his or her advice.

Summary

Teaching patients with low back pain about basic body mechanics is most important. All patients should have this kind of instruction. Knowing how to use the painful back does more to get rid of the pain than anything else.

The material dealt with in this second session is obvious to the leader but less so to the patients. There should be a 10-minute coffee break in the middle of the session.

As far as possible *all* the patients should do *all* the activities explained by the leader.

At the end of the session patients should be encouraged to ask questions.

Before the patients leave, the leader should once again emphasize the vital point that they are responsible for their own cure. This means hard work day after day. "Be good to your back and it will be good to you."

REVIEW OF KNOWLEDGE GAINED

It is highly desirable that the patient should return to the Spine Education Program 3 to 4 weeks after the second session of instruction to test how much knowledge has been retained, (2) to make sure that the patient has been practising the body mechanics that were taught, and (3) to review any exercises and body mechanics that were found to be confusing or difficult.

A good approach is first to ask each patient individually what problems have been encountered and deal with these one by one. It is difficult for some patients to realize that painful exercises must be reduced in number or avoided for a time. This point can be brought home by saying, "When driving your car you come to a red light, you stop till the light changes to green. Pain is your red light. This red light tells you to stop what you are doing, to do less of the activity or to modify it." The activity may be housework, work on the farm, or exercises.

SOME USEFUL AIDS

A Cushion for the Back

Many patients are helped by a firm cushion that can be carried around and placed behind the back in the chair at the office or home, in the car, on an airplane, and in other similar situations. A recommended model is the "Spine-Bac" (Spina Bac, Fimax Inc., P.O. Box 595030, Miami, Florida, 33159). The patient can adjust this to three different positions so that one cushion suits anyone. It can be fastened to the back of the chair with velcro strips.

Supports for the Feet

A folding pocket footstool is useful for many people suffering from low back pain. When sitting in a chair the knees should be slightly higher than the hips. The footstool is a simple way of achieving this. It is also helpful when standing to place one foot on the stool. This allows slight flexion of hip and knee and relaxes the low back. One type of stool is the "Back Easer" (Back Easer Footstool, T. Milburn Co. Ltd., D Floor, 100 Front St. W., Toronto, M5J 1E3). A similar stool used by guitar players can be obtained at many music stores. (Fig. 12-7).

INTENSIVE THERAPY

Spine education as outlined above is sufficient for most patients. A few patients require more intensive therapy for several reasons.

Daily Therapy for 2 to 4 Weeks

Patients from nearby attend daily at Departments of Physiotherapy and Occupational Therapy. Those from a distance stay with friends or relatives or are lodged in a nearby hotel. They spend nearly the whole day in these departments.

Several groups of patients benefit from this type of therapy: patients who do not or cannot understand the education given in the three sessions outlined above, those who have a marked personality disturbance together with a mechanical low back problem, those with very poor posture and marked muscle weakness, those with a Phase II condition (Instability) who may benefit from a 4-week period of muscle building; those who have had low back pain for many years and often several operations, and finally, a similar group who have lost the normal spinal rhythm and whose backs are stiff.

Treatment is given under the supervision of a physiotherapist, an occupational therapist, or both. It varies from patient to patient and the decision as to what modalities are employed is made by the therapist under the guidance and advice of the physician. The following modalities are commonly employed.

Ice. This has been discussed above. It is used in virtually every patient to reduce pain and produce relaxation before other modalities are embarked upon.

Rest and Relaxation. Periods of rest are provided for each patient at intervals during the day. From this each one learns in a practical way how to rest and relax and becomes increasingly aware of the benefits obtained from this simple measure.

Exercises. To begin with, these are the same as those advocated in the Spine Education Program. As the patient progresses, other exercises may be added further to build up the spinal flexor muscles (or occasionally the extensor muscles) or to increase control and power in the rotator muscles. Often the flexors and extensors of the hip and knee also require to be strengthened for the vital part they play in normal function of the lumbar spine. An important part of this plan is the supervision of the therapist who controls, directs, and plans the tempo—the rate at which the patient can progress. Such supervision is especially valuable in dealing with idle patients, those with little self-will, and those not intelligent enough to know when to stop for rest when they experience pain. Rarely, with patients who have spinal instability a 6- to 8-week exercise program may be required.

Rhythm. Most patients learn to regain the normal rhythm of the lumbar spine quite quickly. A few, after prolonged disability and several operations, find great difficulty. Rhythm is certainly as important as muscle power. Fear and uncertainty are great inhibitors of rhythm. This problem is markedly assisted by the performance of rhythmic exercises to move the joints of upper and lower limbs and those of the low back. To obtain a nearly normal range of movement is an important part of regaining rhythm. Some of the reasons for this were discussed in chapter 4 on the perception of pain.

Mobilization. Stiff joints, tight fascial bands (especially tight posterior lumbar fascia), and shortened tight muscles benefit greatly by maneuvers carried out by the therapist to stretch these

Spine Education Program—Intensive Therapy—The Pain Clinic   173

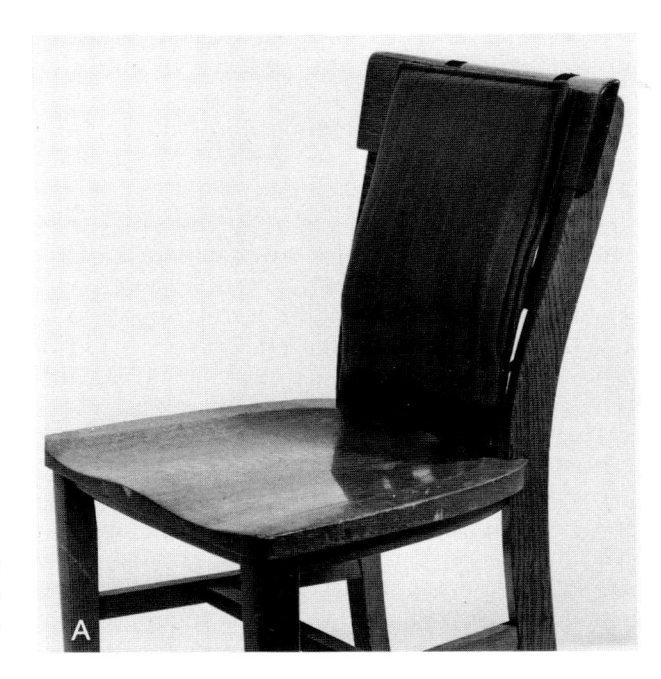

Fig. 12-7. (A) One type of adjustable cushion for the back. (B) The guitar players' stool, patient standing, one foot placed on the stool. (C) The Back-Ease stool, patient sitting, both feet on the stool.

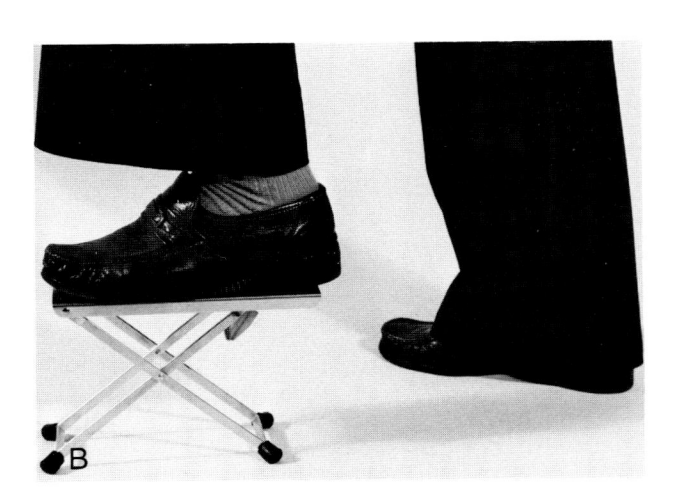

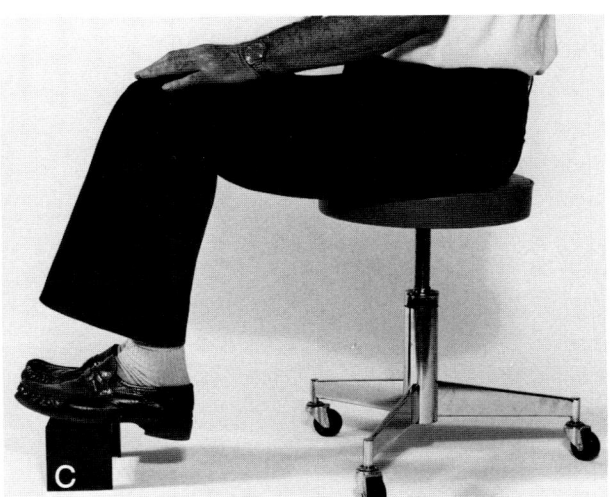

tissues. It is a time-consuming procedure that requires special skill.

Manipulation, discussed at length in chapter 13 is frequently of great benefit and may well be included in this regime of intensive therapy.

Occupational Therapy. There are two aspects of this very important modality of treatment: daily reinforcement of the basic body mechanics taught earlier during the three sessions of the Spine Education Program, and providing patients with specific occupational activities to give them an interest, to take their minds off their pain, and to increase their fitness for a return to work. Carrying out these goals also demands considerable skill, ingenuity, and patience from the therapist.

Psychotherapy. The procedures available to the psychologist in managing patients with low back pain are described fully in chapter 17. Suffice it to say that one or more of these modalities is often incorporated in this regime of intensive therapy.

Assessment of the Patient. Observation of the patient's attitudes, interests, abilities, and disabilities for several hours each day for 2 to 4 weeks enables the therapist to assess patients with a difficult problem more accurately than can be done by physician or therapist in one or more short sessions. The psychologist also has an opportunity to assess the patient further on several occasions.

Review. The physician carries out a final review at the end of this regime of several weeks of treatment. (1) Often he is surprised and delighted at the progress made by a patient he himself was unable to help. (2) The patient with several previous operations, considered a hopeless case, may respond well to this regime. (3) When the patient is one who will never make any effort to help himself, this becomes evident. (4) The prolonged assessment and the response to therapy may help the surgeon to decide if any further operation is advisable and necessary.

THE PAIN CLINIC

Many hospitals now have a well established pain clinic directed by a specially qualified physician and staffed by psychologists, physiotherapists, occupational therapists and social workers. This type of clinic is concerned with the alleviation of pain from many causes and many tissues and organs. This book is not the place for any attempt at a detailed description of the work of the pain clinic. The physician or surgeon managing a case of low back pain will often obtain a great deal of valuable help from the director of this type of clinic in terms of an independent assessment, suggestions for pain medication, treatment of depression, injection techniques (nerve blocks, epidural steroids, sympathetic blocks), and the effect of the team approach used in such a clinic.

13 Manipulation

W. H. Kirkaldy-Willis

INTRODUCTION

Manipulation is an art that requires much practice to acquire the necessary skill and competence. Few medical practitioners have the time or inclination to master it. This modality has much to offer the patient with low back pain, especially in the earlier stages during the phase of Dysfunction. We have seen in previous chapters that the majority of patients are first seen while in this phase. Most practitioners of medicine, whether family physicians, or surgeons, will wish to refer their patients to a practitioner of manipulative therapy with whom they can cooperate, whose work they know, and whom they can trust. The physician who makes use of this resource will have many contented patients and save himself many headaches.

In this chapter we will ask and try to answer the following questions: What is manipulation? How does it work? When is it indicated? and What are the results of treatment? Because this book is written largely for medical practitioners, we will not attempt to describe the details of the technique. Those with a special interest should not only read textbooks on the subject but also be prepared to complete a full apprenticeship with one or more skilled practitioners before embarking on this method of treatment themselves.

WHAT IS MANIPULATION?

The definition given by Sandoz[1,2] is both clear and concise. A manipulation or lumbar invertebral joint adjustment is a passive manual maneuver during which the three-joint complex is suddenly carried beyond the normal physiological range of movement without exceeding the boundaries of anatomical integrity. The usual characteristic is a thrust—a brief, sudden, and carefully administered "impulsion" that is given at the end of the normal passive range of movement. It is usually accompanied by a cracking noise.

The stages of an adjustment are illustrated in Figure 13-1. The central arc on each side of the neutral position represents the range of active movement in one plane such as flexion–extension, lateral bending, or rotation. Passive movement increases the range of movement in both directions and at the end of this, when the slack is taken up, the practitioner feels a resistance, the elastic barrier of resistance. When mobilization is forced beyond this elastic barrier a sudden yielding is felt; a cracking noise is perceived; and the range of movement is slightly increased beyond the physiological limit into the paraphysiological space. At this point a second final barrier of resistance is encountered, formed by the stretched ligaments and capsule; it is called the

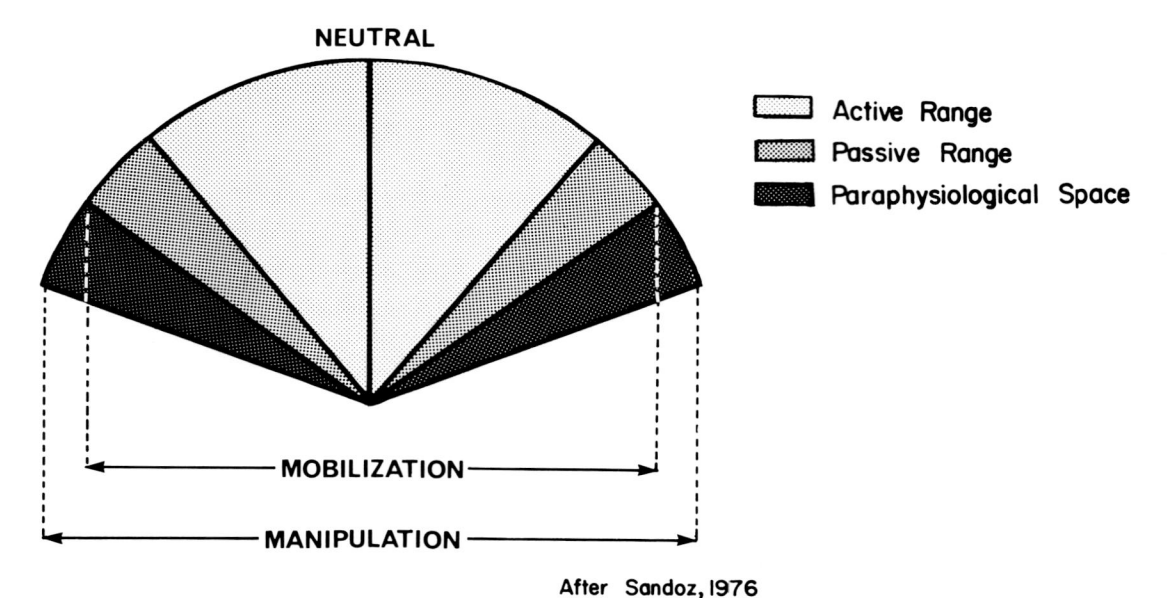

Fig. 13-1. The stages of an adjustment and definition of joint manipulation.

limit of anatomical integrity. Forcing movement beyond this point would damage the ligaments and capsule.

The four zones distinguished in joint adjustment are (1) active movement, (2) passive movement, (3) paraphysiological zone, and (4) pathological zone of movement.

The two barriers are the elastic barrier, overcome by a thrust without damage to joint structures, and the limit of anatomical integrity, which cannot be surpassed without injuring ligaments and capsule.

HOW DOES MANIPULATION WORK?

The Effect of Manipulation on a Normal Joint

Two British anatomists, Roston and Haines,[3] published a paper in 1947 entitled "Cracking in the metacarpo-phalangeal joint." The three phalanges of the middle finger were wrapped in adhesive tape and the tape was attached to a spring dynamometer to indicate the degree of tension applied to the finger. A progressively increasing force was applied to distract the metacarpo-phalangeal joint. Radiographs were taken at intervals to record changes in the joint space. In this experiment, the force was applied by a machine and not manually and by progressive traction rather than by a thrust, but the conditions may be considered comparable with those in a spinal adjustment.

The results of the experiment are shown in Figure 13-2. The tension is recorded on the abscissa and the separation of the cartilage surfaces on the ordinate. The initial separation of 1.8 mm is due to the thickness of the cartilages. The separation increases gradually up to a tension of 8 kg. At this point the surfaces jump to a separation of 4.7 mm and a cracking noise is heard. Increasing tension to 18 kg produces a further joint separation up to 5.4 mm. On reduction of the tension the joint surface separation is again approximately 2 mm, a distance slightly more than the initial separation of 1.8 mm. The ways in which the results of this experiment may be correlated with intervertebral joint adjustment are shown in Figure 13-3.

Three phenomena occur at the same time as the elastic barrier is passed: the articular surfaces separate suddenly; a cracking noise is heard; a radiolucent space appears within the joint. These occurrences can be explained as follows. Normally a small negative pressure is present in a joint

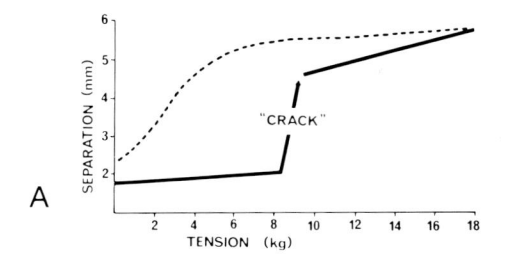

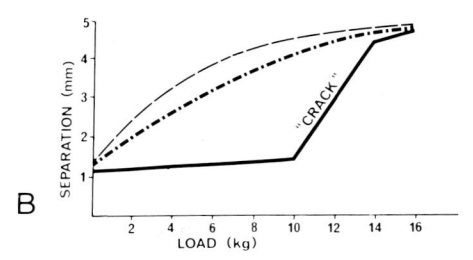

Fig. 13-2. (A) Effect of Manipulation on a normal joint. A "crack" is heard at 9 kg of tension, with separation of the cartilage surfaces. Increasing tension produces some further separation of the surfaces. When the tension is released (the dotted line), the separation of the surfaces decreased but does not quite return to normal. (After Roston JB, Haines RW: Cracking in the metacarpophalangeal joint. J Anat 81:165, 1947.) (B) Following the "crack" (lower solid line) the joint separation returns nearly to normal after 15 minutes (upper curve). On reloading immediately after "cracking," the joint separation follows the middle curve. No "crack" is heard. Modified from Sandoz R: Some physical mechanisms and effects of spinal adjustments. Ann Swiss Chirop Assoc 6:91, 1976, after Unsworth A, Dowson D, Wright V: Cracking joints, a bioengineering study of cavitation in the metacarpophalangeal joint. Ann Rheum Dis 30:348, 1971.

space; it maintains the cartilage surfaces in apposition and is one of the factors that maintain stability of the joint. With axial traction the synovial folds and capsule tends to invaginate toward the center of the joint. When the joint surfaces are forced apart beyond the elastic barrier (beyond the limit of invagination of soft tissues), gases are suddenly released from the synovial and tissue fluid to form a radiolucent cavity seen in the radiograph. The released energy is thought to be responsible for the cracking noise (Fig. 13-4).[4]

Manipulation also stimulates the mechanoreceptors (see chapter 4) with an effect both on the segmental muscles at the level of the intervertebral joint and on the pain mechanism (see below).[2]

The Therapeutic Effect of Manipulation on the Abnormal Joint

Reference to the discussion of pathology and pathogenesis in chapter 3 will make it clear that though we know much about the changes that take place, we still know very little about the way in which lumbar spinal disorders are initiated at the start of the degenerative process. Currently we know equally little about the effects of spinal adjustment. However, it is possible to postulate the ways in which this form of treatment may work in different spinal lesions.[5,6]

In the posterior joint syndrome the joint may lock, entrapping a synovial fold, or a minor subluxation of facets may be present. Via the arthrokinetic reflex the segmental muscles are in a state of hypertonic contraction and this splints the joint. Stimulating small nerve fibers results in pain. An adjustment (manipulation) that separates the articular surfaces may release entrapped synovial folds. It may also reduce a 1- or 2-mm subluxation. By stretching the segmental muscles it may relieve the state of hypertonicity. Joint movement, previously restricted, becomes almost normal, and local and reflex pain is often relieved.[7]

In the sacroiliac syndrome local and reflex pain is present and movement is restricted. In our present state of knowledge it is difficult to envisage how synovium can be entrapped or how subluxation can occur in a joint that has very small range of movement. Adjustments directed specifically to this joint, however, often relieve the symptoms. Possibly the effect is produced by stretching the posterior muscles and relieving the joint fixation and by stimulating mechanoreceptors.

In the quadratus lumborum syndrome the muscle is in hypertonic contraction at one level. It is postulated that when the lesion is not treated quickly, fibrosis develops within the affected portion of the muscle. The thrust of the adjustment is directed to stretching the tight segment of muscle.

Herniation of the Nucleus Pulposus. Many theories have been propounded to explain the way in which manipulative adjustments may re-

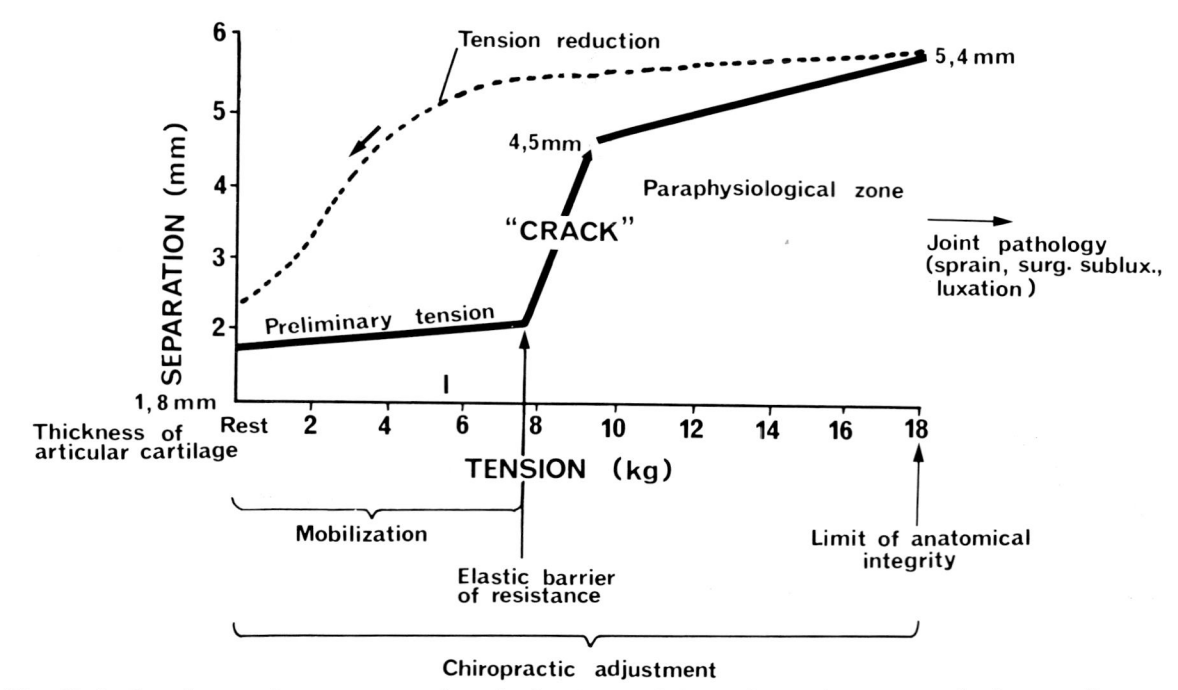

Fig. 13-3. Correlation of experiments described in Figs. 13-2A and B with intervertebral joint adjustment. (After Sandoz R: The significance of the manipulative crack and of other articular noises. Ann Swiss Chirop Assoc 4:47, 1969.)

lieve the patient with this condition of back and leg pain. The author has in the past been doubtful of the value of this therapeutic modality. Availability of the high resolution CT scanner and soft tissue imaging make it possible now to visualize accurately the site and size of a disk herniation and to assess the effects of different forms of treatment by repeat scanning after a period of time. Before long the physician should be in a position to say what form of treatment is most effective.

De Sèze[8,9] believes that lumbago develops because a fragment of the nucleus pulposus becomes incarcerated within an annular tear with resultant bulging of the annulus and pressure on the sinuvertebral nerve. His adjustment exerts rotatory traction on the spine as follows: The lumbar spine is flexed with the patient lying on the side so that the disk space is opened posteriorly. The upper shoulder is rotated backward and the lower shoulder pulled forward. Lateral flexion causes the disk space to open on the upper side. The shoulder girdle and the pelvis are further rotated in different directions to produce torsion. A thrust is delivered. The way in which de Sèze and others think that these manipulations work is shown in Figure 13-5.

Levernieux's experiments[10] on spines obtained at autopsy are of considerable interest. He injected an opaque dye into the disk, then placed the specimen in a traction device, and obtained radiographs before, during and after traction.

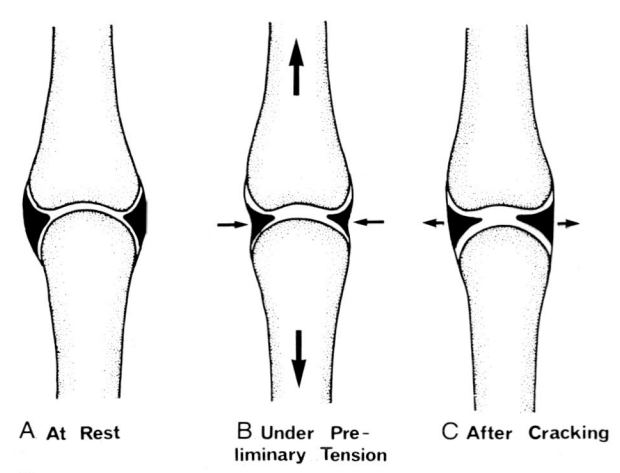

A At Rest   B Under Preliminary Tension   C After Cracking

Fig. 13-4. Effect of traction on a joint.

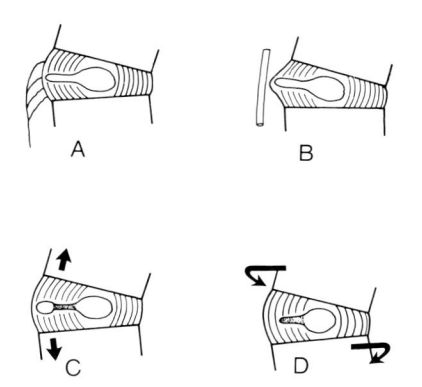

Fig. 13-5. Explanation of the way in which manipulation may reduce pressure of a disk herniation on a nerve. (A) Herniation with irritation of branches of sinuvertebral nerve. (B) Herniation with pressure on a spinal nerve. (C) Traction separates the vertebral bodies and allows the herniated material to return to the nucleus. (D) Rotation encourages further return of herniated material to the nucleus. Modified from Sandoz R: Some physical mechanisms and effects of spinal adjustments. Ann Swiss Chirop Assoc 6:91, 1976, after de Sèze S: Les manipulations vertebral. Sem Hôp Paris 1:2313, 1955.

When the disk was disrupted internally, the dye passed from front to back of the disk and sometimes protruded into the spinal canal. During traction the disk space became wider and the dye passed toward the center of the disk. When traction was discontinued, a part of the contrast medium was retained in the center of the disk (Fig. 13-6).

Chrisman and coworkers[11] found that 51% of patients with sciatica improved clinically on side posture manipulation but that no change in the myelographic appearance occurred (Fig. 13-7).

Matthews and Yates,[12] using epidurography before and after manipulation in cases of acute lumbago, demonstrated that the bulge seen at the back of the disk was smaller in size following treatment.

Sandoz considers that traction for an internal derangement of the disk may aid in reducing sequestered nuclear material but that it is difficult to see how traction can be of benefit in cases when the disk is extruded. He thinks that the aim of treatment should not be to reduce the herniation,

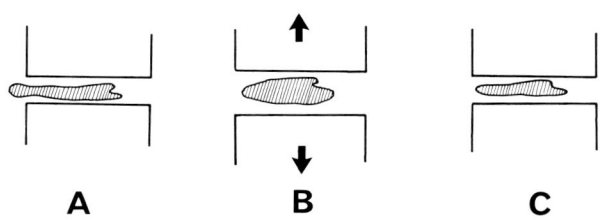

Fig. 13-6. Effect of traction after diskography. A. Disk Herniation: dye protruding backwards (to the left). B. On traction the protruding disc material returns to the centre of the disk. C. On relaxing the traction the disc material tends to remain in the centre of the disk. After Levernieux J: Les tractions vertebrales. L'expansion, Paris, 1960.

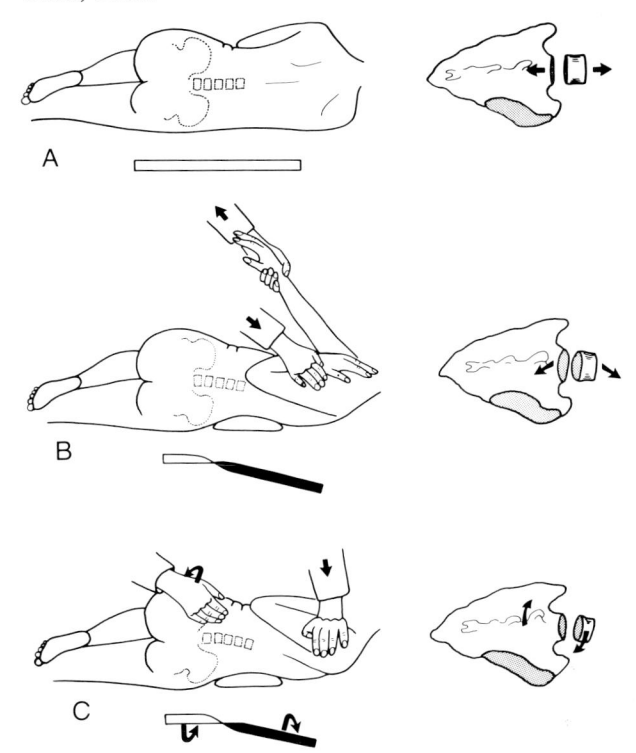

Fig. 13-7. The three stages of the mechanism of side-posture adjustment. (A) Flexing the pelvis and thigh opens the disk space posteriorly. (B) The upper shoulder is rotated backward and the lower shoulder is rotated forward to create a turning moment. The pillow under the lower flank causes lateral flexion of the lumbar spine. The disk spaces are opened on the upper side. (C) Rotation of the pelvis and shoulder girdles in opposite directions produces a torque in dorsal and lumbar spines. The effect of this adjustment is a helicoidal traction exerted on the upper posterolateral portion of the motion segment.

but to ease the disco-radicular conflict. Figure 13-8 demonstrates the antalgic posture assumed for a herniation lateral to the nerve and for one medial to the nerve. He postulates that manipulation in the direction of this antalgic posture benefits the patient by shifting the inflamed nerve away from the herniation.[1,13]

We have to admit that most publications on the role of manipulation for a disk herniation deal mainly with theoretical concepts. On the other hand it is not reasonable to condemn the procedure out of hand. During the past 30 years the author has not encountered any patient with a disk herniation who was made worse by manipulation. We have employed this modality of treatment only in subacute cases where only minimal neurological deficit is present. Certainly it should never be used in the presence of a cauda equina syndrome.[11-16]

Lateral Canal Stenosis with Spinal Nerve Entrapment. The way in which this takes place by anterior subluxation and/or enlargement of a superior articular process has been described at length in chapters 3, 8, and 9, Pathology, Clinical Syndromes and Lesions and Diagnosis. In patients with dynamic recurrent lateral stenosis, adjustment of the spine into flexion and axial rotation in the pain-free direction open up the lateral canal and foramen and may be of benefit (Fig. 13-7). When the stenosis is fixed because gross degenerative changes have occurred, it is not easy to see how manipulation can be of assistance.[1,5,7,11,12]

Central Stenosis. Manipulative adjustments are rarely indicated, but this form of treatment has a place in management. Flexion of the lumbar spine increases the diameter of the spinal canal. Impingement of posterior articular processes on the cauda equina may sometimes be reduced by flexion and rotation.

Retrospondylolisthesis is a common sequela of degenerative disease. This is reduced in flexion and accentuated in extension. Thus a manipulation—carried out with the patient lying on his side with the painful side uppermost—into flexion, opening up of the disk on the painful side, and rotation can be expected to help some patients.

Degenerative Spondylolisthesis. The forward slip of the upper on the lower vertebra is accentuated in flexion. It is thus logical to think that manipulation into extension may be of assistance.

Isthmic Spondylolisthesis. It is difficult to envisage the way in which this lesion can be alleviated by spinal adjustment. Frequently it is complicated by a posterior joint syndrome one level above the lesion or by a sacroiliac syndrome. Thus, improvement in the patient's symptoms results, not from any effect on posterior joints or disk at the level of the slip, but from the effect of manipulation on these other joints. The author recalls patients not benefitted by decompression and/or fusion, who were relieved of their back and leg pain by manipulation directed to the sacroiliac joint.[17]

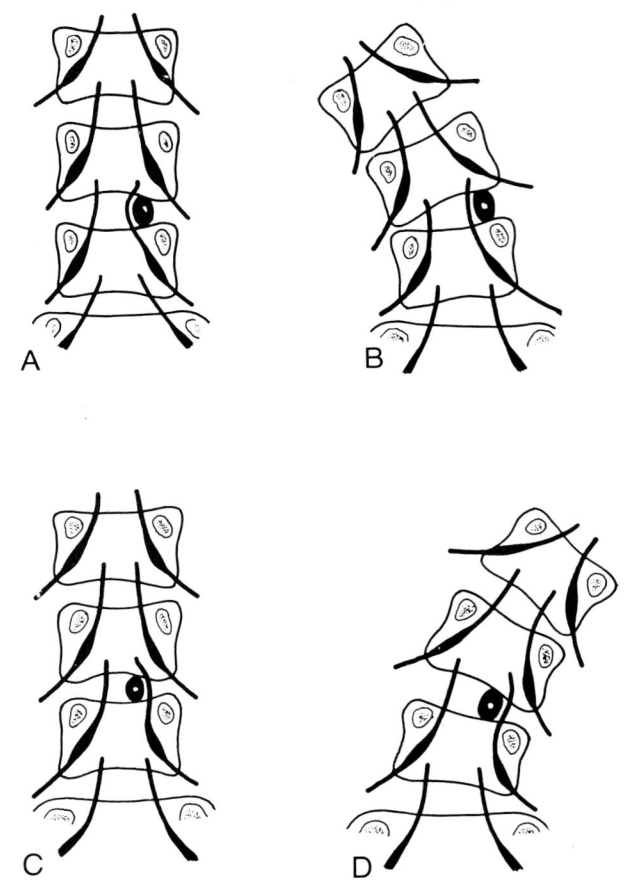

Fig. 13-8. Explanation of direction of scoliosis in patients with a disk herniation. (After Armstrong JR: Lumbar Disc Lesions. Livingstone, Edinburgh and London, 1965.) (A) Herniation lateral to spinal nerve. (B) Bending (scoliosis) to the left moves the nerve on the right away from the herniation. (C) Herniation medial to spinal nerve. (D) Bending to the right moves the nerve away from the herniation and reduces the neuro–diskal conflict.

Instability. Patients with this phase of disease may expect temporary relief of back and leg pain. It is unreasonable to expect that relief will last for more than a short period of time. In some patients Instability at the L4–5 level may be accompanied by Dysfunction at the L3–4 or L5–S1 level and the latter may be helped considerably by manipulative adjustment.

The Effect of Manipulation on the Mechanoreceptors. Until now we have been concerned with the mechanical effect of manipulation on various clinical lesions and syndromes. While discussing the perception of pain in chapter 4, we saw that stimulation of the mechanoreceptors, supplied by large fibers in the posterior joint capsule, the ligaments, and the annulus fibrosus had the effect of closing the gate for the perception of pain. It is reasonable to postulate that stimulating these sensory fibers by manipulation is a very important part of the way in which this modality is effective.

THE INDICATIONS FOR MANIPULATION

Some idea of these has been given as we discussed the ways in which we think manipulation affects the different lesions that were encountered. In defining the indications it is convenient to identify the categories in which manipulation is clearly and definitely the treatment of choice and those in which it is less clearly indicated.

Definite and Certain Indications

1. Dysfunction with a posterior joint and/or sacroiliac syndrome
2. Quadratus lumborum syndrome
3. Posterior joint or sacroiliac syndrome complicating isthmic spondylolisthesis

Less Certain Indications

1. Dysfunction complicating Instability
2. Lateral canal stenosis (dynamic)
3. Dysfunction complicating degenerative stenosis
4. Disk herniation (small)

THE RESULTS OF TREATMENT

During the past 6 years 283 patients with low back pain and leg pain have been treated by manipulation by Drs. J. D. Cassidy, R. Milne, S. Mior, and M. MacGregor, under the supervision of the author.

The patients were graded as follows:

Grade I. Symptom free and with no restrictions for work or other activities

Grade II. Mild constant pain or intermittent pain with no restrictions for work or other activities

Grade III. Improved but restricted in their activities by pain

Grade IV. Symptoms not significantly affected by manipulation

[The results, calculated separately for each of the conditions treated, are given in Tables 13-1 to 13-7; they are summarized in Table 13-8.

It is important to point out, first, that these patients are a select group taken from a specialized Low Back Pain Clinic, reserved for patients who have not responded to simple conservative measures; second, that they had all suffered from low back pain for many years and, third, that they were in Grade IV (disabled by pain) at the start of treatment.

Comment

The best results were obtained in patients with Dysfunction due to a posterior joint or sacroiliac syndrome or a combination of these. Some patients with Instability were improved. The author is of the opinion that improvement was due to treatment of Dysfunction that was present with the Instability. Fifty percent of patients with lateral entrapment were markedly improved and as a result did not require operation. Thirty-six percent of patients with central stenosis were significantly improved. These were patients who were not fit for operation. Rightly or wrongly it was decided not to attempt manipulation in patients with a disk herniation. It is evident that many patients, especially those in the phase of dysfunction, were greatly improved by this form of treatment.

Table 13-1. Sacroiliac Syndrome

Number of patients	69
Average duration of symptoms	7.9 years
Length of follow-up (av)	10.3 months
Results	
Grade I	72%
Grade II	20%
Grade III	3%
Grade IV	4%

Table 13-2. Posterior Joint Syndrome

Number of patients	54
Average duration of symptoms	5.6 years
Length of follow-up (av)	9.2 months
Results	
Grade I	64%
Grade II	15%
Grade III	9%
Grade IV	12%

Table 13-3. Combined Posterior Joint and Sacroiliac Syndrome

Number of patients	48
Average duration of symptoms	9.8 years
Length of follow-up (av)	13.9 months
Results	
Grade I	67%
Grade II	21%
Grade III	6%
Grade IV	6%

Table 13-4. Posterior Joint and/or Sacroiliac Joint Syndrome with Lumbar Instability

Number of patients	31
Average duration of symptoms	7.7 years
Length of follow up (av)	8.0 months
Results	
Grade I	26%
Grade II	19%
Grade III	29%
Grade IV	26%

Table 13-5. Fixed Lateral Entrapment

Number of patients	60
Average duration of symptoms	7.2 years
Length of follow up (av)	14.0 months
Results	
Grade I	25%
Grade II	25%
Grade III	17%
Grade IV	33%

Table 13-6. Dynamic Lateral Entrapment

Number of patients	10
Average duration of symptoms	11.5 years
Length of follow up (av)	12.6 months
Results	
Grade I	40%
Grade II	10%
Grade III	20%
Grade IV	30%

Table 13-7. Central Stenosis

Number of patients	11
Average duration of symptoms	16.9 years
Length of follow up (av)	7.0 months
Results	
Grade I	18%
Grade II	18%
Grade III	18%
Grade IV	46%

Table 13-8. Statistical Summary

Patient Status	Improved	Not Improved
No previous operation	157	58
Previous operations	44	24
Proximal leg symptoms	70	15
Distal leg symptoms	77	51
No leg symptoms	54	16
Mild degenerative changes	107	35
Severe degenerative changes	89	45

CONCLUSION

Assessment of the results of treatment shows that manipulation has very considerable value in carefully selected patients. It is essential to make an accurate diagnosis before embarking on treatment. This includes defining both the phase and the clinical lesion. The most definite indication is to treat Dysfunction. The majority of patients seen are in this phase.

No patient in this series was made worse by manipulation though in some patients it was discontinued because it was not helping the patient.

From the discussion of the natural history of the degenerative process (chapter 1), it will be appreciated that this process is often a continuing one and therefore we cannot expect a permanent cure from manipulation or from any other modality, including operation.

ACKNOWLEDGMENT

The author acknowledges his great debt to Dr. J. D. Cassidy for knowledge obtained regarding the role and the value of manipulation in disorders of the lumbar spine and for much hard work in compiling the results of his treatment of our patients set out in Tables 13-1 to 13-8.

REFERENCES

1. Sandoz R: Some physical mechanisms and effects of spinal adjustments. Ann Swiss Chirop Assoc 6: 91, 1976
2. Sandoz R: Some reflex phenomena associated with spinal derangements and adjustments. Ann Swiss Chirop Assoc, 7: 45, 1981
3. Roston JB, Haines RW: Cracking in the metacarpophalangeal joint. J Anat 81: 165, 1947
4. Sandoz R: The significance of the manipulative crack and of other articular noises. Ann Swiss Chirop Assoc 4: 47, 1969
5. Maigne R: Douleur d'origine vertébrale et traitment par manipulations. L'expansion, Paris, 1968.
6. Maigne R: Orthopaedic Medicine. Springfield, IL, Charles C Thomas, 1972
7. Cassidy JD: Narrowing of disc spaces with recurrent posterior joint subluxation following chemonucleolysis in the lumbar spine. J Can Chirop Assoc 24: 22, 1980
8. de Sèze S: Les accidents de la detérioration structurale du disque. Semin Hôp Paris 1: 2267, 1955
9. de Sèze S: Les attitudes antalgiques dans la sciatique discoradiculaire commune. Semin Hôp Paris 1: 2291, 1955
10. Levernieux J: Les tractions vertébrales. L'expansion, Paris, 1960
11. Chrisman OD, Mittnacht A, Snook GA: A study of the results following rotary manipulation in the lumbar intervertebral disc syndrome. J Bone Joint Surg 46A: 517, 1964
12. Matthews JA, Yates AH: Reduction of lumbar disc prolapse by manipulation. Br Med J 3: 695, 1969
13. Armstrong JR: Lumbar Disc Lesions. Livingstone, Edinburgh and London, 1965
14. Cyriax JH: Lumbago, mechanism of dural pain. Lancet 1: 427, 1945
15. Sandoz R: Degenerative conditions of the lumbosacral spine. Ann Swiss Chirop Assoc 1: 77, 1960
16. Sandoz R: Newer trends in the pathogenesis of spinal disorders. Ann Swiss Chirop Assoc 5: 93, 1971
17. Cassidy JD, Potter GE, Kirkaldy-Willis WH: Manipulative management of back pain patients with spondylolisthesis. J Can Chirop Assoc 22: 15, Mar, 1978

14 Supports and Braces

W. H. Kirkaldy-Willis

INTRODUCTION

The aim of treatment is freedom from pain through regained movement. Therefore, rigid braces and casts are used as little as possible. In this chapter the following supports are described:
1. The Elasticon garment, which gives support without restricting movement
2. The lumbosacral corset used in elderly patients with advanced generalized spondylosis
3. The chair back brace employed in elderly patients with advanced generalized spondylosis and sometimes following spinal fusion
4. The light cast jacket spica, applied for 3 months to immobilize the lumbar and lumbosacral spine after a spinal fusion.

THE ELASTICON GARMENT*

For the past 15 years the author has used an elastic type of supporting garment, the Elasticon, to treat patients with acute, subacute, and chronic low back strains and disk herniations and has found it to be of considerable help to them. This garment has also been used by patients recovering from surgery for disk herniation and central and lateral spinal stenosis. It is complementary to a program of instruction in low back care and exercises.

While rigid supports and braces have their place in treating fractures, infection, neoplasms, osteoporosis, marked generalized degenerative spondylosis, and scoliosis, the situation is entirely different in low back pain that is caused by repeated minor trauma and to many localized degenerative lesions.

In treating painful conditions of other joints, such as shoulder, hip or knee, it is well recognized that freedom from pain closely depends on a return to near normal movement. A stiff joint that is not ankylosed is frequently a painful joint. In treating strains and injuries to the lumbar spine the desirability of obtaining near normal movement has not generally been appreciated.

Physicians and others skilled in techniques of mobilizing the lumbar spine are well aware of the benefit of returning normal movement to a stiff and painful three-joint complex at one level. And so is the patient. In discussing the role of the Elasticon, emphasis is placed on both the need for some support and the desirability of allowing almost full spinal movement during treatment, as tolerated by the patient. The degree of comfort that is obtained is considerable, equivalent to that supplied by a tensor bandage for minor injury to the collateral ligaments of the knee.

---

*Manufactured by Camp Company, Trenton, Ontario, Canada and by Camp International Inc., Jackson, Michigan, U.S.A.

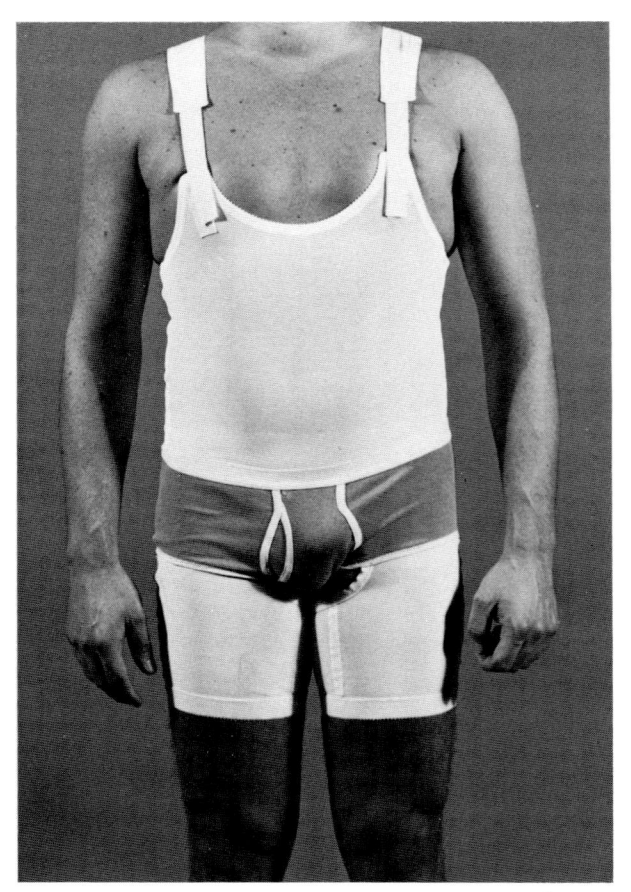

Fig. 14-1. The Elasticon from the front. Note the two shoulder straps fastened with velcro strips. These can be adjusted to make the garment fit more loosely or more tightly.

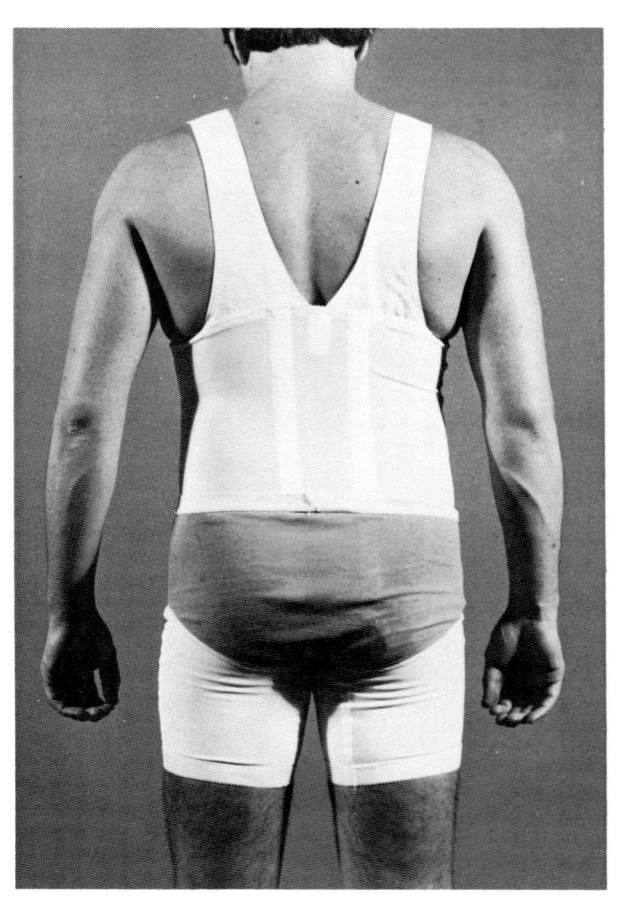

Fig. 14-2. The Elasticon from behind. Note the two spiroflex metal strips, one on each side of the midline.

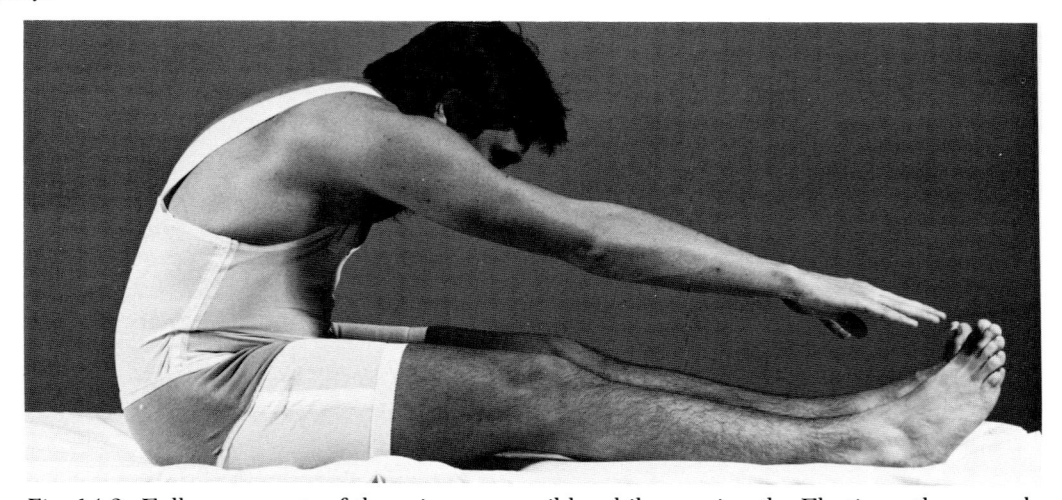

Fig. 14-3. Full movements of the spine are possible while wearing the Elasticon: thus muscle activity is not impeded.

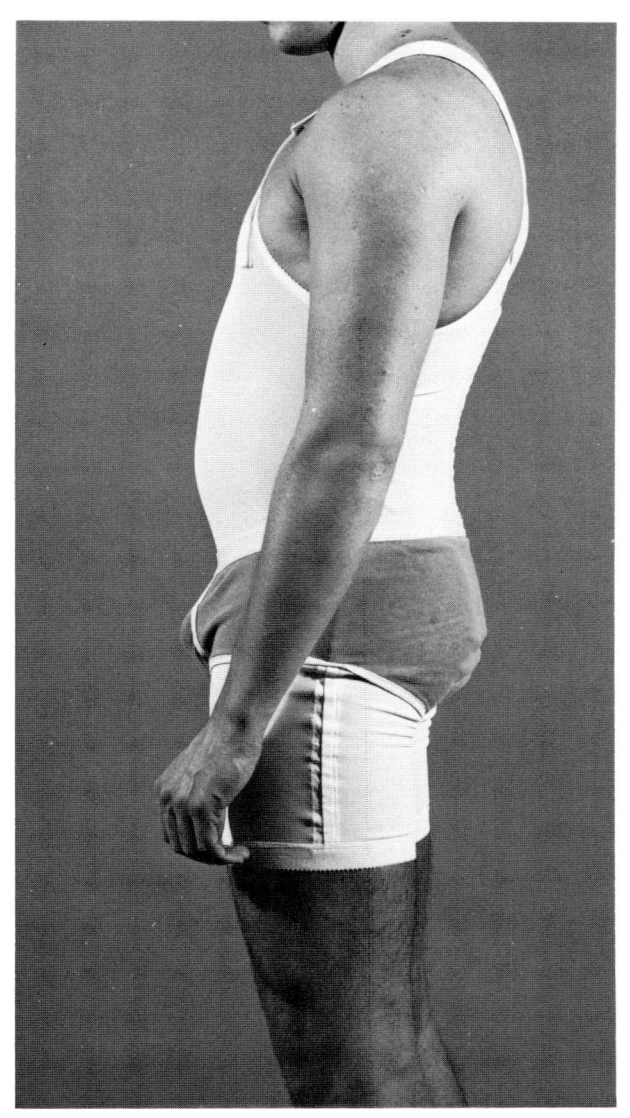

Fig. 14-4. Side view of the patient. Note the lumbar lordosis.

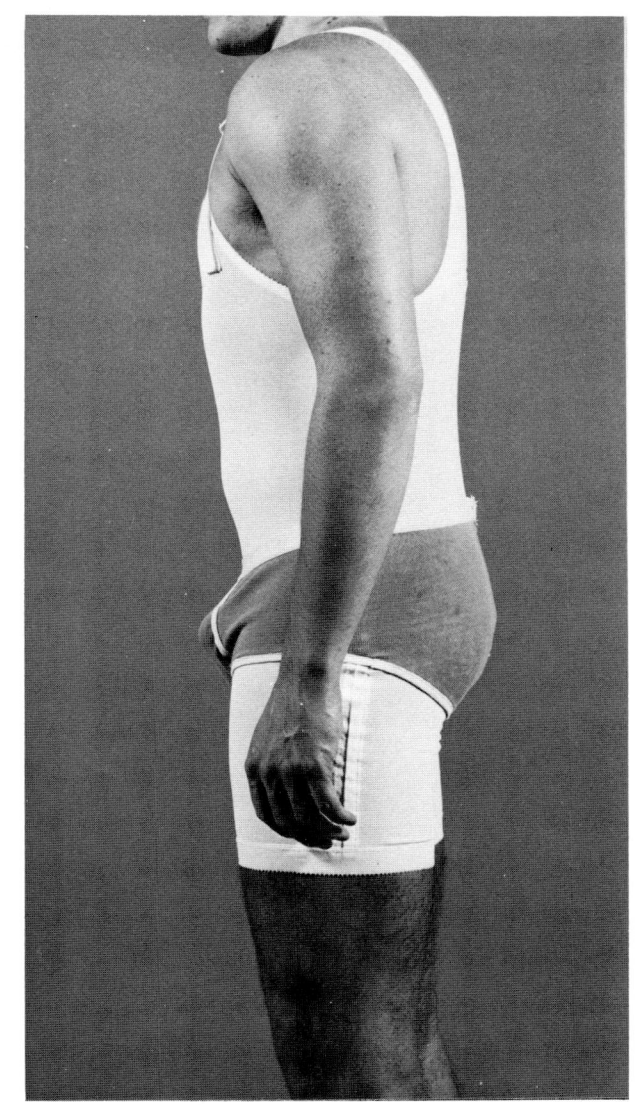

Fig. 14-5. Side view of patient. The lordosis is corrected by pelvic tilting. The Elasticon helps to pull in the abdominal muscles.

Description

Designed to resemble a garment rather than a corset, the Elasticon is made of two-way stretch lycra spandex material. It is supplied in four sizes. The essential components are:

1. An encircling cylinder of two way stretch material extending from the nipple line to the level of the greater trochanter
2. Two spiroflex spring supports sited on either side of the midline at the back
3. Two thigh pieces reaching halfway from hip to knee to prevent the bottom of the cylinder from rolling up
4. Two shoulder straps, fastened by velcro strips on each side in front, to prevent the top of the cylinder from rolling down and to allow adjustment of the garment
5. The length of the main elastic supporting cylinder is longer in front than at the back. This tends to draw the lumbar spine into flexion (Figs. 14-1 to 14-5).

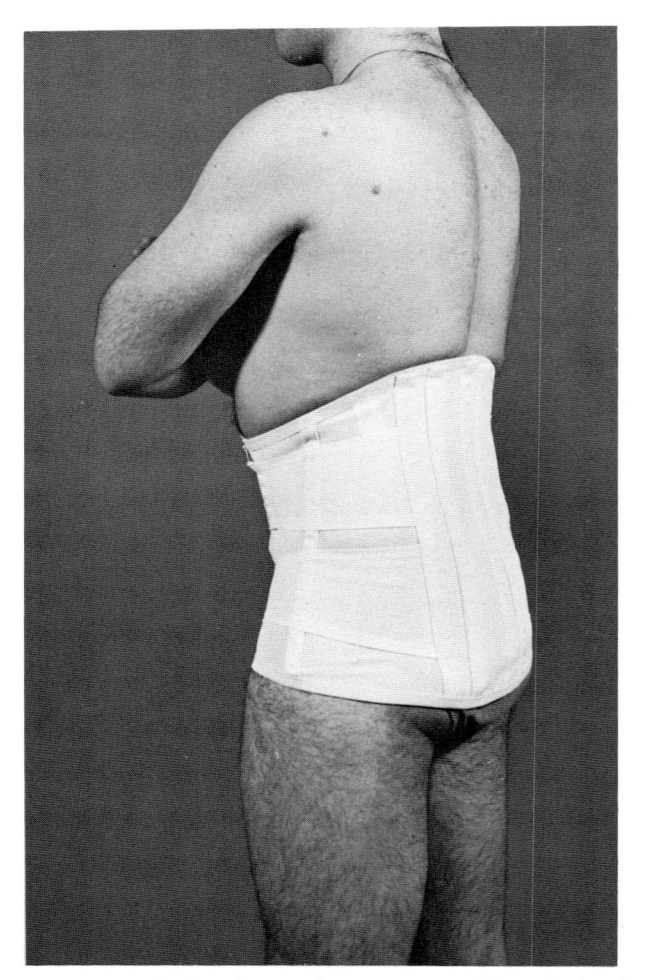

Fig. 14-6. The lumbosacral corset viewed from behind and from the side.

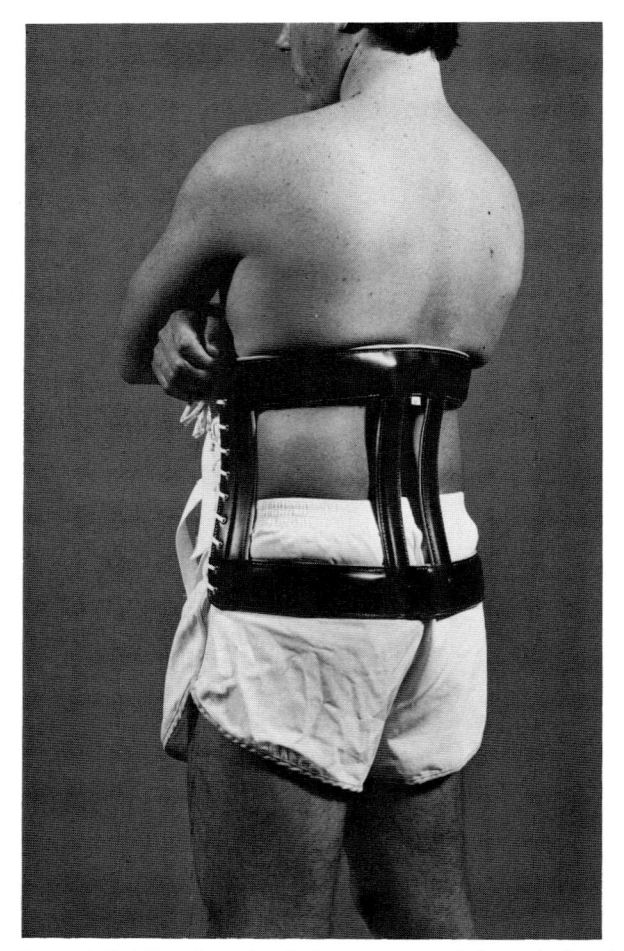

Fig. 14-7. The chair back brace viewed from behind and from the side.

The Ways in Which It Functions

1. It gives support to the painful area, spread over several segments above and below the site of pain.
2. It helps the patient to look upon the lumbar spine as a unit.
3. The elastic material exerts pressure on the abdomen. This tends to reduce the lumbar lordosis and to increase the intra-abdominal pressure.
4. It permits almost full movement of the lumbar spine in all directions and thus allows full muscle activity.
5. The result is that the patient experiences increased comfort and is reassured without developing dependence on the garment.
6. It enables the patient to increase activity more quickly and to indulge in activities that would otherwise not be possible without pain.

Discussion

The majority of patients for whom the Elasticon is prescribed find it considerably helpful.

Those recovering from an acute low back strain, from a herniation of the nucleus pulposus, or from a diskectomy find that they can pursue their activities of daily living more easily, with more confidence and less pain. Among these activities are

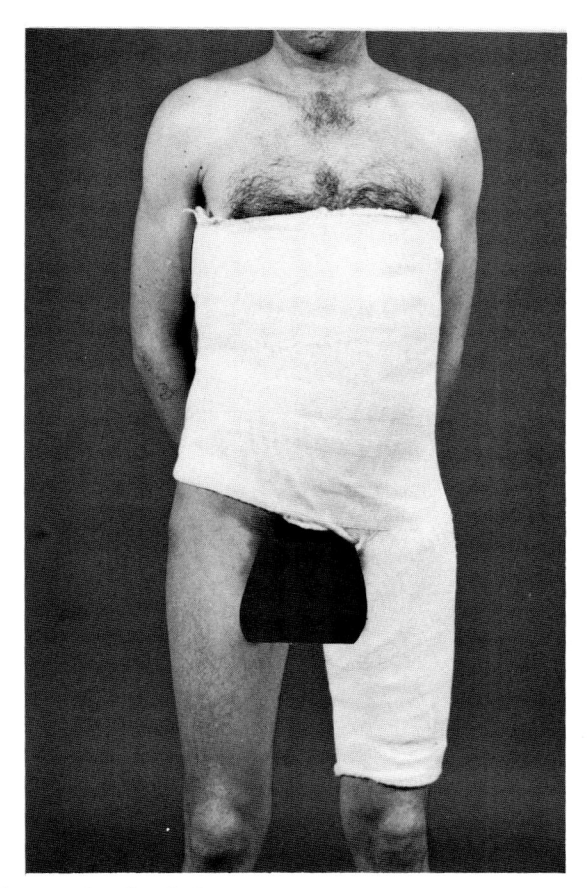

Fig. 14-8. The light cast jacket spica seen from the front.

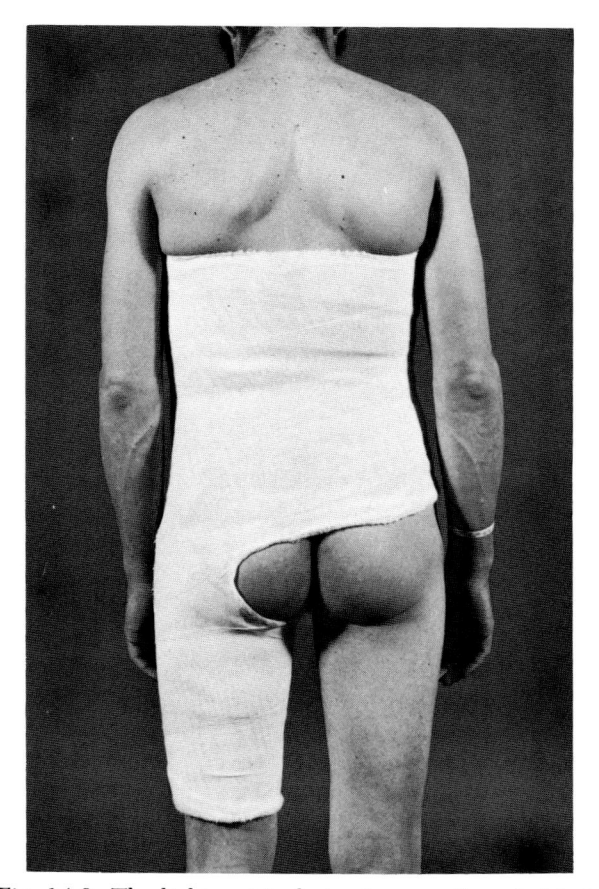

Fig. 14-9. The light cast jacket spica seen from behind.

getting in and out of a car and taking long car or plane journeys. Initially, it is more effective for such patients to carry out pelvic tilting and exercises to strengthen the abdominal muscles while wearing the garment. Most patients gradually discard the support after 3 to 5 months, wearing it only for long journeys by car, for golf or tennis, or during a particularly arduous day of work. A few patients continue to wear the garment indefinitely. This does no harm because almost full muscle activity is still possible.

Other patients suffering from generalized degenerative disease of the lumbar spine and those who have had a decompression for spinal stenosis often continue to wear the Elasticon indefinitely.

The present design of the Elasticon makes it more suitable for men. Women usually prefer a light elastic body stocking. This is almost as effective, though it has no spiroflex spring supports at the back.

THE LUMBOSACRAL CORSET

This garment is made of elastic material with cotton front and back panels. It extends from about 7 inches above the waist line to 2 inches above the greater trochanter. It encircles the lower chest and abdomen. It is fastened by snap fasteners in front (Fig. 14-6).

This type of corset reduces the movement of the lumbar and lumbosacral spine but does not eliminate movement completely.

In the writer's experience it is useful in two situations: (1) For elderly patients with generalized spondylosis that results in low back pain. The reduction of movement gives relief from the pain, and lack of muscle activity is no great disadvantage in such patients. (2) For patients after spinal fusion who have been immobilized in a body jacket for 3 months and require further protection.

THE CHAIR BACK BRACE

This support is more rigid than the lumbosacral corset. It is made of slightly malleable metal, covered by leather or similar synthetic material, fastened by buckles in front and tightened by laces or stays (Fig. 14-7). It is employed in the same situations as the lumbosacral corset (see above) but when more rigid and complete immobilization is deemed advisable. The upper part of the lumbar spine is more completely immobilized than the lower. The immobilization produced by this support is not in the writer's opinion sufficient to treat a patient during the first 3 months following a spinal fusion.

THE LIGHT CAST JACKET SPICA

This is made in the cast room from "light cast" bandages. It encircles the chest and abdomen from the nipple line to the groin. One hip and one thigh are incorporated as far as the knee. A jacket spica made from this material is lighter, stronger, and more durable than one made with plaster of paris bandages (Figs. 14-8, 14-9).

This type of cast is employed after all lumbar or lumbosacral spinal fusion operations and is worn for 3 months to produce the highest possible rate of fusion by almost complete immobilization.

15 Gravity Lumbar Reduction

C. V. Burton

The modern resurgence of medical interest in the management of low back pain has reflected legitimate concerns that the quality of care in this area has been less than optimal in the past. This impression has only been further enhanced by data documenting the surprisingly low efficacy of low back surgery over past decades.

In view of these concerns, it is encouraging to report that there has been a recent knowledge explosion in this particular area of medicine over the past few years. This has been due in large part to studies that have attempted to understand the reasons for previous poor results and to the concomitant advent of new and highly sophisticated diagnostic tools, of which noninvasive high resolution computed tomographic (CT) scanning, with soft tissue differentiation capability, is a primary example.[1,2,3]

While this information has done a lot to advance the quality of existing surgical and nonsurgical therapy, it has also made evident the need for more innovative and effective treatment modalities. The Gravity Lumbar Reduction Therapy Program (GLRTP) developed at the Sister Kenny Rehabilitation Institute in Minneapolis has reflected this need made evident by the careful study of many patients who had not improved with "routine" modes of therapy.

It has become clear that any individual's best opportunity to maintain successful biped ambulation on Earth (a relatively high gravity planet) is to be born with a symmetrically developed and well supported spinal column so that loading and stress can be evenly distributed. Should the owner of this quality spine then maintain normal body weight and good muscle tone and observe prudent body postures and dynamics, the likelihood of experiencing low back pain is markedly decreased.[4] Unfortunately, we cannot choose our parents and most of us function in a basically sedentary environment. Therefore, it is not surprising that 80% of us have at least one significant episode of disabling back pain during our lives and that in 1981 worker compensation costs in the United States for low back problems alone represented an expenditure of about $16 billion.

It has become progressively apparent that if the force of gravity could be moderated on the low back, particularly in the case of individuals whose spines are subject to uneven loading and stress and thus are liable to focused areas of advanced "wear and tear," it would be beneficial. The ideal situation from the standpoint of loading is a gravity-free environment (as in outer space), but on Earth our choices are limited. One reasonable approach is to float in water. As Archimedes pointed out, a floating body is essentially weightless. For this reason and from the standpoint of effective exercise for stomach and back muscles, swimming is a particularly beneficial activity for the lumbar spine. Recently interest has focused on the use of inverted body traction techniques in which the individual hangs head down supported by the ankles as a means of creating anti-gravity forces on the body and benefiting the back. While it is unlikely that significant distractive force is actually created in the back (as compared, for example, with that in the knee joints) these traction techniques *do* appear to be of value as physical fitness modalities that, by maintaining good organ and muscle support, may contribute to maintaining a healthy back.[5]

Excessive acute and chronic stress-related injury to the low back produces degeneration of lumbar disks and zygapophyseal joints leading to segmental instability and pain. In the disks the degeneration of the nucleus pulposus and annular tearing of the annulus fibrosus creates a situation where the body endeavors to absorb this injured tissue, decrease interspace volume, and create an "auto-fusion" by subperiosteal bone deposition leading to bridging osteophytes. In the lucky individual this stabilization occurs without compression of exiting spinal nerves by lateral spinal stenosis.[6] There are many cases, however, where the body is not able to absorb sufficient degenerated disk material before annular tears coalesce into radial fissures and the abnormal nuclear material is forced toward and into the spinal canal, producing the classic back and leg pain of a herniated disk with associated clinical symptoms that reflect either irritation or compression (or both) of the dorsal or ventral nerves.

Since the introduction by Walter Dandy in 1929[7] of the concept of the lumbar disk and its surgical removal, (later popularized by Mixter and Barr)[8] disks have been often considered to be "routine" surgical fare. It is only in recent years that less stringent means of successful treatment have entered into general medical and surgical consciousness. When one considers that some neurosurgeons who specialize in treating low back problems estimate that 80% or more of patients who have had a diskectomy could have been adequately treated without surgery, the need for change becomes compellingly evident.[9]

The Sister Kenny Institute Gravity Lumbar Reduction Therapy Program (GLRTP) was clinically introduced in 1976.[10] It was developed specifically as a nonsurgical treatment program for "virgin" (no previous back surgery) back–leg pain patients with acute contained disk herniations who were not overweight and could tolerate the mild discomfort of wearing a chest harness. Selecting the rib cage as the point of fixation made it possible to focus the force of gravity (involving 40% of body weight) on the lumbar spine in a progressive and controlled fashion over significant periods of time. The initial theory regarding mechanism of action was that the distractive force would create negative pressure within the abnormal disk and allow sufficient reduction of the disk out of the spinal canal to alleviate nerve irritation or compression. It was theorized that through daily intermittent use of this treatment modality the injured annulus and herniated disk would allow the deposition of reparative beta collagen as a healing process. Following 6 years of clinical experience with GLRTP at our Institute and approximately 500 other institutions, it would appear that the original predictions remain substantiated.[11,12]

Key elements in the successful application of GLRTP relate to the amount of force employed and the gradual and progressive manner in which it is directed to the lumbar spine. There are many potential means of producing tissue distraction. Body tissue adapts to gradual change without injury as opposed to more sudden influences, which are traumatic and may produce greater patient liability than benefit.

Our medical staff believes that patients should not be treated with bed rest, analgesics, etc. for more than a week before starting the GLRTP. We regard this program as initial conservative treatment for selected patients who are not overweight. Patients presenting as acute neurologic emergencies (e.g., profound neurologic deficit such as complete foot drop or bowel or bladder impairment) are still considered to be immediate surgical candidates.

At this point our radiologic staff under the direction of Dr. Kenneth Heithoff has performed over 18,000 high resolution CT scans of the lumbar spine. This highly accurate and informative sophisticated diagnostic study has essentially replaced myelography at our Institute and is performed on all patients presenting with objective neurologic deficit. In this way information from the history and physical examination can be directly correlated with objective information regarding the specific nature of the pathology and can also rule out other entities such as cysts, conjoint nerve roots, tumors, and lateral entrapment. This clinical–diagnostic correlation corroborates an initial impression of nerve-specific diskogenic disease.

When used as part of a comprehensive back care program in an environment of well-informed and trained allied health personnel the GLRTP program has been of particular value in managing the following three entities:

1. Disk "bulging" producing distention of the annulus and posterior longitudinal ligament. This entity produces pain by stimulating branches of the sinuvertebral nerve. A dorsal ramus pain syndrome typically referred to the low back, hips, and knees is produced. Pain is rarely referred as far as the ankles.
2. A herniated disk, in which nuclear material extends beyond the annulus but is contained by the posterior longitudinal ligament (sometimes called a "roof disk"). Compression of a spinal nerve either exiting or traversing the interspace produces sciatic pain that radiates to the toes and feet and neurologic findings that are associated with this compression.
3. A herniated disk in which nuclear material extends beyond the annulus and is beginning to erode through the posterior longitudinal ligament but has not yet become a free protrusion.

Experience has shown that when herniated disk material extrudes past the posterior longitudinal ligament (free protrusion) or migrates in the spinal canal (sequestered fragment) the application of gravity traction *accentuates* pain and neurologic deficit rather than alleviating it. This phenomenon occurs during the first few days of treatment and is most important to document, because it signals the need to discontinue the GLRTP program and consider more aggressive treatment modalities such as chemonucleolysis or surgery. Chemonucleolysis is now regarded as the last conservative measure employed prior to surgery and it also serves well as an alternative to GLRTP for patients with significant disk problems who cannot use the traction because of obesity, cardiopulmonary disease, or chest harness intolerance. In comparing the various treatments available, it is important to compare potential mortality and morbidity as well as cost. GLRTP is highly cost-effective, and the most significant adverse reaction documented on our clinical service to date has been chest harness irritation to skin and ribs.

High resolution CT scanning with soft tissue differentiation capability, paricularly of the type described by Heithoff, serves well not only to clarify the initial nature of the disk pathology (and associated pathologic processes) but also to provide serial follow-up, thus supplying objective measurements to correlate with clinical observations and the neurologic examination.

The point to be made is that patient treatment must be based on the clinical situation rather than on diagnostic studies. Information provided by sophisticated CT scanning basically serves only to confirm the diagnosis *already* made on clinical grounds or to suggest that it is in error. Pathologic changes frequently seen on CT may be benign for a given patient.

TECHNIQUE

As created at the Sister Kenny Institute, the GLRTP approach has been a two-phase program:

In-Patient

Patients are admitted to the hospital, fitted with a chest harness, and placed in a self-operated electrical tilt bed (Fig. 15-1). Starting at 30° tilt and progressing at an increase in angle of 5° per day (total time in traction 4 hours per day performed in multiple episodes), the patients usually reach their goal of either 70° or 90° in 8 days (depending on ability and tolerance). Although patients are basically on complete bed rest they actively exercise while in traction and attend therapeutic swimming once or twice a day. During this phase of treatment an educational and instructional program is directed to program participants by our occupational, physical, and recreational therapy staff. In addition to publications and audio-visual review, patients attend low back school and are given individual instruction in appropriate body mechanics and dynamics.

Approximately 5% of patients find the traction too uncomfortable to the abdomen or chest wall

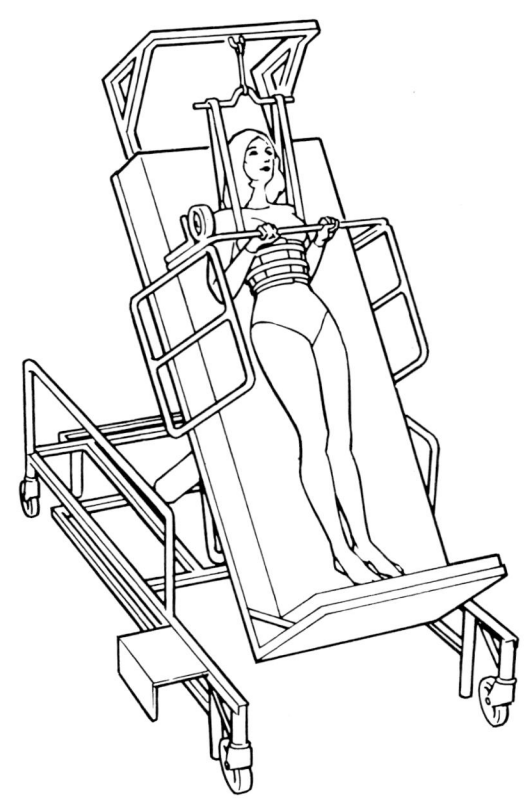

Fig. 15-1. The inpatient program is initiated by fitting the patient with a specially designed chest harness and utilizing a patient-controlled electrically operated tilt bed (or modified Stryker Circ-O-Lectric bed). The traction angle is gradually increased on a daily basis. The safety strap system is not shown in this drawing. (Courtesy of the Institute for Low Back Care.)

to continue. Those whose back and leg pain or neurologic deficit are made worse are typically found to have either a free disk protrusion or a chronic calcified disk. Initial rib "soreness" is common. During the first few days of treatment the physician has a unique opportunity to observe the patients' reaction to the stress of starting this program. More meaningful information is often conveyed by this alone than by many other diagnostic studies.

Out-Patient

Prior to discharge from the hospital, patients are provided with maintenance units and instructed in their use. The maintenance program

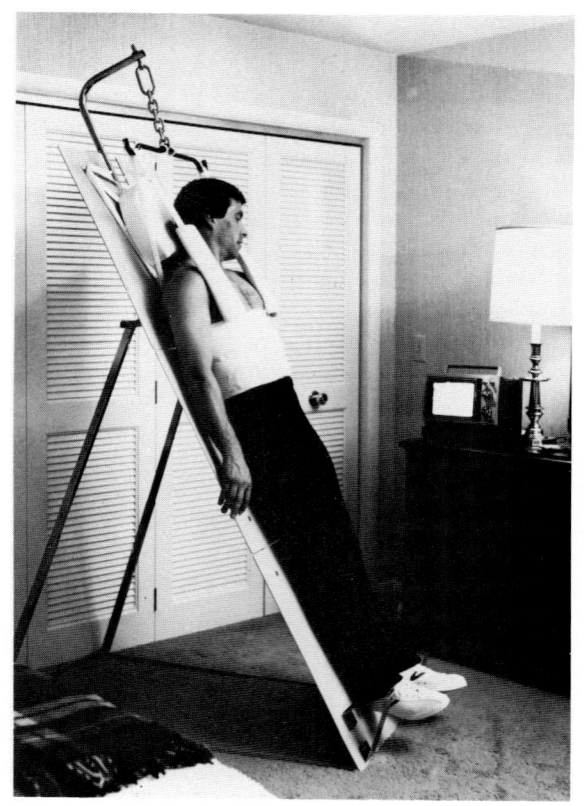

Fig. 15-2. A 60° maintenance unit. During the one hour, twice a day traction episodes, patients are encouraged to use the time productively in other pursuits. (Courtesy of Camp International.)

utilizes either a 60° or 90° support frame (Figs. 15-2, 15-3) and involves 1 hour of traction twice a day. During this phase of treatment, which may continue from 3 to 12 months, patients return to normal activities or to gainful employment. Progress is assessed on outpatient visits to our clinic.

Efficacy

In determining the efficacy of any treatment modality it is always advantageous to obtain "hard scientific documentation." This is a lot easier to say, however, than to accomplish in many conservative treatment modalities where it is difficult to compare both the patient pathology and the exact consistency of the treatment being applied. While double-blind controlled studies would be

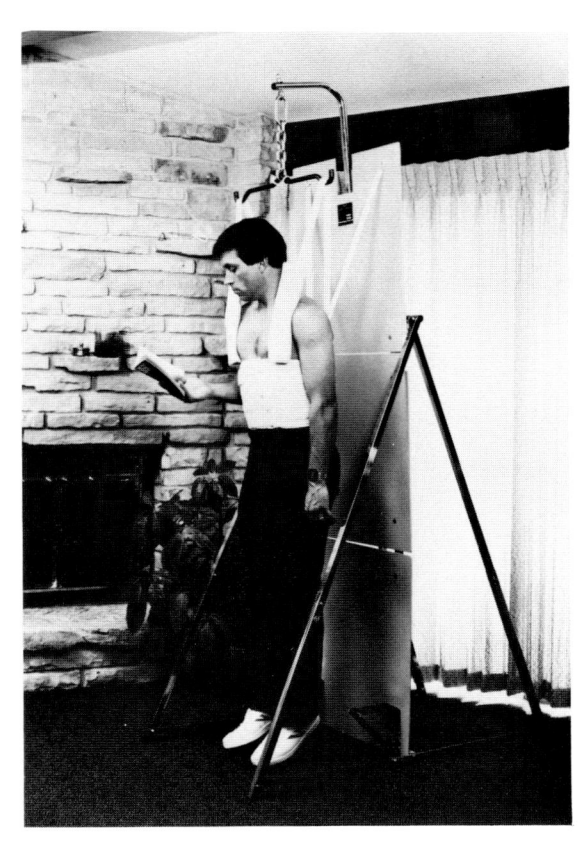

Fig. 15-3. A 90° free-standing traction unit. If an attic or basement is convenient, patients can affix traction and safety bolts and hang directly from these. (Courtesy of Camp International.)

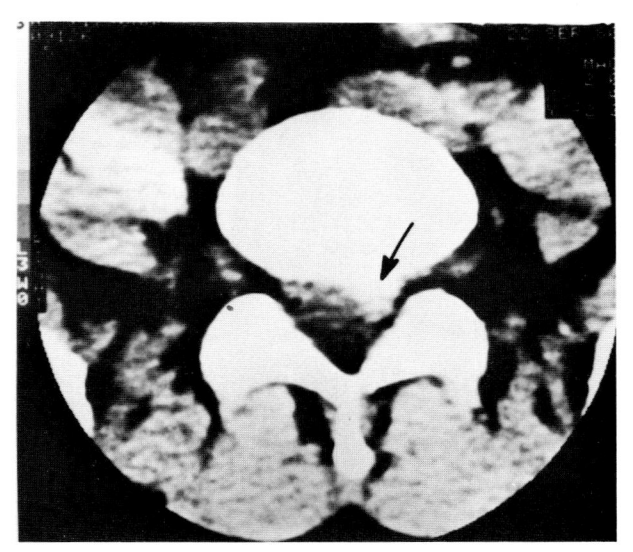

Fig. 15-4. The arrow points to a large disk herniation projecting into the canal at the L5–S1 level and compresing the left S1 nerve root, which has been obliterated.

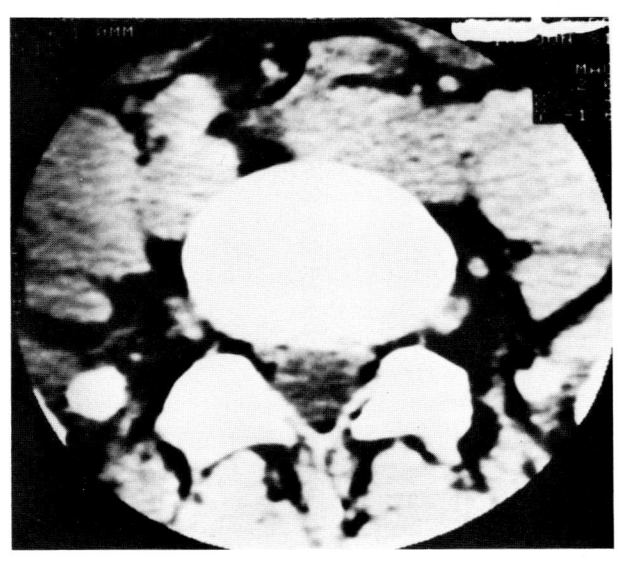

Fig. 15-5. Following 8 months of gravity lumbar reduction treatment, the patient's neurologic status has returned to normal and repeat CT examination reveals that the disk herniation has been essentially resolved. Both S1 nerve roots and epidural veins are identifiable. This patient was originally referred for a surgical diskectomy.

ideal, they are extremely difficult to construct for therapies such as traction, as reflected by the dearth of such studies. As recently noted in Medical World News regarding many of the newer treatment modalities, "Controlled trials? None, just as there are none to substantiate the claims made for most disputed therapies."

The situation is not, however, as bleak as it may appear. Figures 15-4 and 15-5 represent a CT scan on a patient with a large herniated disk who was treated with GLRTP and a repeat scan after 8 months, respectively. CT offers an objective means of documentation in addition to corroborating clinical findings and allows each patient to serve as his or her own controlled study. Over the 6 years in which the GLRTP program has been in use at the Sister Kenny Institute, it has been the definitive treatment modality in approxi-

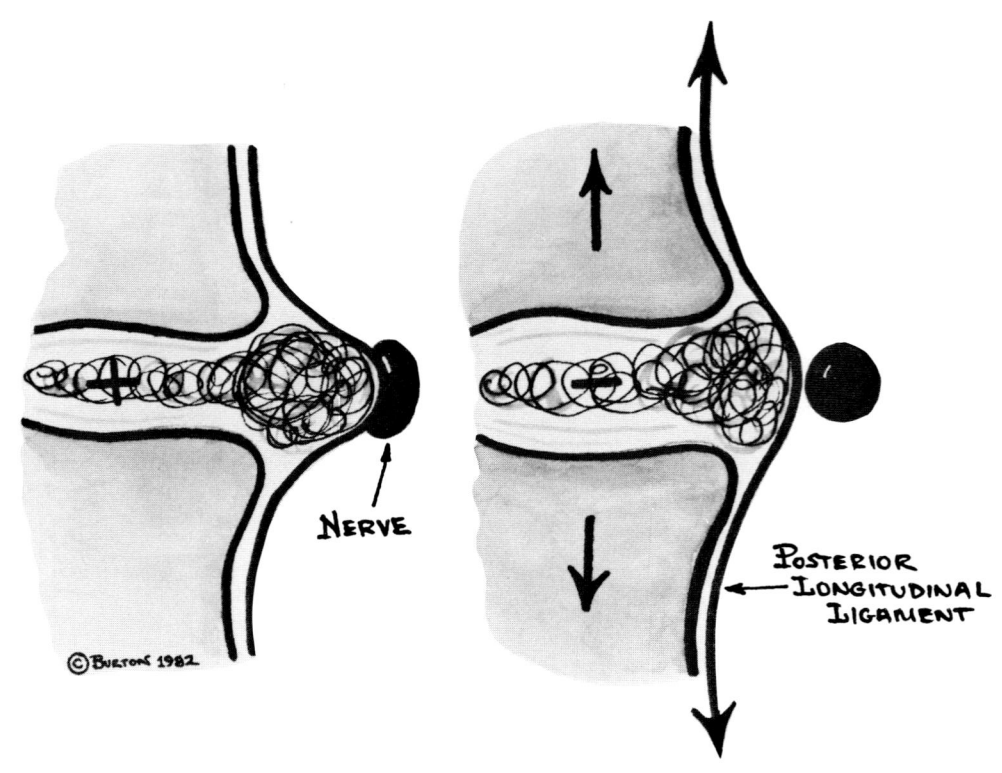

Fig. 15-6. CT scanning shows that the application of axial traction on the vertebrae, annulus fibrosus, and longitudinal ligaments causes the protruding disk to diminish in volume but rarely to return to its normal state. The clinical problem relates to distention of annular and ligamentous dorsal ramus nerve fibers and spinal nerve compression. It is believed, on the basis of biomechanical calculation, that significant intradiskal negative pressures may be produced. The intermittent reduction appears to allow reparative processes to reestablish support.

mately 70% of patients who have initiated the hospital in-patient program. Only 5% of patients are unable physically to tolerate the traction itself. The remaining patients usually go on to chemonucleolysis or surgery.

Figure 15-6 demonstrates what has been consistently observed in follow up CT scans on GLRTP patients. These data indicate that the substantial change is in spinal nerve compression and that the reduction in disk protrusion is of secondary importance.

INVESTIGATIONAL AREAS

The primary application of GLRTP has been to treat the acute contained herniated disk. The following conditions are currently being explored as other possibly valuable applications for the therapy: acute lumbosacral strain, early spondylolisthesis, early scoliosis, and spinal nerve compression secondary to some cases of lateral spinal stenosis.

CONTRAINDICATIONS AND PRECAUTIONS

The GLRTP program is contraindicated in patients whose obesity precludes use of a chest harness, those with chronic pulmonary disease in whom the harness would compromise function, patients with some types of cardiovascular disease, and some patients who have had previous abdominal surgery or hiatus hernia, where abdominal compression produces significant pain. GLRTP has been studied in patients with the failed back surgery syndrome. In only a few cases has improvement been noted, and this cannot, therefore, be recommended as a basic application, although additional study on the subject is continuing.

COMPLICATIONS

Potential complications from the use of GLRTP relate to misuse of components or loss of support during traction. For these reasons a security strap system should always be employed to avoid the possibility of patient injury. No noteworthy patient morbidity has occurred in patients treated at our Institute.

SUMMARY

The Sister Kenny Institute GLRTP represents a safe, cost-effective, and clinically valuable means of treating patients with acute contained disk herniations. Patients are incapacitated for only short periods of time and then continue treatment while also returning to gainful activities. This treatment modality is extensively used on a daily basis at our Institute and represents an exciting, new, and innovative means of conservatively treating low back pain patients.

ACKNOWLEDGMENTS

Development of the Sister Kenny Institute Gravity Lumbar Reduction Therapy Program has, in many areas, been a joint effort of the Institute with Lossing Orthopedic and Camp International. Particular appreciation is expressed to Gail Nida, R.N. for her untiring efforts to create means by which medical professionals are better able to use this program for their patients' benefit, to Kenneth Heithoff, M.D. for giving us access to the fourth dimension as reflected by high resolution CT scanning and to William Kirkaldy-Willis, M.D. who has served us all as friend, medical pioneer, and mentor. His devotion to excellence in knowledge of the lumbar spine has been an important stimulus to our institution and to all of us associated with it.

REFERENCES

1. Heithoff KB: High resolution computed tomography in the differential diagnosis of soft-tissue pathology of the lumbar spine, Computed Tomography of the Lumbar Spine. Edited by Genant HK, Chafetz N, Helms CA. San Francisco, Univ. of California Press, 1982
2. Heithoff KB: Pathogenesis and high resolution computed tomographic scanning of direct bony impingement syndromes of the lumbar spine, Computed Tomography of the Lumbar Spine. Edited by Genant HK, Chafetz N, Helms CA. San Francisco, Univ. of California Press, 1982
3. Lifson A, Heithoff KB, Burton CV, Ray CD: High resolution CT scan in diagnosis of lumbar spine lesions, Modern Neurosurgery. Edited by Brock M. Berlin-Heidelberg, Springer-Verlag, 1982
4. Burton CV: Conservative management of low back pain. Postgrad Med 70: 168, 1981
5. Martin MR: Cum Gravity: Living with Gravity. San Marino, Essential Publishing, 1979
6. Kirkaldy-Willis WH, Wedge JH, Yong-Hing K, et al: Pathology and pathogenesis of lumbar spondylosis and stenosis. Spine 3: 319, 1978
7. Dandy WE: Loose cartilage from intervertebral disc simulating tumor of the spinal cord. Arch Surg 19: 660, 1929
8. Mixter WJ, Barr JA: Rupture of the intervertebral disc with involvement of the spinal canal. N Engl Med 211: 210, 1934
9. Finneson BE: Low Back Pain, vol 2. Philadelphia, JB Lippincott, 1980
10. Burton C, Nida G: The Sister Kenny Institute Gravity Lumbar Reduction Therapy Program. Publication No. 731. Minneapolis, Sister Kenny Institute, 1982
11. Burton C, Nida G: Be Good to Your Back. Publication No. 738. Minneapolis, Sister Kenny Institute, 1980
12. Oudenhoven RC: Gravitational lumbar traction. Arch Phys Med Rehab 59: 510, 1978

16 Surgical Techniques

K. Yong-Hing

Although operations on the lumbar spine for backache are not difficult to master, there is no place for the occasional spinal surgeon. This is not because exceptional technical expertise is required but rather because of the more difficult and important aspect of selecting the correct patients and operations in a complex syndrome that often affects demanding patients. In addition, not all surgeons have the temperament required for maneuvering in the small deep space between two laminae.

The desired goal of the operation—decompression, fusion, or both—has been dealt with in chapter 11. The means of achieving the goal and the surgical approach and technique will be described here. Certain assumptions will be made: (1) An accurate diagnosis has been made. (2) Proper conservative treatment has failed. (3) The patient has been correctly selected as suitable for operation.

The principles of operating on the lumbar spine are the same two as for any operation: to deal with the lesion that causes the symptoms and to prevent intra- and postoperative complications.

PREVENTION OF COMPLICATIONS

Complications are prevented by careful technique, a clear knowledge of the anatomy of the spinal canal, and especially a constant awareness of all the possible complications.

Nerve Root Damage

A good surgical exposure helps to prevent accidental damage to nerve roots and makes strenuous retraction of the roots unnecessary. We do not recommend routine extensive exposures by making long incisions, stripping four or five vertebrae of paraspinal muscles or excising several laminae, ligaments, and posterior joints because such exposures increase the risk of late instability and adhesions. We aim for the minimum exposure necessary to explore the spinal canal thoroughly and execute the planned procedure safely.

We previously recommended exploring the lateral recess on the asymptomatic side at the time of a diskectomy. If lateral stenosis was present, we recommended prophylactic decompression to prevent spinal nerve entrapment from the inevitable settling of the disk space after the disk was excised. This routine bilateral exploration is now unnecessary if the CT scan demonstrates a normal lateral recess on the asymptomatic side.

If only one side is to be explored, the spinous process can be cut at its base and retracted to increase the view of the depths of the canal (see below) without sacrificing the process and interspinous ligaments (Fig. 16-1).[1]

Magnifying glasses and an operating headlamp with adjustable focus are recommended during that part of the operation in which the nerve root is being exposed, manipulated, and decompressed.

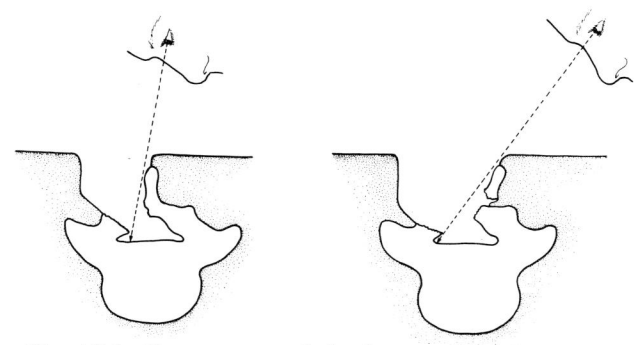

Fig. 16-1. Osteotomy and displacement of the spinous process improves the view during unilateral exposure.

Bleeding

Excessive bleeding can convert a straightforward operation into an awful "snatch and grab" exercise because only intermittent glimpses of the nerve roots are obtained. Bleeding must be diminished by properly positioning the patient (see below) and injecting a hemostatic solution. Elevation of the paraspinal muscles should be meticulously subperiosteal and care must be taken to cauterize the muscular branches of the lumbar arteries as they are encountered.[2] Bipolar diathermy should be tested on subcutaneous fat and adjusted before it is used on epidural vessels, and then only after the dura and nerve root are retracted away from its tip. Temporary packing with patties and Gelfoam in the epidural space further controls bleeding and increases the exposure in the spinal canal. Routine hypotensive anesthesia is unnecessary, but blood should be available for replacement if difficulty is predicted. We recommend cross matching 1 or more liters for reexplorations and spinal fusions.

Wrong Side and Level

To avoid operating on the wrong side or the wrong level the surgeon should develop and routinely practice a series of checks. I check the recorded notes, myelogram, and CT scan, and I doublecheck the side with my first assistant before starting. To avoid operating on the wrong level I routinely expose the sacrum and identify it by both visual examination and palpation. I apply a Kocher forceps to the L5 spinous process to elicit movement in relation to S1. Occasionally, I also obtain a lateral X-ray with the Kocher forceps on a spinous process to confirm the level. I always do this if a transitional vertebra is present and when operating on the upper lumbar spine.

Damage to Dura and Large Vessels

At the start of the operation the X-ray films should be examined for defects in the posterior elements (spina bifida occulta); if defects are present, special care should be taken to avoid accidental penetration into the spinal canal during elevation of the paraspinal muscles. The dorsal surface of the normal sacrum can be surprisingly thin and easily penetrated. During both the first entry into the canal and excision of the ligamentum flavum the dura should be protected from the scalpel blade with patties or a blunt dissector.

Damaging the aorta, vena cava, and iliac vessels is a risk during diskectomy from a posterior approach, and the dura and nerve roots are at risk during diskectomy from an anterior approach. These serious complications are avoided by constant awareness of the depth of any instrument that is placed in the disk space. The average midline anteroposterior (AP) diameter of the lumbar disk space is 2.5 to 3.0 cm, but laterally this measurement is smaller. Use of curettes and rongeurs with marks on the metal at graduated intervals are recommended. Placing a red mark at 2.5 cm is a good safety precaution. During the maneuvers in the disk space, the "feel" of the instrument on the bone of the endplate will avoid penetration beyond the confines of the annulus (Figs. 16-2, 16-3).

Postoperative Adhesions

Gentle handling and retraction of the tissues in the spinal canal decrease the risk of postoperative adhesions and arachnoiditis. Controlling of bleeding by bipolar diathermy during the operation and removing hematoma by a closed suction drain in the first 2 days following surgery decrease the severity of this complication. Free fat grafts measuring 0.5 to 1.0 cm in thickness are taken from subcutaneous fat either at the edge of the incision or, rarely, from a separate buttock incision

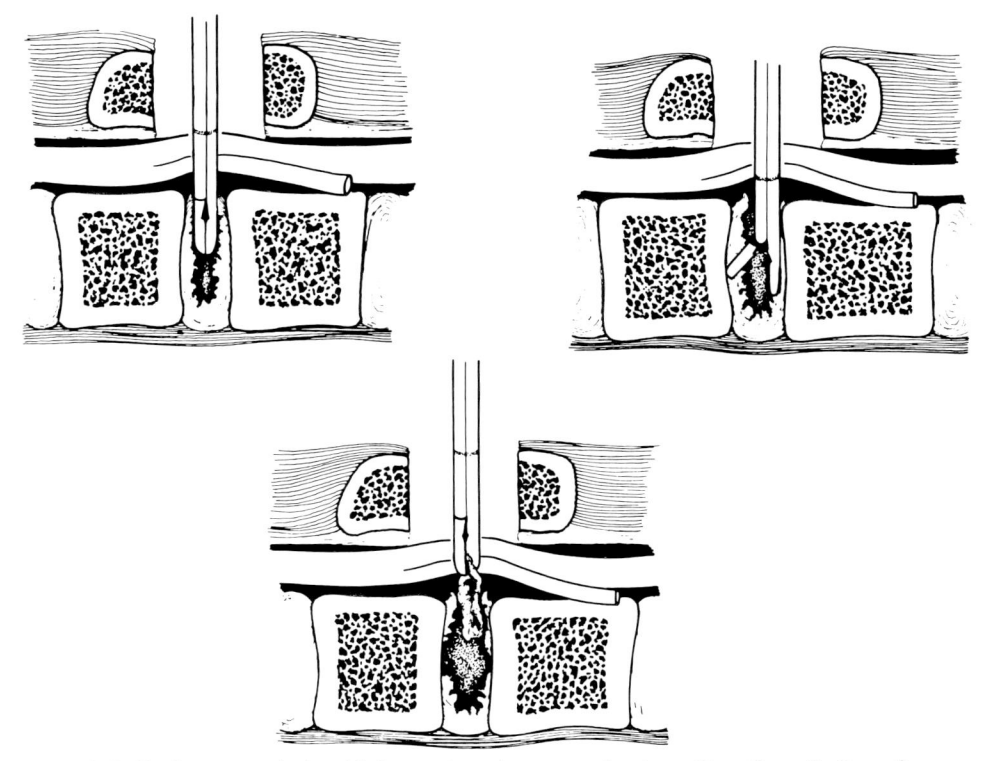

Fig. 16-2. Disk removal. Avoid damaging the nerve by inserting the pituitary forceps with its jaws closed. Avoid damaging the great vessels by referring to depth mark scored on forceps.

and are placed over the exposed dura.[3] Two to four absorbable sutures are placed through the edge of the graft and nearby soft tissues to hold the graft against the dura and prevent its displacement. All Gelfoam used for temporary packing is removed before the wound is closed (Fig. 16-4).

Wound Infections

Routine prophylactic antibiotics are unnecessary. We give high dose intraoperative broad-spectrum intravenous antibiotics during the more difficult and longer procedures, if a break in aseptic technique occurs or during reexplorations that were previously infected. No antibiotic is given after completion of the operation. At intervals during the operation and before wound closure the entire wound is irrigated with a dilute antibiotic–saline solution.

SURGICAL APPROACHES

The lumbar spine can be approached from in front or from behind (Fig. 16-5).[4]

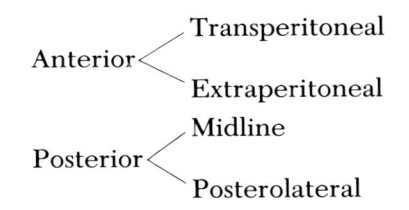

Anterior
- Transperitoneal
- Extraperitoneal

Posterior
- Midline
- Posterolateral

Anterior Transperitoneal Approach

This approach can be used for L5–S1 fusion. The level of bifurcation of the aorta is not always the same. Fusion at L4–L5 through this approach is more difficult and the anterior extraperitoneal approach is preferred. The transperitoneal approach can also be used for osteomyelitis and for

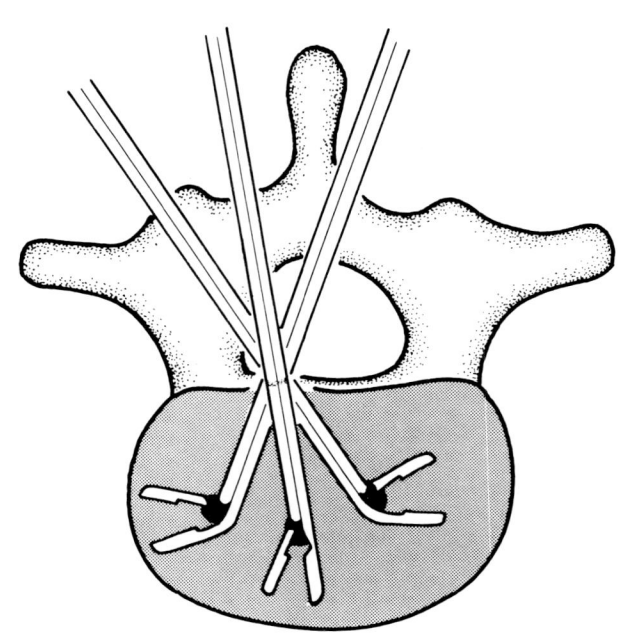

Fig. 16-3. Use straight and angled pituitary forceps with marks on metal to indicate a measured depth.

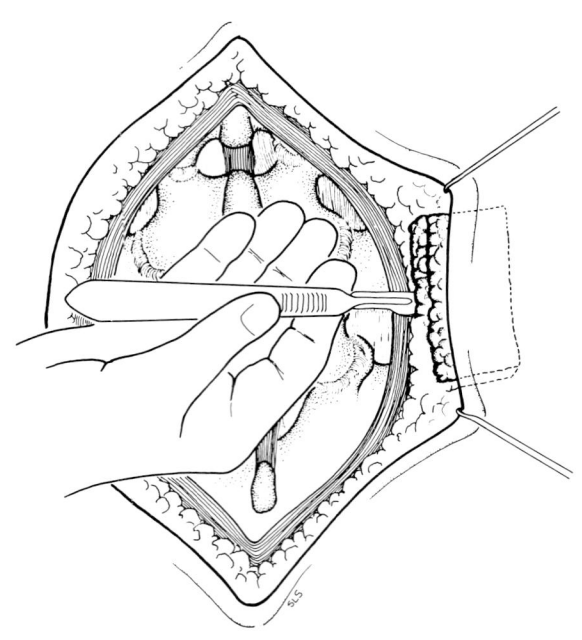

Fig. 16-4. Free fat graft taken from the wound edge used to cover the dura and prevent adhesions.

tumors involving the L5 or S1 vertebral bodies.[5]

As with the retroperitoneal approach the transperitoneal approach cannot be used if decompression of the neural elements is necessary. It involves all the hazards of a laparotomy. The real risk of sterility (not impotence) due to retrograde ejaculation is unknown. Also unknown is the relative risk of this complication in the transperitoneal as compared with the retroperitoneal route. The risk seems to have been exaggerated in earlier publications.[6,7]

General anesthesia with muscle relaxation is used. The patient is positioned supine, 10 to 15° head down (to displace the intestines cephalad and to decrease venous bleeding) with a 5 to 10° break in the table at the level of the iliac crests in order to displace the spine nearer to the anterior abdominal wall (Fig. 16-6).

A midline longitudinal, paramedian, or Pfannenstiel incision is made. If a midline incision is used, the anterior peritoneum is split with the linea alba. The intestines are packed off cranially and laterally with saline-soaked packs behind abdominal retractors. The bifurcation of the aorta and, below it, the sacral promontory are identified (Fig. 16-7).

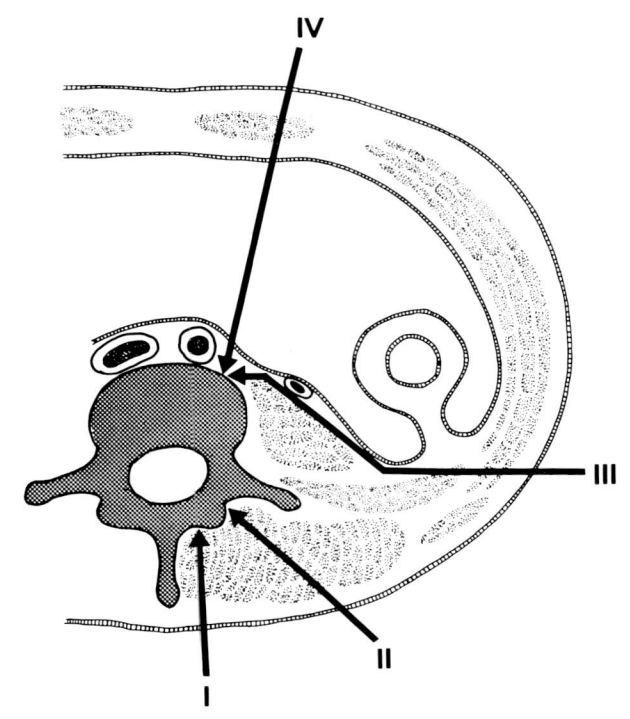

Fig. 16-5. Surgical Approaches. (I) Posterior midline. (II) Posterolateral. (III) Anterior extraperitoneal. (IV) Anterior transperitoneal. (After Rathke FW, Schlegel KF: Surgery of the Spine. Philadelphia, WB Saunders, 1979.)

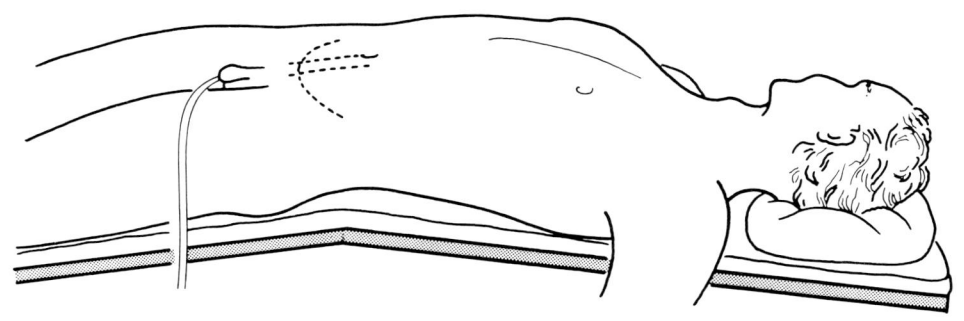

Fig. 16-6. Anterior transperitoneal approach. Note 10° head down position and 10° break in table. The choice of incisions is shown.

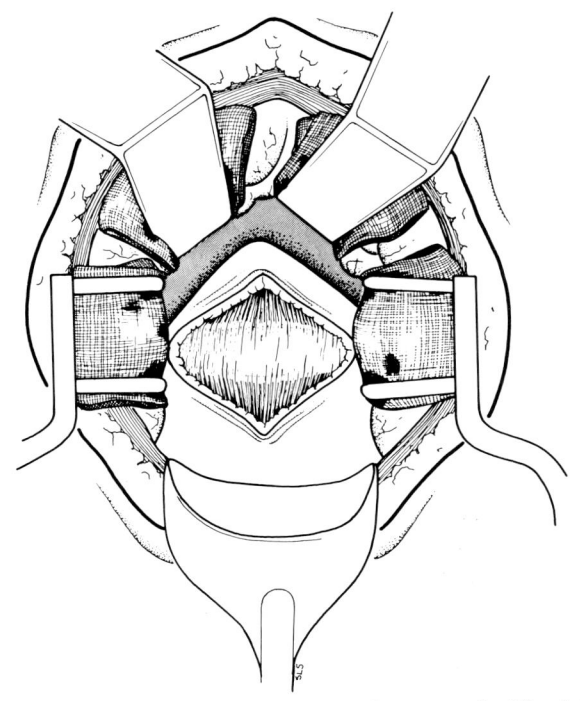

Fig. 16-7. Anterior transperitoneal approach. The bifurcation of the aorta and, below it, the sacral promontory are identified. The peritoneum is split vertically to avoid injuring the presacral plexus.

Anterior Extraperitoneal Approach

This approach provides wide exposure and all operations on the vertebral bodies and disks from L2 to S1 can be accomplished through it. It is better than the transperitoneal approach for interbody fusion if both the L4–L5 space and the L5–S1 space are to be fused. It has the advantage that an iliac bone graft can be taken through the same skin incision. Care must be extended to protect the aorta on the left side, the inferior vena cava on the right side, and—proceeding more distally on both sides—the common iliac vessels. In the presence of an inflammatory process the ureter may adhere to the scar tissue and require careful dissection.[5-7]

General anesthesia supplemented by muscle relaxants is used. For the upper lumbar spine the patient is placed in the left lateral position with the right hip and knee flexed and the left extremity straight. The table is broken at 10° at the level of the iliac crests and in addition is tilted 10° head down to displace the intestines cranially and decrease bleeding (Fig. 16-8). To approach the lower lumbar spine the supine position is used and again the table is broken 10° at the iliac crests and tilted 10° head down (Fig. 16-9).

All or part of an oblique incision extending from the anterior to the posterior midline is employed. The line of the incision is midway between the umbilicus and symphysis pubis and midway between the costal margin and iliac crest. Alternatively, the lower lumbar spine may be approached by a paramedian incision.

The external oblique aponeurosis and muscle are divided in the direction of their fibers. The internal oblique is divided transversely in the line of the incision. The transverse abdominis is carefully nicked to avoid cutting the peritoneum, which is then pushed away from the abdominal wall and vertebral bodies with blunt dissection using a swab-on-forceps. Any perforation of the peritoneum should be repaired immediately to prevent extension of the tear or omission of this

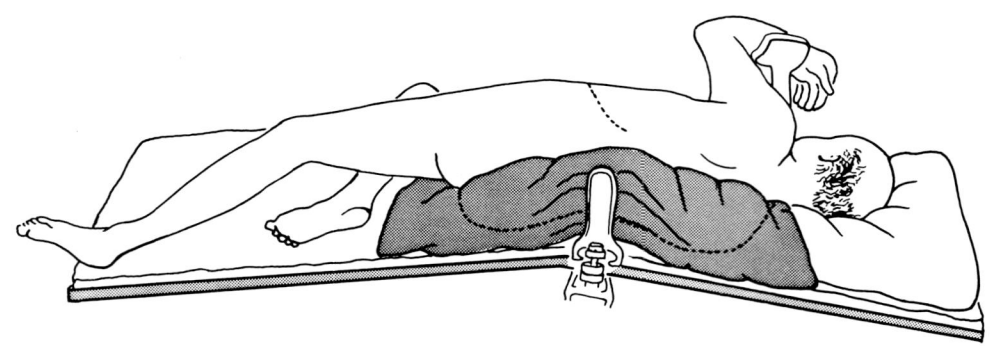

Fig. 16-8. Anterior extraperitoneal approach. Positioning and skin incision for operations on the upper lumbar levels.

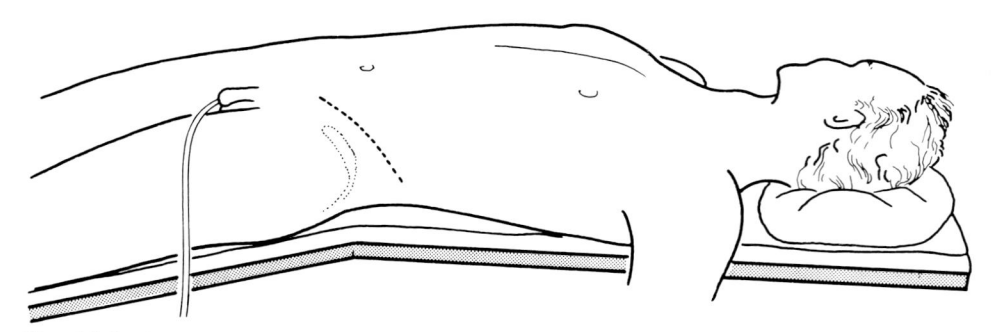

Fig. 16-9. Anterior extraperitoneal approach. Positioning and skin incision for operations on the lower lumbar levels.

repair later on. The ureter is reflected medially with the peritoneum. Three columns formed by the aorta, vertebral bodies, and the psoas muscle come into view (Figs. 16-10 to 16-13).

Posterolateral Approach

The posterolateral approach provides good exposure of the transverse process and pars interarticularis.[8] We recommend it for posterolateral fusion in spondylolisthesis. Decompression of the nerve roots is easily accomplished through this approach. Access to the posterolateral quadrant of the vertebral body and disk space after osteotomy of the transverse process is possible but very restricted. Operating anterior to the plane of the transverse process endangers the aorta, vena cava, or common iliac vessels depending on the side and level.

The patient is anesthetized, intubated, and positioned prone as for a posterior midline approach (see below). The subcutaneous fat and paraspinal muscles are infiltrated with a hemostatic solution in the line of the planned incision. A longitudinal incision is made 5 to 7 cm lateral to the midline, and the dorsolumbar fascia is incised in line with the incision. Retraction is made easier by extending the fascial incision in J-fashion (Figs. 16-14, 16-15). The lateral third of the paraspinal muscle mass is then split longitudinally, generally in line with the muscle fibers, by a combination of blunt dissection and diathermy knife (Fig. 16-16). Careful attention should be given to controlling bleeding muscle branches as they are encountered, if a continuous ooze is to be avoided.

An alternative is to make the skin incision a little more lateral and make the deep dissection between the paraspinal muscle mass and quadratus lumborum. This is not recommended, since it offers no advantage and poor exposure.

A large periosteal elevator is used to strip the muscles from the transverse process laterally and

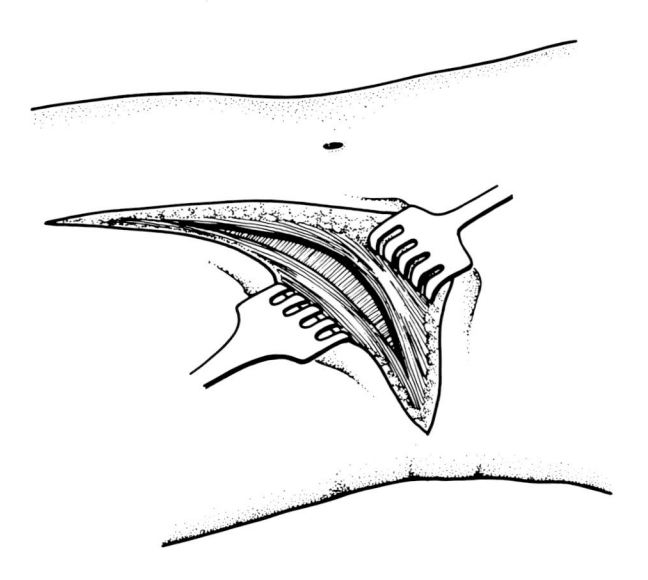

Fig. 16-10. External oblique aponeurosis and muscle fibers are incised in line of incision. (After Rathke FW, Schlegel KF: Surgery of the Spine. Philadelphia, WB Saunders, 1979.)

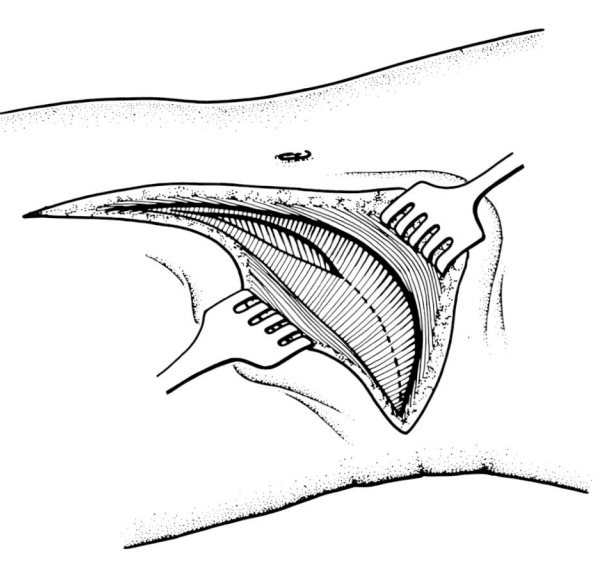

Fig. 16-11. Internal oblique muscle is divided transversely. (After Rathke FW, Schlegel KF: Surgery of the Spine. Philadelphia, WB Saunders, 1979.)

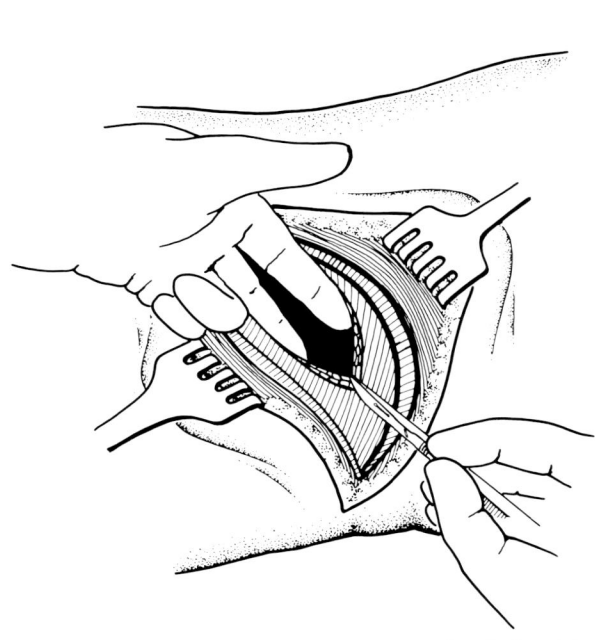

Fig. 16-12. Transversus abdominis is divided taking care not to cut the peritoneum.

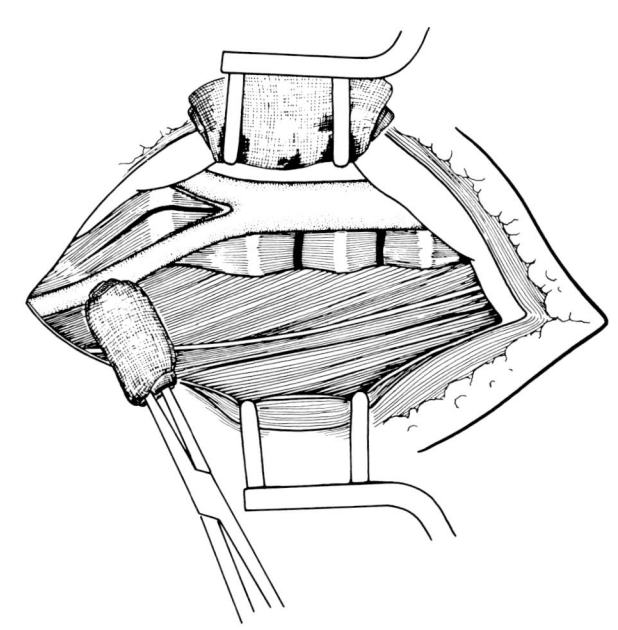

Fig. 16-13. Three columns formed by the aorta, vertebral bodies, and the psoas muscle. The ureter is pushed medially with the peritoneum. The genitofemoral nerve is seen on the psoas muscle.

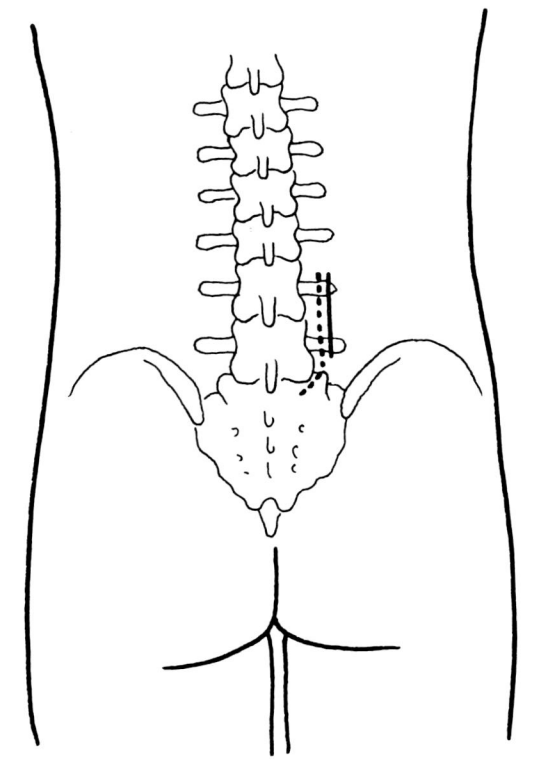

Fig. 16-14. Posterolateral approach. Skin (solid line) and fascial (broken line) incisions.

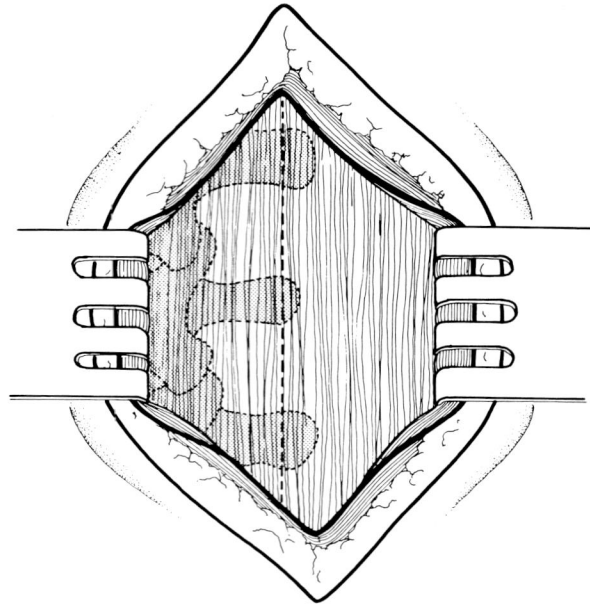

Fig. 16-15. Posterolateral approach. The dorsilumbar fascia is incised (dotted line).

the posterior joint and lamina medially. For limited procedures on the posterolateral quadrant of the vertebral body and disk, the anterior surface of the transverse process is carefully stripped of periosteum with an elevator, taking care to keep the instrument in contact with bone throughout the maneuver (Fig. 16-17). The transverse process is excised to its base with rongeurs or a guarded osteotome. The posterolateral aspect of the vertebral body comes into view when a long retractor is inserted and braced against the lateral surface of the vertebral body (Figs. 16-18, 16-19).

Posterior Midline Approach

The posterior elements, transverse processes, spinal canal, disk space, and vertebral bodies can be exposed for diskectomy, laminectomy, partial facetectomy, posterolateral fusion, or posterior interbody fusion by using the posterior midline approach.

Operations through this approach are carried out under general anesthesia and endotracheal intubation. Several positions—sitting, lateral, knee-to-chest (rabbit position)—have been used but we prefer the semi-flexed prone position on a modified Hastings frame. We continue to experiment with other positions, frames, and bolsters, but we have found none as satisfactory as the Hastings frame.[9]

The original Hastings frame was made of wood. We use a simplified metal version with the patient in the same position as Hastings described, i.e., with the knees and hips flexed 110 to 120°. The patient's weight is borne on the chest—which rests on a firm padded washable cube—the buttocks, and the knees. The spine should be 10° head down. The advantages of this position and frame are that the dependent position of the abdomen, together with the 10° head-down position, serves to decrease the pressure in the vena cava and to minimize epidural bleeding. The spine is slightly flexed to increase the interlaminar space. The knees and hips are not in such an excessively flexed position as to predispose to deep vein thrombosis (Fig. 16-20).

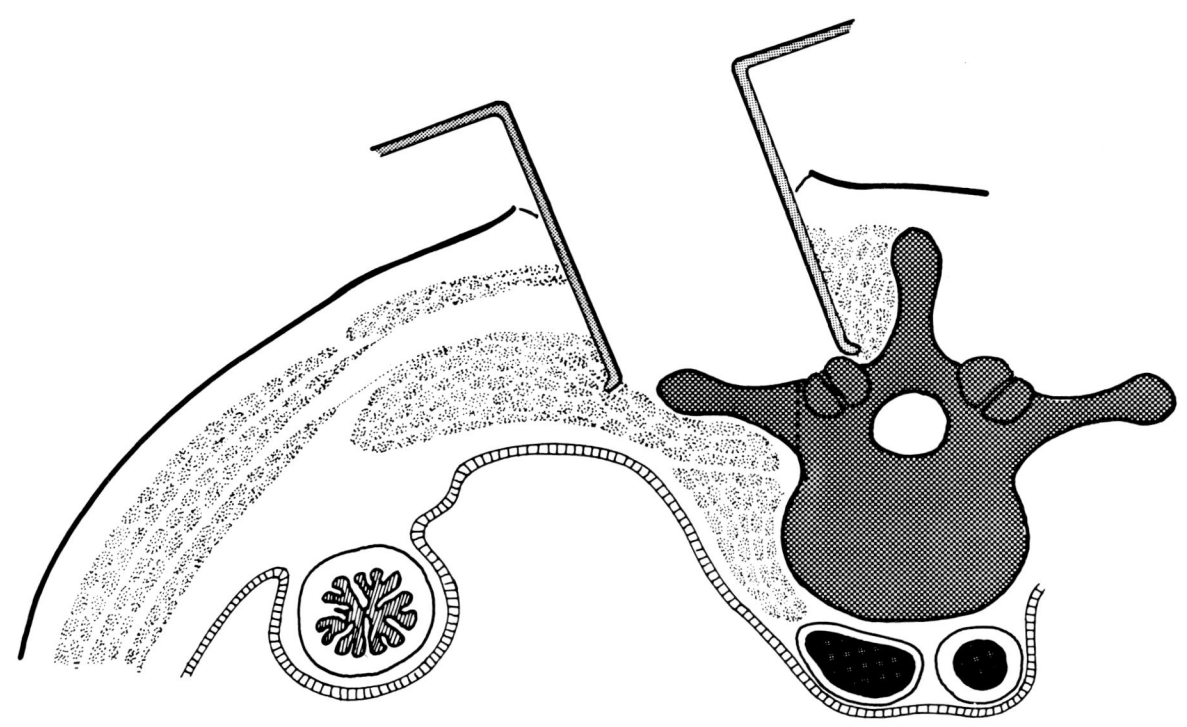

Fig. 16-16. Retraction and exposure. The transverse process may be osteotomized (dotted line) to approach the posterolateral quadrant of the disk or vertebral bodies for limited procedures.

Special precautions are important to prevent serious complications.
1. Avoid pressure on the eyes to prevent blindness.
2. Avoid excessive neck extension or rotation to prevent nerve root or spinal cord injury.
3. Avoid pressure over the ulnar nerve at the elbow and peroneal nerve at the knee to prevent paralysis.
4. Avoid excessive abduction of the shoulders to prevent brachial plexus traction injury.

The patient may move on bolsters and frames during the operation. We have had one case of femoral nerve palsy caused by pressure of blanket bolsters in the groin. Fortunately, this disappeared spontaneously after 4 days. Bolsters probably increase the risk of deep vein thrombosis by pressing on the femoral vein.

Crock's sausage is an excellent and versatile bolster that is useful for patients with special problems such as stiff joints in the lower extremities or gross obesity. It is economically made and consists of a plastic-covered roll of firm material that can be bent into a U-shape. The bend in the U supports the sternum and clavicles. The roll is thick enough to allow the obese abdomen to be dependent. A break in the table at the level of the iliac crests reduces the lumbar lordosis (Fig. 16-21).

A midline longitudinal incision that is centered over the level to be explored is made. Only as many laminae as necessary to complete the planned procedure safely are exposed. For example, the L4 to S1 laminae are exposed for L5–S1 diskectomy. The subcutaneous fat and paraspinal muscles are infiltrated with a hemostatic solution using 22-gauge 6-inch needles. First, the skin is infiltrated through two punctures. It is then incised to expose the deep fascia and is retracted with self-retaining Gelpi retractors. The paraspinal muscles are then infiltrated by inserting the needles 5 cm lateral to the spinous processes in fan-like directions. The needle is inserted level with the spinous process deep enough to strike

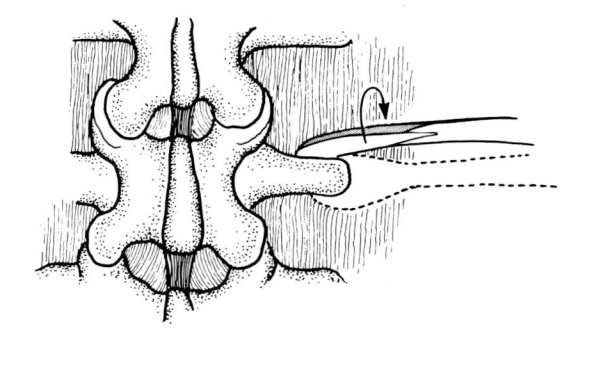

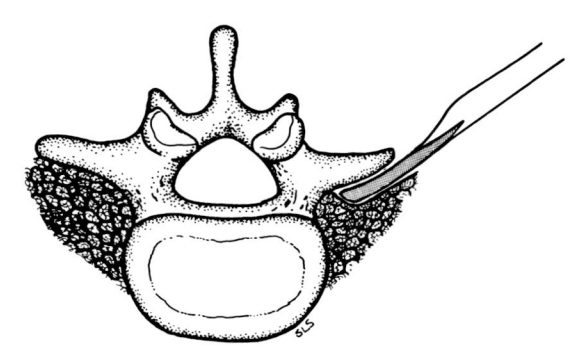

Fig. 16-17. The anterior surface of the transverse process is carefully stripped of periosteum.

Fig. 16-18. The anterior structures are protected and the transverse process is osteotomised at its base. (After Rathke FW, Schlegel KF: Surgery of the Spine. Philadelphia, WB Saunders, 1979.)

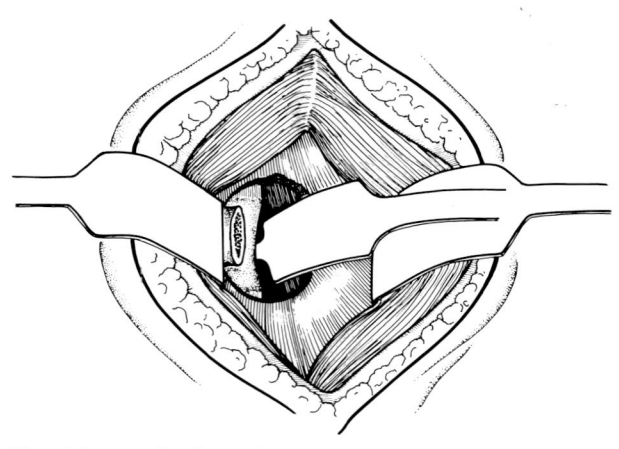

Fig. 16-19. The lateral surfaces of the vertebral body and disk are exposed. A blunt ended Hohmann retractor is braced against the vertebral body and protects the great vessels.

the posterior joint or transverse process and then retracted 1 cm before the injection is started. The injection is continued as the needle is withdrawn. This is repeated at every level that is to be exposed and on both sides for bilateral approaches. This technique avoids puncturing the skin in more than two places. The deep fascia is longitudinally incised close to the spinous processes to be exposed. A large periosteal elevator is inserted against the surface of the spinous process and the muscles are stripped subperiosteally. With the elevator held in one hand to stretch the musculotendenous fibers of origin, they are divided close to the bone with a scalpel in the other hand. The spinous processes should be exposed distally-to-proximally, because the orientation of the muscle fibers that originate from the spinous processes facilitates this maneuver. A gauze pack is inserted and the elevator is used to push the pack and muscles laterally to expose the posterior joints. This step is repeated at each level and on both sides in bilateral exposures. A good habit to cultivate is to insert no more than one pack for each spinous process—making sure to remove the same number in the next step. The packs are removed and Gelpi self-retaining retractors inserted. Bleeders in muscle are cauterized. Fat, torn periosteum, and frayed tags of muscle are removed to denude completely the laminae and ligamenta flava in the entire field. A bone rongeur is best

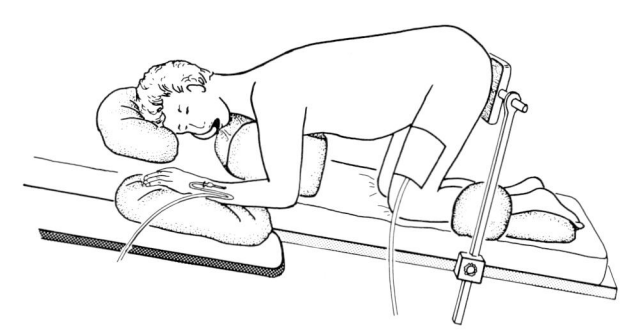

Fig. 16-20. The Modified Hastings Frame. Take care to prevent injury to the eyes, cervical spine, brachial plexus, ulnar nerve, and peroneal nerve (see text).

suited for this step. This procedure is repeated on both sides for bilateral exposures.

For a unilateral exploration in obese or muscular patients the surgeon's view can be improved by temporary displacement of the spinous process.[1] The spinous process is osteotomized, with a curved osteotome and mallet, where the process flares outward at the apex of the spinal canal. One or more spinous processes may be osteotomized. Gelpi retractors placed on the interspinous ligaments displace the spinous process or processes to expose both the lamina on the side to be explored and half the lamina on the opposite side (Fig. 16-1).

The L5–S1 junction is then identified by visual examination, palpation, probing with a blunt dissector, forcibly moving the L5 spinous process, and, in many cases, a lateral X-ray with a metal marker on the L5 spinous process.

DISKECTOMY

Central and lateral stenosis may be present in association with a disk herniation.[10] If present, the stenoses are dealt with as discussed below after the herniation is excised. If a CT scan has shown normal central and lateral canals, the exploration is confined to the side of the herniation with or without osteotomy of the spinous process. If central or lateral stenosis is present, a bilateral approach is made and the stenosis dealt with as described below. In the event that no CT scan is available, the myelogram will also determine if central stenosis is present. However, the possibil-

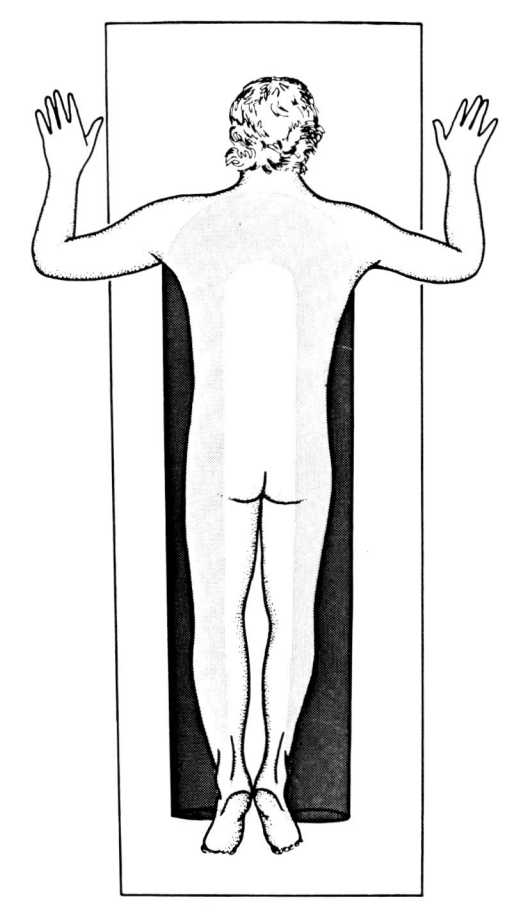

Fig. 16-21. Crock's Sausage. A useful bolster for patients with stiff lower extremity joints or obesity.

ity of missing lateral stenosis on the asymptomatic side is real and we recommend bilateral exploration, intraoperative measurement of the lateral recesses with graduated probes, and lateral decompression if the canals are narrow. The CT scan is obviously invaluable in avoiding unnecessary bilateral explorations.

Technique

A posterior midline approach is made and the level to be explored is identified. The upper edge of the ligamentum flavum is partly detached from its attachment to the anterior surface of the upper lamina with a curette using a controlled scraping and pushing motion. The exposed lower edge of this lamina is then excised using Kerrison rongeurs. The safest place to start the incision into the ligamentum flavum is in the midline where it is tented away from the underlying dura. A small patty or narrow dissector is then inserted through the opening to displace anteriorly and protect the dura and epidural fat. The ligamentum flavum is then excised in one piece to expose the interlaminar space on one side. The opening is widened by excising one-third of the superior and inferior laminae. Pressing gently on the dura with a blunt dissector may detect the fullness caused by a disk herniation felt through two thicknesses of dura. The surgeon dons headlight and magnifying glasses and with a bayonet nontoothed forceps and a blunt Penfield dissector explores the lateral recess. The nerve root lying medial to the pedicle is identified and retracted. Any difficulty retracting the root suggests that it is compressed by a disk herniation or entrapped in a narrowed lateral recess. Care should be taken not to confuse a nerve root stretched over an anteriorly placed herniation for the bulge of the herniation itself. The best precaution is always to identify the nerve root before incising the annulus fibrosus (Fig. 16-22). Epidural vessels are cauterized with bipolar diathermy at a low setting, taking care not to diathermize the nearby dura or nerve root inadvertently. Patties can be packed anterior and lateral to the dura both proximally and distally in the canal to control bleeding further and to retract the dura. Once the nerve root is confidently identified, it is retracted and a cruciate incision is made in the bulging annulus. The loose fragments of disk material are extracted with pituitary rongeurs. To avoid accidental avulsion of the root in the jaws of the rongeur, the latter is inserted through the annulus incision with the jaws closed and opened only when it is in the disk space. To avoid accidental damage to the retroperitoneal great vessels, the surgeon should take the special precautions described above. Ring curettes are inserted to scrape the endplates gently and the procedure with pituitary rongeurs is repeated (Figs. 16-2, 16-3).

The nerve root should be freely mobile and easily retracted. Difficulty retracting the root may indicate that residual compression by migrated disk material or lateral stenosis is present, and a search should be made by probing the canal and foramen proximally and distally. The method of enlarging the lateral recess and foramen is described below.

At intervals throughout the procedure the entire wound is irrigated with a topical antibiotic diluted in saline. All patties, Gelfoam, and packs are removed and a free fat graft is placed over the exposed dura and sutured loosely to nearby soft tissue such as a posterior joint capsule. A closed suction tube drain is placed deep to the muscles and brought through a stab incision in the skin. A water-tight closure of the edges of the dorsilumbar fascia is made with interrupted sutures of absorbable material. Another tube drain is placed in the subcutaneous fat, which is apposed with a layer of absorbable sutures. The skin is closed with subcuticular stainless steel.

Postoperative Care

A neurological examination is carried out in the recovery room and any new deficit noted. The findings serve as a baseline. The patient is nursed supine for 24 hours. Intramuscular narcotic analgesics and antiemetics are given as required. Difficulty with micturition is frequent in males and if simple measures fail, a small catheter is inserted to be removed in 2 to 3 days. On the 2nd postoperative day the patient is stood up at the bed side twice for 5 minutes each time. Thereafter, the patient stands and walks for increasing periods that are interspersed with rest periods in bed. The

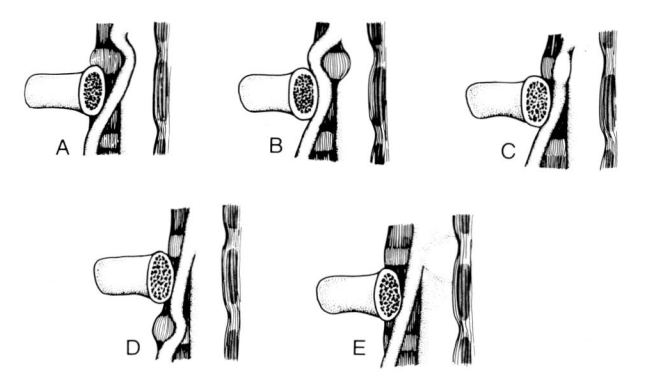

Fig. 16-22. The disc herniation may lie in one of several positions. Always identify the nerve root before incising the presumed herniation.

wound dressing is not removed unless excessive pain, tenderness, or fever raises the suspicion that a wound infection is present. The drains are removed without disturbing the dressing on the 2nd postoperative day. The sutures are removed on the 10th day and the patient can usually go home by the 14th day after surgery. No braces are prescribed.

The patient starts low back exercises (pelvic tilting and half sit-ups) at this stage and is seen at 4- to 6-week intervals initially. Light work is started at 6 to 8 weeks and heavy work at 12 to 16 weeks. Patients are encouraged to continue daily exercises indefinitely.

CENTRAL CANAL DECOMPRESSION

The narrowed central canal is unroofed by a wide laminectomy that extends laterally on both sides as far as the facet joints. The number of laminae to be excised is determined by the clinical picture, the number of narrow levels seen on the CT scan or myelogram, and the reestablishment of normal dural pulsation during the operation.

In severe central spinal stenosis, the nerve roots of the cauda equina are tightly crowded within the dura in a small bony canal. In addition the interlaminar spaces are narrow and the bone is hard. The risk of damaging the cauda equina by clumsy probing, excessively large instruments, or tight packing is great.

Technique

A posterior midline approach is made and the paravertebral muscles are elevated on both sides of all the vertebrae with narrow canals. Starting with the most distally involved vertebra, the spinous process is excised with angled double-action bone shears. The epidural space is entered by incising the ligamentum flavum as described for diskectomy. If the canal is exceedingly small, the lamina is excised piecemeal with a rongeur. First the posterior cortex of the lamina is removed, leaving the thin anterior cortex intact. A toothed rongeur makes this step easy. The anterior cortex is then removed piecemeal with small Kerrison rongeurs. This precaution is important in central stenosis because of the crowded space, the small amount of epidural fat present and the dramatic immediate bulging of the dura as more of the lamina is excised. This procedure is repeated for all the vertebrae with narrowed canals (Figs. 16-23, 16-24).

The wound is then irrigated with antibiotic diluted in saline and a free fat graft is loosely sutured to cover the exposed dura. The wound is drained and closed as described for diskectomy (Fig. 16-25).

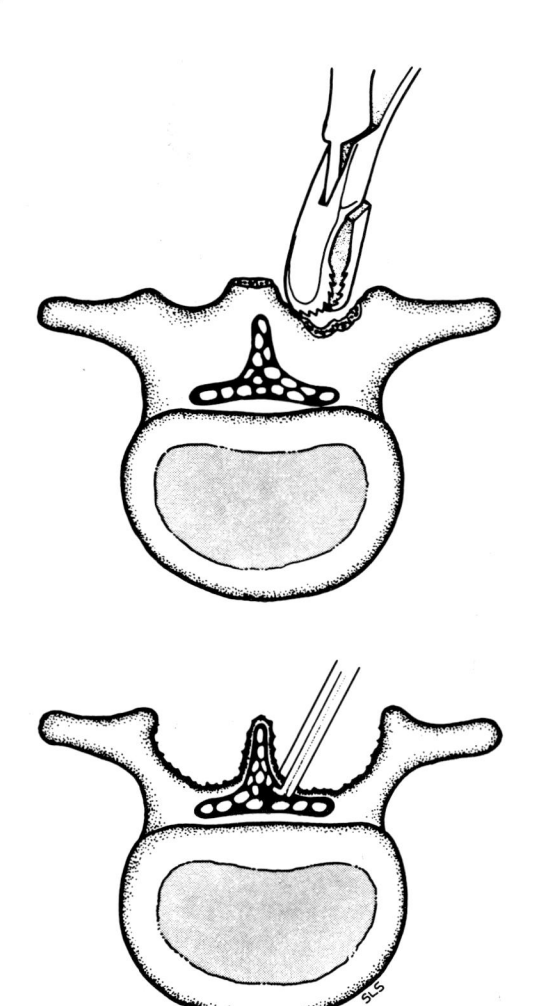

Fig. 16-23. Central spinal stenosis. Thin the thick hard lamina with a toothed rongeur before using a Kerrison rongeur. This prevents damage to the nerve roots, which are crowded into a small canal.

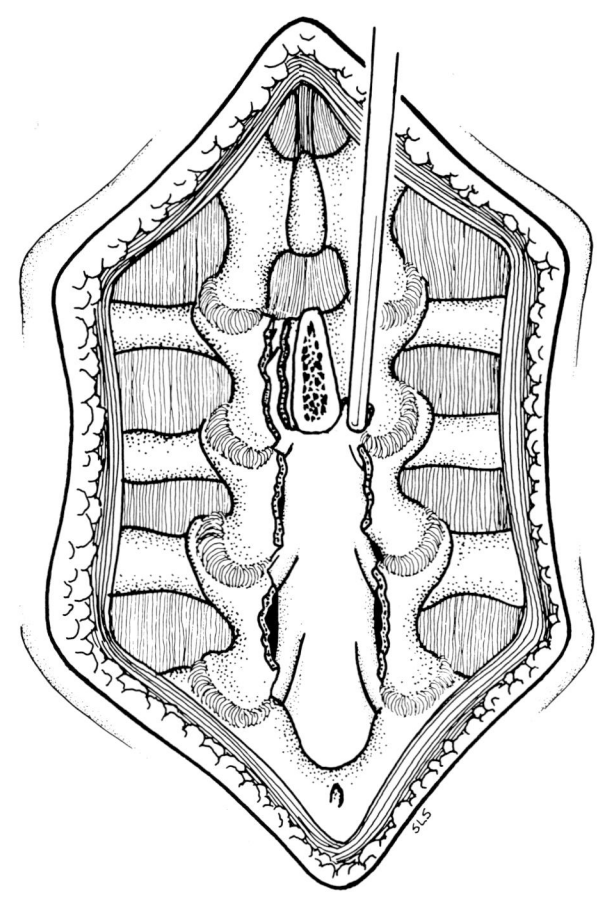

Fig. 16-24. Three level laminectomy for central spinal stenosis.

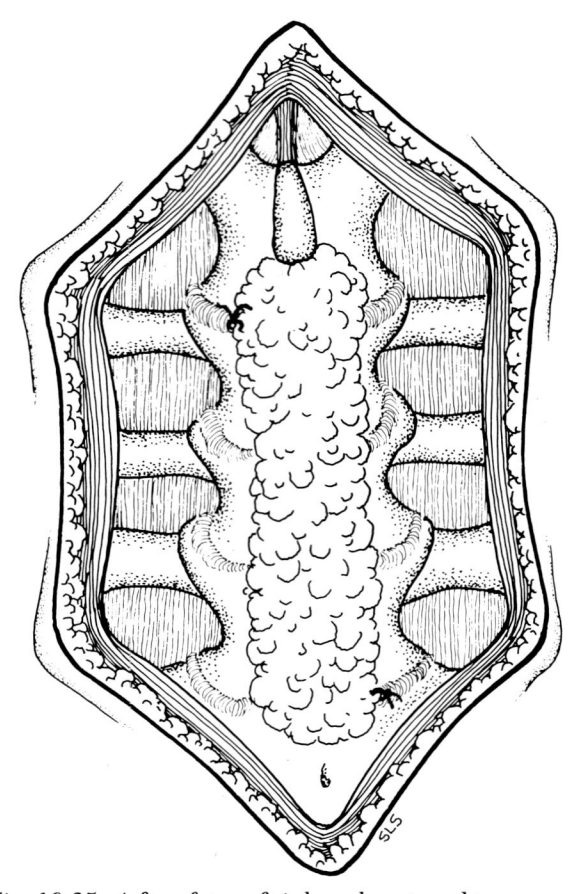

Fig. 16-25. A free fat graft is loosely sutured to prevent its displacement.

Postoperative Care

Care is the same as after diskectomy, but these patients experience less discomfort in the immediate postoperative period and so require less analgesia.

LATERAL CANAL DECOMPRESSION

When lateral stenosis is present on one side, the opposite side is often narrowed enough to cause symptoms or, if asymptomatic, to require prophylactic decompression. At any one level four nerve roots (two pairs) should be explored.[10] For example, at the L5–S1 level exploration should include the pair of L5 "exiting" and the pair of S1 "transversing" roots. Blunt-ended probes measuring 3, 4, 5, and 6 mm are used to measure the diameter of the lateral recesses and the foramina. The L5 roots are decompressed by excising the tips of the superior articular processes of S1 vertebrae and the S1 roots are decompressed by bilateral partial medial facetectomy (Fig. 16-26).

Technique

A posterior midline approach is made. The paraspinal muscles are elevated bilaterally and the involved intervertebral space identified. The ligamentum flavum is excised and the interlaminar space widened by excision of the upper and lower lamina edges and spinous processes.

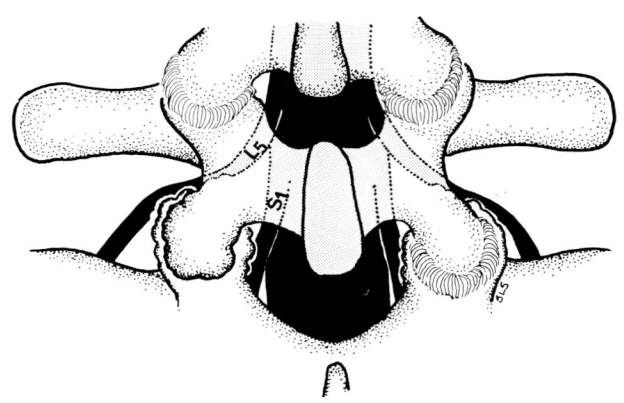

Fig. 16-26. At any one level four nerve roots (two pairs) can be explored.

The medial third of the inferior articular process is cut with a narrow osteotome and mallet. This step exposes the joint cartilage on the superior articular process. The medial third of the superior articular process is osteotomized with the same osteotome while the nerve is retracted and a flat dissector is placed in the recess to protect the nerve from injury. While the nerve is still being retracted, the most lateral part of the recess is widened by shaving the anterior surface of the superior articular process with a Sonic curette (Sonic Surgery, Quintron Inc.). The size of the recess is remeasured and if still narrow, it is widened further. The same procedure is repeated on the opposite side (Figs. 16-27 to 16-29).

On occasion the major narrowing is at the foramen. Further decompression should be effected by excising the lower medial edge of the pedicle with the use of the Sonic curette and Kerrison rongeurs.

The exiting nerve is explored by undermining the inferior edge of the upper lamina. The nerve root should be seen exiting under the pedicle. In the event that the tip of the superior articular process is entrapping the exiting root the tip is osteotomized with the Sonic curette to permit free passage of the nerve (Fig. 16-30).

The wound is irrigated at intervals during and at the completion of the operation with antibiotic diluted in saline. A free fat graft is positioned to cover exposed dura and loosely sutured to nearby soft tissue such as a posterior joint capsule. The wound is drained and closed as for diskectomy.

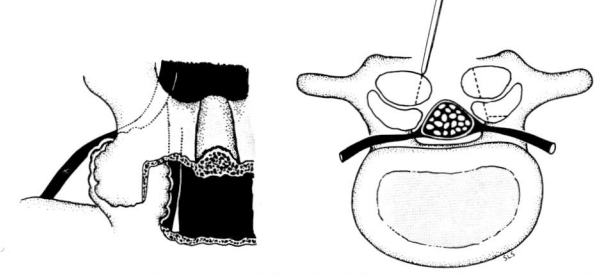

Fig. 16-27. The medial third of the L5 inferior articular process is osteotomized.

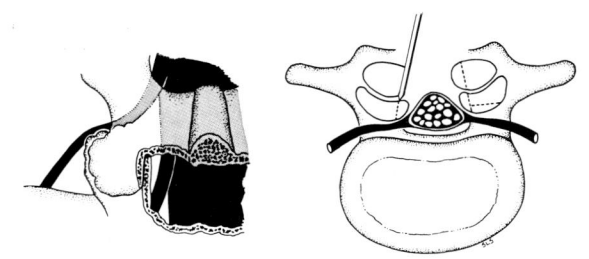

Fig. 16-28. The medial third of the S1 superior articular process is osteotomised. The nerve root should be retracted and protected.

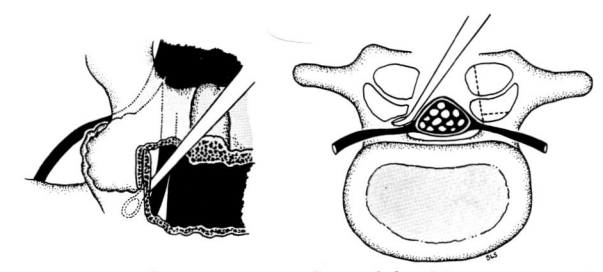

Fig. 16-29. The anterior surface of the S1 superior articular process (roof of the lateral recess) is shaved with a curette.

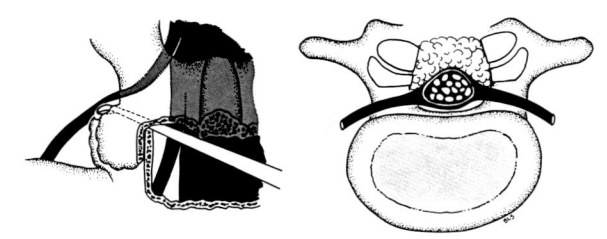

Fig. 16-30. The tip of the S1 superior articular process is removed to decompress the exiting L5 nerve. A free fat graft is loosely sutured to cover the dura.

Postoperative Care

Care is the same as that described for diskectomy.

REEXPLORATIONS

Reexploration after previous surgery through the same approach can be pleasantly simple or exceedingly difficult. The scar may be tough enough to require a new scalpel blade after every few scalpel strokes. Heterotrophic bone in the scar is occasionally present. The dura may adhere densely to the laminectomy membrane and may tear easily. A few precautions should be observed and a few tips may simplify the operation.

Technique

Blood should be cross-matched in case excessive bleeding occurs. The preoperative plain X-ray films should be studied to determine the extent of previous laminectomies and the myelogram should be searched for postsurgical pseudomeningoceles so that problems can be anticipated.

The original skin incision is used. The deep fascia is incised. The deep dissection is started in relatively normal tissues proximal, distal, and lateral to the previous laminectomy. Attention is directed at the most distal *intact* vertebra, which is stripped of muscles with an elevator. The same is done for the *intact* lamina just proximal to the previous laminectomy. The approximate depth of the dura below the laminectomy membrane can then be estimated, and the scar is incised down to this level without cutting the dura, for the length of the laminectomy. The blunt elevator is used to extend the dissection laterally to just beyond the lateral bony limit of the previous laminectomy, whether this is the lamina, posterior facets, or pedicle. Attention is directed at the lateral edge of the laminectomy membrane where the dissection becomes subperiosteal. The dissector is used to push the laminectomy membrane and encased dura off the sides of the bony canal. Roots often encased in scar tissue are exposed by blunt dissection using a Penfield dissector. The root and dura can then be retracted to expose the disk.

No attempt should be made to separate the central part of the laminectomy membrane from the dura, since this is unnecessary and increases the risk of tearing the dura (Fig. 16-31).

Postoperative Care

No special care is necessary.

SPONDYLOLISTHESIS

The surgical treatment of spondylolisthesis depends on several factors (Table 16-1).
1. Age
2. Degree of slip

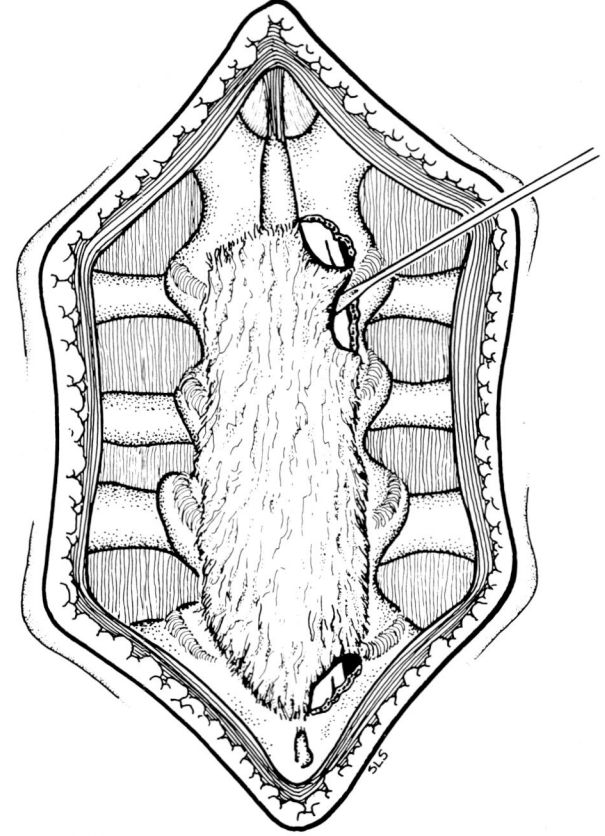

Fig. 16-31. Re-exploration. No attempt is made to separate the laminectomy membrane from the dura. The nerve roots are dissected out by starting at the proximal, distal, and lateral edges of the membrane.

Table 16-1. Surgical Treatment of Isthmic Spondylolisthesis

Age	Leg Symptoms	Grade	Operation
Child	Yes	I, II	Fusion L5–S1
		III, IV	Fusion L4–S1
	No	I, II	Fusion L5–S1
		III, IV	Fusion L4–S1
Adult	Yes	I, II	Decompression and fusion L5–S1
		III, IV	Decompression and fusion L4–S1
	No	I, II	Fusion L5–S1
		III, IV	Fusion L4–S1

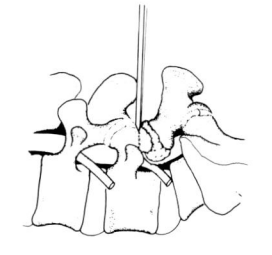

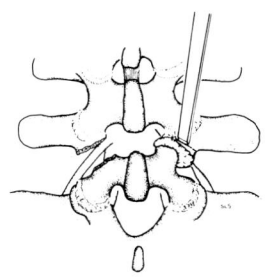

Fig. 16-32. Decompression for spondylolisthesis. Removing the rattler is optional, but the fibrous tissue and bone proximal to the pars defect must be excised in order to decompress the nerve.

3. Presence or absence of leg symptoms
4. Integrity of the disk above the proposed fusion

We concur with Wiltse's experience in regard to the need for decompression in some adults but rarely in children and adolescents.[11] We do fusion alone, or decompression and fusion but rarely a decompression alone.

In the more severe degrees of slip it is technically difficult to place grafts for posterolateral fusion between the L5 and S1 posterior elements and transverse processes. The pseudarthrosis rate for one-level fusion is unacceptably high, so we extend the fusion to L4.

The method of decompression is different for a posterior midline and posterolateral approach. In a midline approach we excise the entire "rattler"—a spinous process, laminae, and pars defect. It is extremely important to excise the mass of fibrous tissue, cartilage, and bone on the cephalad side of the pars defect. We do this with Kerrison rongeurs or with osteotome and mallet. At completion of the decompression the pair of exiting nerve roots should be easily visible from behind without the need for retraction. In a bilateral paraspinal approach the pair of exiting roots are decompressed by excising the fibrous tissue and approximately 0.5 cm of bone on either side of the defect without excising the entire lamina and spinous process, or rattler (Fig. 16-32).

In the adult for whom a one-level fusion is being considered, a diskogram of the next proximal disk should be obtained and if it is abnormal, the fusion should be extended to include this level. Instability, lateral stenosis, and disk herniation at this level should be searched for on stress radiograms and the CT scan.

We have not attempted to reduce the subluxation. Recently we have been assessing the results of posterior interbody fusion for spondylolisthesis.[12]

SPINAL FUSION

The principles for successful arthrodesis apply to the spine as much as elsewhere.
1. Large areas of decorticated bone must be present at the site.
2. Cancellous bone graft must be abundant.
3. Bone contact and compression are desirable.
4. Immobilization must be prolonged until fusion has taken place.

POSTEROLATERAL FUSION

Techniques

If a posterior midline approach is used, a transverse cut is made in the dorsilumbar fascia without cutting the underlying paraspinal muscles. This facilitates the strong retraction that is necessary to expose the transverse processes as far as their tips. At the end of the operation, this transverse fascial incision is repaired and seems to cause no detectable defect (Fig. 16-33). Bone graft is taken from the posterior iliac crest through a separate oblique or transverse incision. In muscular or obese individuals this approach offers a restricted

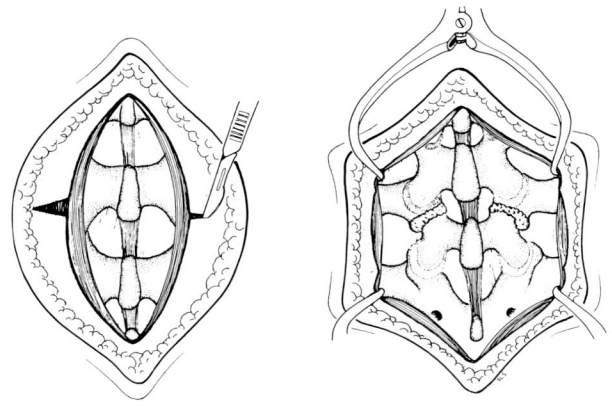

Fig. 16-33. Posterolateral fusion. A transverse cut in the dorsilumbar fascia permits strong retraction of the muscles to expose the transverse processes. The cuts are repaired before wound closure.

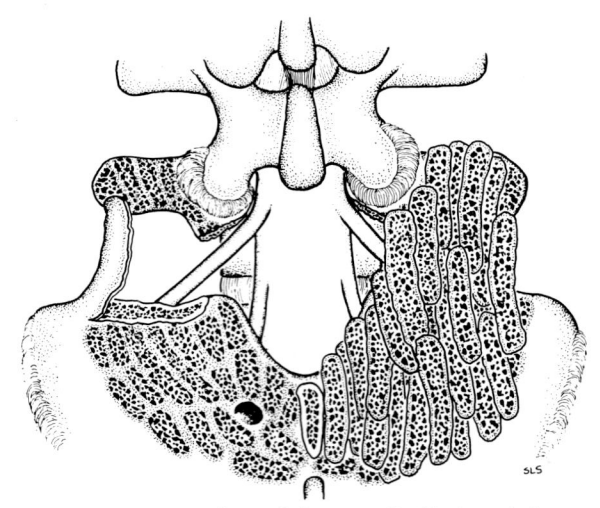

Fig. 16-34. Posterolateral fusion. (Left) Avoid damaging the posterior joint and sacroiliac joint during decortication. (Right) Avoid placing bone graft on exposed nerves.

view and is not recommended. If a bilateral paraspinal approach is used, one of the two incisions is used to harvest the bone graft from the posterior iliac crest. Thereafter the operation is the same. This approach is highly recommended.

The posterior articular and transverse processes are completely denuded of periosteum with an elevator. Care should be exercised during this procedure to avoid damaging the posterior joint at the level above the planned fusion. The dissection should extend to the tips of the transverse processes and should be kept in a plane posterior to the transverse processes, except for one maneuver that will now be described. Once the posterior surface of the transverse process is stripped, the anterior surface is stripped using a flat elevator with a peeling action starting at the superior edge of the transverse process. The instrument is kept constantly flat against the surface of the process. This extra stripping provides more bare bone and stimulates more new bone formation. However, the temptation to place bone graft anterior to the transverse processes should be resisted (Fig. 16-17). A sharp, curved gauge is used to raise "shingles" of cortico-cancellous bone on the posterior surface of the transverse process. The same process of denuding and shingling is done to the upper and posterior surface of the sacrum far laterally without interfering with the capsule of the sacroiliac joint. A generous block of bone is elevated from the flat upper surface of the lateral sacral mass. The graft is made long enough to span 2.5 cm to the L5 transverse process when it is hinged on itself. Free cancellous bone graft is then placed over and between the denuded surfaces. If a midline approach was used, a free fat graft is carefully trimmed, positioned, and sutured over the exposed dura to prevent encroachment onto the bone graft (Fig. 16-34).

Postoperative Care

The post operative care is the same as after diskectomy up to the 10th day. Then the sutures are removed and a body spika that extends from nipples down to the thigh on one side but permits free hip flexion on the other is applied with the patient standing. All patients should be able to walk in the spika with a cane or crutches. The spika is worn for 12 weeks and then a chair back brace is worn during the day until fusion occurs—usually an additional 8 weeks.

POSTERIOR LUMBAR INTERBODY FUSION

Cloward published clear step-by-step illustrations of this procedure, but we suggest that anyone planning to do this operation should first be taught by observing a practised operator.[12] He has designed a set of instruments, many of which are indispensable for the operation. The operation takes a long time, especially when autogenous bone graft is taken at the same session. Lin has described minor modifications to Cloward's operation.[13]

The advantage of this operation over anterior interbody fusion is that either diskectomy or decompression can be done through the same approach as the fusion. At least theoretically it is advantageous for the bone graft to be under compression. The possibility of posterior migration of the graft with serious consequence cannot be ignored, although this seems rare.

More epidural dissection, retraction, and cauterization is required than for other operations. The average spinal surgeon seeing the procedure for the first time may be taken aback by the amount of cauterization that is necessary to make the procedure possible. Postoperative perineural fibrosis is probably severe after the Cloward technique, but any role it may have in causing symptoms is uncertain. It may not be of consequence if a successful fusion eliminates movement at the operated level. Our experience is too recent to allow us to recommend this procedure.

Technique

This description is a little different from that of Cloward. The patient is positioned prone and an oversized bone graft is taken from the posterior iliac crest through a transverse incision. Use an oscillating power saw rather than osteotome to avoid cracks that weaken the graft. A posterior midline approach using a midline skin incision is made. If the fusion follows excision of a disk herniation, the canal is approached through the interlaminar space. For spondylolisthesis, the approach is made after the "rattler" has been excised. In either case we completely excise the ligamentum flavum.

When the operation is for disk disease, the interlaminar space is widened by removal of the superior and inferior margins of the adjacent laminae, partial medial facetectomy, and retraction with a laminar spreader. Epidural vessels are liberally cauterized and the charred remains are excised

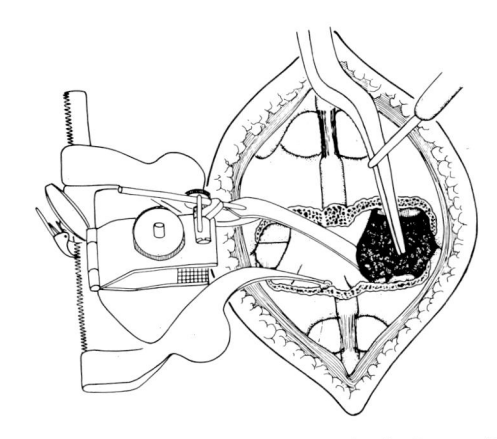

Fig. 16-35. Posterior lumbar interbody fusion. Epidural vessels are cauterized with cutting diathermy set at a low current. (After Cloward RB: The Cloward Technique. In Low Back Pain. 2nd Edition, Edited by Finneson BE. Philadelphia, JB Lippincott, 1980.)

with scissors. A self-retaining nerve root retractor is placed on the root and dura, which are retracted to the midline. The cauterized vessels are pushed aside to expose the annulus anteriorly. Bleeding vessels are pushed off with patties and packed temporarily with Gelfoam behind more patties. It is important not to proceed further until good hemostasis and good exposure of the annulus are obtained (Fig. 16-35). A rectangle of annulus is excised. The bony ledge or shelf of the posterior superior margin of the lower vertebral body that "overhangs" the interspace is removed with a narrow osteotome. The endplates and disk material are removed with alternate use of straight and curved osteotomes, curettes, and pituitary rongeurs. Bleeding from the endplates can be extensive and can require temporary packing with Gelfoam or Surgicel (Figs. 16-36 to 16-41). Blocks of cortico-cancellous bone taken from the iliac crest are cut to the measured size of the "disk space" and jammed into the space. The first grafts are moved medially to enlarge the laterally adjacent space so that the second or third graft can be inserted. This maneuver is carried out with a pair of blunt ended "chisels" using three maneuvers. The same is repeated on the opposite side. A free fat graft is sutured to nearby soft tissue to cover the dura (Figs. 16-42 to 16-47).

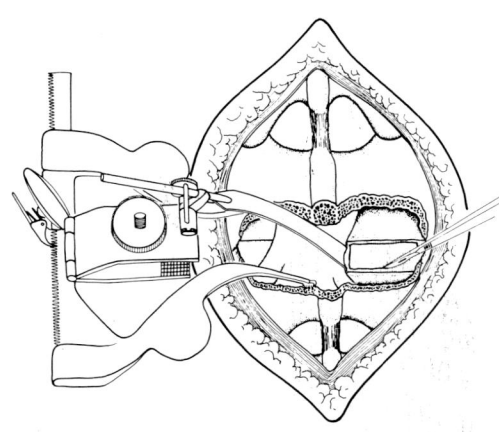

Fig. 16-36. Posterior lumbar interbody fusion. A window of posterior longitudinal ligament and annulus is excised. (After Cloward RB: The Cloward technique. In Low Back Pain. 2nd Edition. Edited by Finneson BE. Philadelphia, JB Lippincott, 1980.)

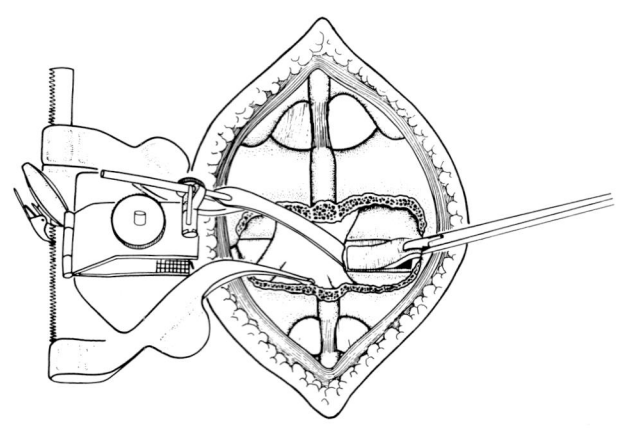

Fig. 16-37. Posterior lumbar interbody fusion. (After Cloward RB: The Cloward technique. In Low Back Pain. 2nd Edition. Edited by Finneson BE. Philadelphia, JB Lippincott, 1980.)

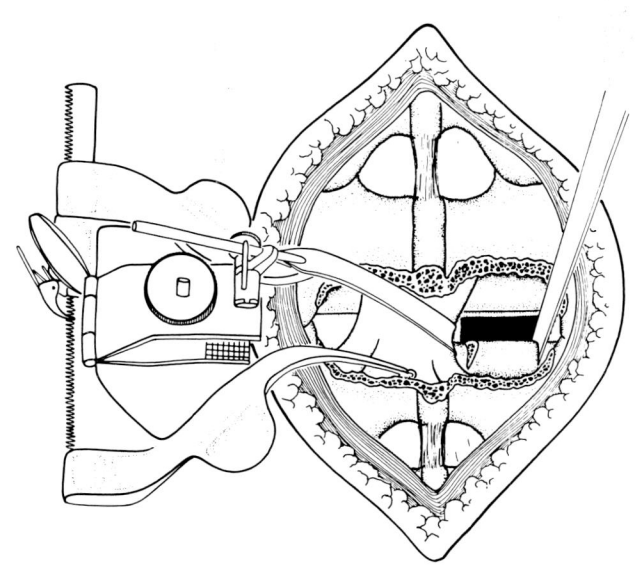

Fig. 16-38. Vertical cuts in the superior edge of the lower vertebra. (After Cloward RB: The Cloward technique. In Low Back Pain. 2nd Edition. Edited by Finneson BE. Philadelphia, JB Lippincott, 1980.)

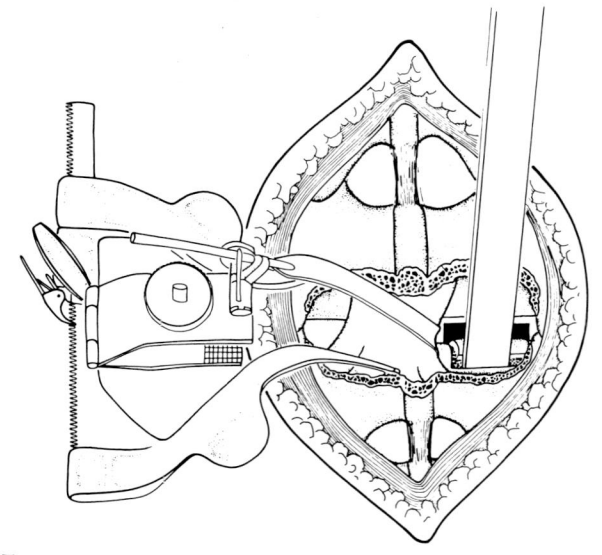

Fig. 16-39. The superior edge of the lower vertebra is removed. (After Cloward RB: The Cloward technique. In Low Back Pain. 2nd Edition. Edited by Finneson BE. Philadelphia, JB Lippincott, 1980.)

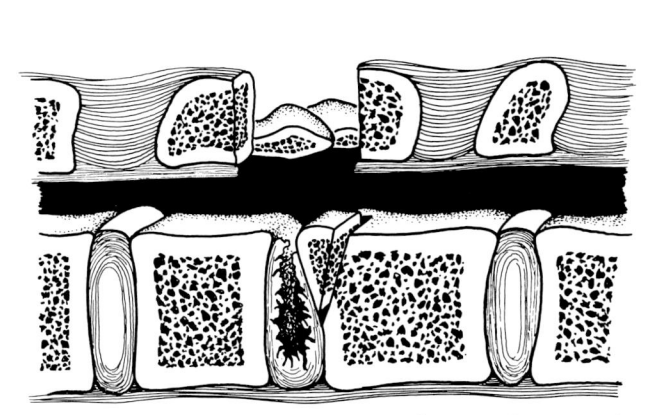

Fig. 16-40. The wedge of removed bone is shown. (After Cloward RB: The Cloward technique. In Low Back Pain. 2nd Edition. Edited by Finneson BE. Philadelphia, JB Lippincott, 1980.)

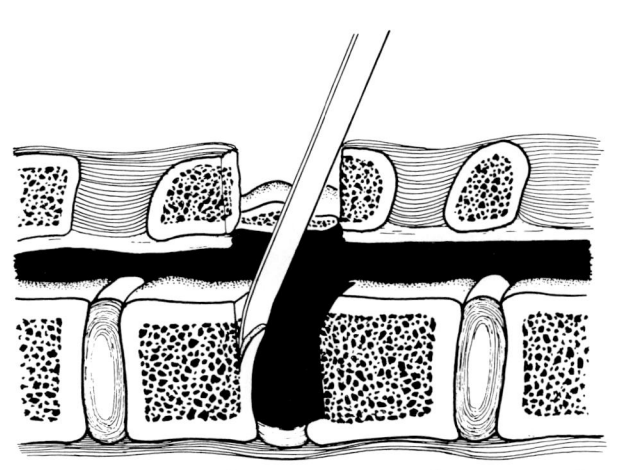

Fig. 16-41. A curved osteotome is used to remove the endplates. (After Cloward RB. The Cloward technique. In Low Back Pain. 2nd Edition. Edited by Finneson BE. Philadelphia, JB Lippincott, 1980.)

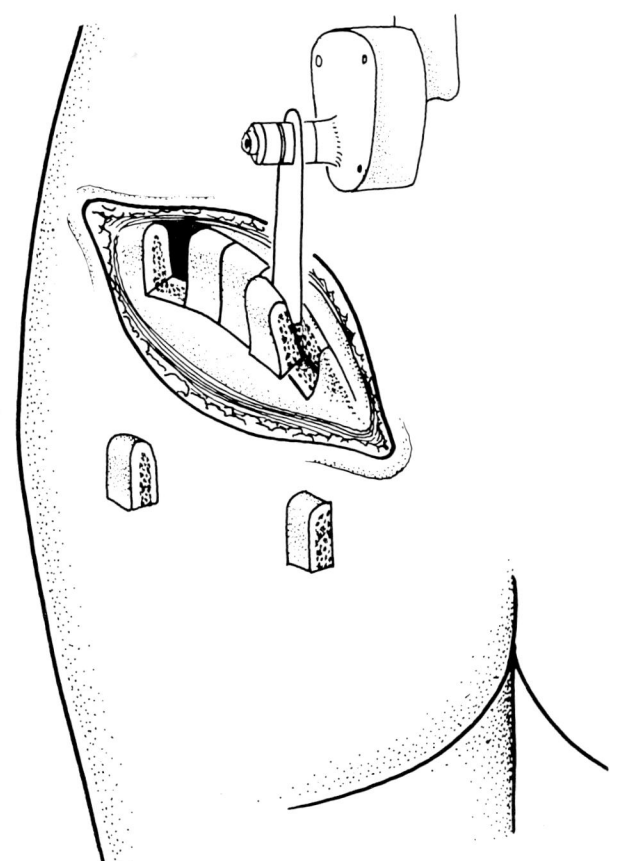

Fig. 16-42. Oversized partial and full thickness corticocancellous bone graft is removed with an oscillating saw through a separate skin incision.

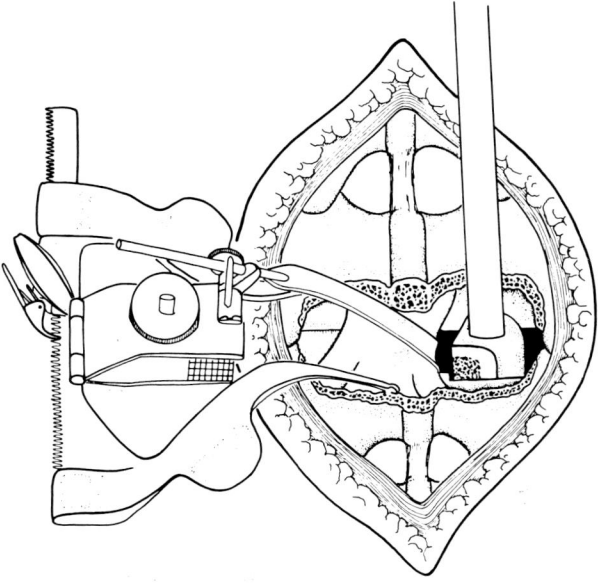

Fig. 16-43. A slightly oversized graft is punched into the space. (After Cloward RB: The Cloward technique. In Low Back Pain. 2nd Edition. Edited by Finneson BE. Philadelphia, JB Lippincott, 1980.)

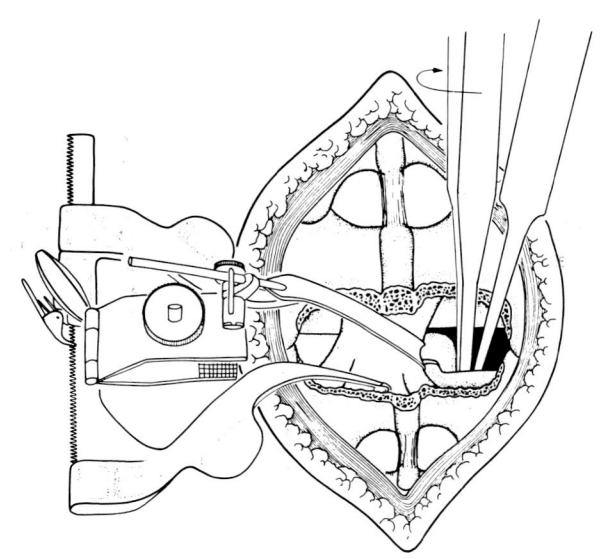

Fig. 16-44. The graft is moved medially with Cloward's blunt chisels.

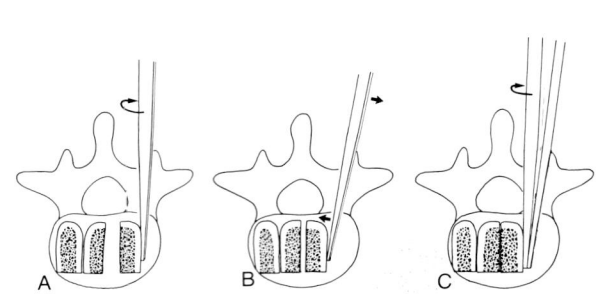

Fig. 16-45. Techniques for moving the graft medially. (A) Twisting. (B) Levering. (C) Twisting with a second chisel.

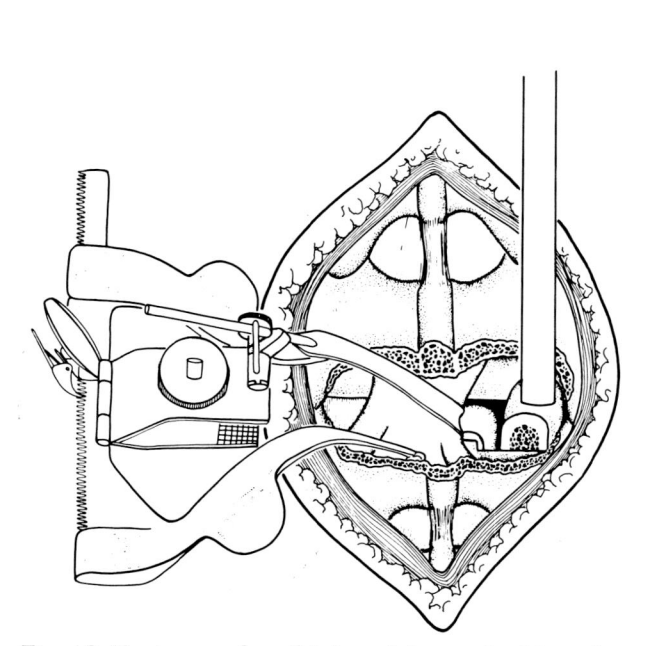

Fig. 16-46. A second or third graft is punched into the space. (After Cloward RB: The Cloward technique. In Low Back Pain. 2nd Edition. Edited by Finneson BE. Philadelphia, JB Lippincott, 1980.)

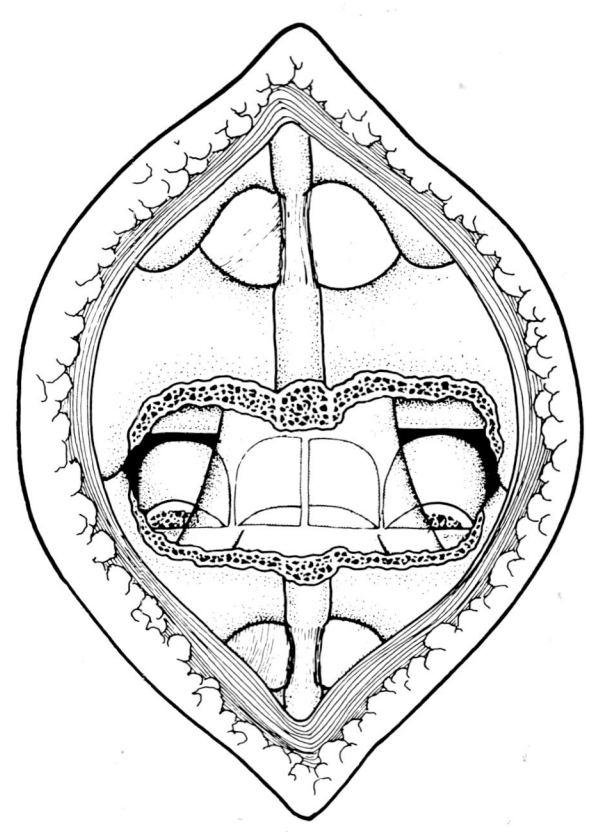

Fig. 16-47. The completed operation. (After Cloward RB: The Cloward technique. In Low Back Pain. 2nd Edition. Edited by Finneson BE. Philadelphia, JB Lippincott, 1980.)

Postoperative Care

Cloward does not recommend braces or casts when the procedure is for disk disease and recommends a chair type steel brace for 30 days for spondylolisthesis.

ANTERIOR INTERBODY FUSION

Technique

The help of two good assistants is important. An anterior retroperitoneal or transperitoneal approach is made. The aorta and its bifurcation are identified. When L5–S1 fusion is planned, two long narrow blunt-ended retractors are placed, one to retract the common iliac vessel and viscera to the right and the other to retract the iliac vessels to the left. The disk excision and grafting are carried out between these two retractors, which protect the vessels from damage. A flap of anterior longitudinal ligament and anterior annulus fibrosis hinged on the right is raised with a scalpel. When the disk space is extemely narrow, this step is impossible and instead a horizontal incision in the annulus is made (Fig. 16-48). The disk material is removed piecemeal under direct vision with curettes and pituitary rongeurs as far posterior as the posterior longitudinal ligament. Work on

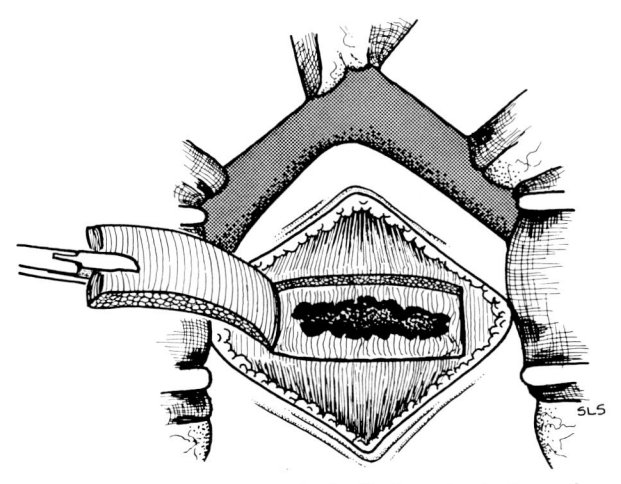

Fig. 16-48. Anterior interbody fusion. A window of annulus is incised and hinged to the patient's right.

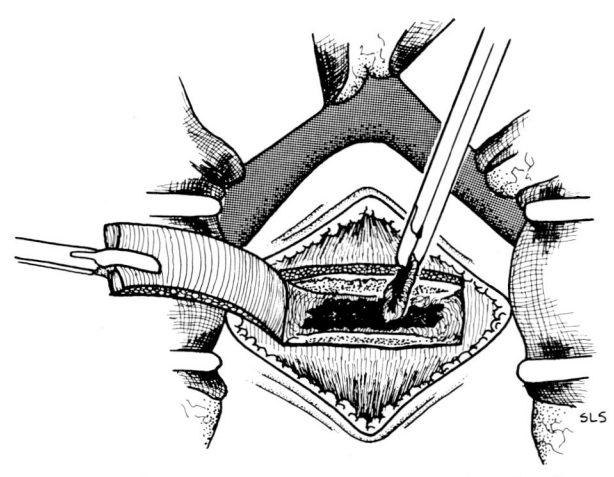

Fig. 16-49. The disk is removed piecemeal under direct vision with pituitary forceps. The endplates are removed with curved osteotomes.

the bone is postponed until the disk is completely cleared posteriorly and laterally. The endplates are then excised to bleeding cancellous bone using straight and curved osteotomes. Bleeding may be brisk and the space may have to be packed temporarily with Gelfoam or Surgicel (Figs. 16-49). Full thickness iliac crest grafts are then punched into the space. During their insertion, they are guided and stabilized by punches that are placed into the disk space to fill openings not yet filled with graft. Once the last graft is in place, all the grafts are counter-sunk 2 to 3 mm deep to the anterior edge of the vertebral body, and the break in the table is straightened to hold the grafts in between the vertebral bodies. The flap of anterior ligament and annulus is replaced and sutured with heavy Dexon (Figs. 16-50, 16-51).

To fuse L4–L5 or L3–L4 the lumbar spinal vessels above and below the disk are identified and ligated. The same retractors are used, one to retract to the right and protect the aorta and the other to retract the viscera in a cephalad direction. The disk excision and bone grafting are the same as described for the L5–S1 level.

At the end of the procedure the retroperitoneal space is drained with a closed suction tube drain and the abdominal muscle layers are closed with interrupted Dexon sutures.

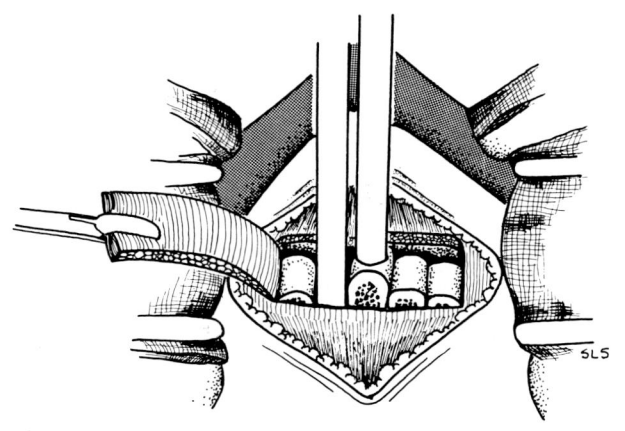

Fig. 16-50. Slightly oversized cortico-cancellous bone grafts are punched into the space. Punches in the unfilled spaces prevent the grafts from tilting during their insertion.

Postoperative Care

A nasogastric tube is routinely inserted and oral intake is delayed until bowel sounds return or flatus has been passed. The care is the same as for diskectomy except that a plaster spika that immobilizes the hip on one side is fitted to be worn continuously for 12 weeks. If the fit of the graft in the interspace is judged insecure, the patient is kept horizontal in an ordinary bed for 6 weeks. Log-rolling 45° each way is permitted. The patient is then permitted to walk in a plaster spika for 6 weeks.

DISKOGRAPHY

The indications for diagnostic lumbar disk injections are controversial. The most common indication we find is to assess the condition of the disk above a proposed spinal fusion (Fig. 16-52).

The resistance to the injection, the volume of fluid accepted, and the X-ray appearance are reliable criteria for differentiating between a normal and abnormal disk. We have not found any reliable indicators for distinguishing if a particular abnormal disk causes the complaints. In our experience, the patient's reports of pain on injection of saline, contrast fluid, or local anesthetic have not been as reliable as other authors claim.[14-16]

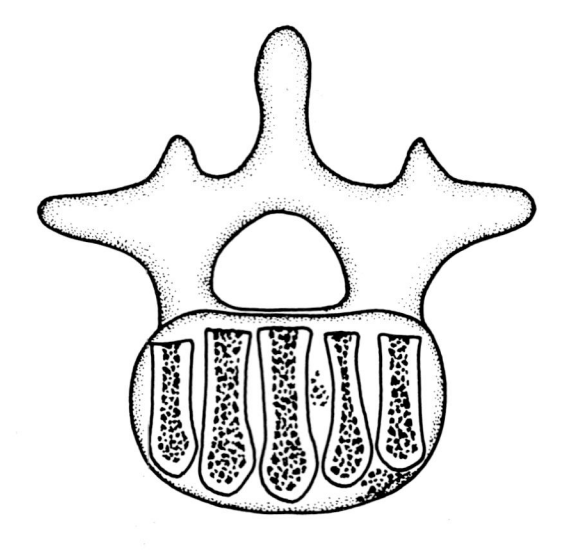

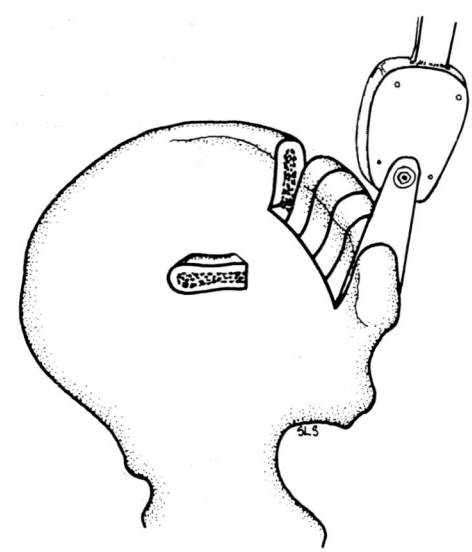

Fig. 16-51. Bone grafts are cut with a power saw to prevent cracks and are counter sunk behind the edge of the intervertebral space.

An abnormal disk accepts the injection with small resistance, a quality that is quickly learnt after only a few injections. The abnormal disk accepts more than 0.5 ml of fluid. Radiographs show that the contrast is confined to the center of the normal disk, though the shape may vary. The dye tracks extensively into the periphery of the abnormal disk, and outside the confines of the disk if the annulus is ruptured (Fig. 16-52).

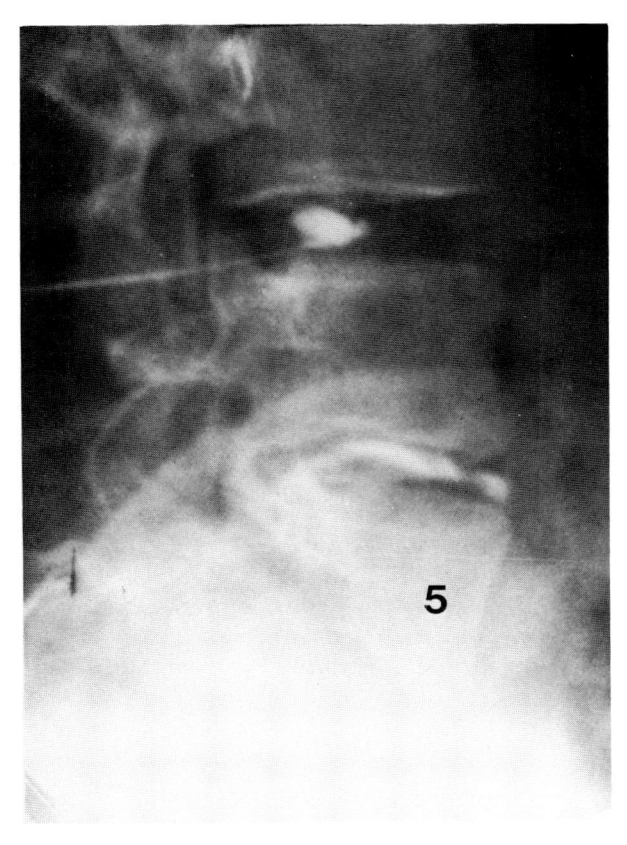

Fig. 16-52. A normal diskogram at L3–4 and an abnormal diskogram at L4–5. A fusion was planned for L5–S1 spondylolisthesis, but was extended one level higher.

Technique

After the patient is mildly sedated, the procedure is carried out in the Radiology Department under local anesthesia with aseptic technique and two-plane X-ray fluoroscopy guidance. It is helpful to have an articulated spine in the room at the time. The posterior midline transdural approach is easier and is used more often than the posterolateral extradural approach. For either approach, the patient is positioned on the side with a folded sheet placed under the flank to straighten the spine. The position is adjusted so that a true lateral and anteroposterior view of the spine is obtained before starting.

In the posterolateral approach, a 6-inch 18-gauge needle is inserted 8 cm lateral to the midline and is angled 45 to 60° toward the midline at the level of the disk. For the more difficult L5–S1 level it is often necessary to pierce the skin further from the midline (9 to 10 cm to avoid striking the posterior joint, which is larger and in a more lateral position.

The "bent needle" technique is useful if difficulty is encountered at the L5–S1 level.[17] A 4-inch 18-gauge needle is inserted 10 cm lateral to the midline and 60° to the sagittal plane. The needle is advanced and adjusted so that its tip is ajacent to the posterior aspect of the disk space. A 6-inch 22-gauge needle is then introduced through the lumen of the 18-gauge needle. The terminal ¾ inch of the 22-gauge needle is first bent so that the bevel lies on the convex side of the curve; thus when it emerges from the 18-gauge needle, it curves towards the disk space.

The needle direction is adjusted as necessary to place the tip equidistant from pedicles on the AP view and in the center of the disk equidistant from the endplates on the lateral view. When direction is changed, the needle tip must be withdrawn close to the skin before it is redirected and reinserted (Fig. 16-53). Renografin 60 is injected, and the fluoroscope is used to check that sufficient dye for a good image has been injected. The needle is removed and permanent lateral and AP films are made. The latter is taken with the patient supine with hips and knees flexed and the X-ray beam directed 20° cephalad.

In the posterior transdural approach, a 4-inch 18-gauge needle is inserted between the two spinous processes in the midline and advanced as far as the ligamentum flavum. The direction is adjusted as necessary. A 6-inch 22-gauge needle is passed through the shorter needle and its tip is advanced through the two layers of dura and into the disk. The remainder of the procedure is as described for the posterolateral approach.

CHEMONUCLEOLYSIS

Complications following chymopapain injection are rare, unpredictable, and potentially lethal. A repeat chymopapain injection is contraindicated in patients who have been injected previously.

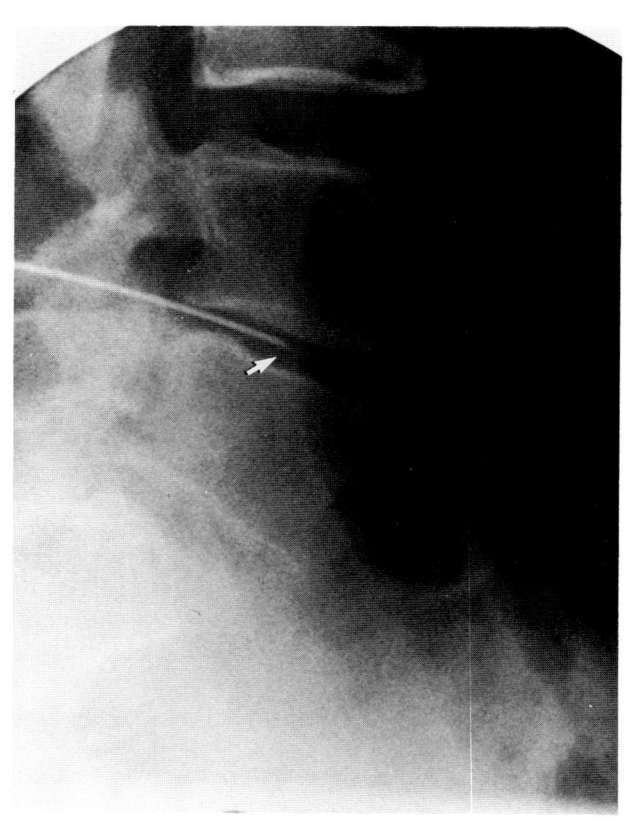

Fig. 16-53. Correct placement of the needle tip.

Technique

Until recently we gave the injection in the operating room under general anesthesia with endotracheal intubation. McCulloch has recently reported his large experience of chemonucleolysis under local anesthesia.[18] Anaphylactic shock can be diagnosed more rapidly in a conscious patient, and it can be treated more easily in the absence of the pharmacological effect of general anesthetic agents. We have since changed to using local anesthesia in our center.

Aseptic technique and two-plane image intensifier guidance are used. The posterolateral extradural approach (as described above for diskography) is always used to avoid penetrating the dura and prevent leakage of chymopapain into the subarachnoid space. Preparations are made before injection to treat a possible anaphylactic reaction. A secure intravenous line is established and pulse rate and blood pressure are monitored. Hydrocortisone, epinephrine, aminophylline, and diphenhydramine are immediately available. An anaesthetist with intubation and ventilation equipment must be present during the injection.

The use of contrast material is kept to a minimum. Only a drop or two is injected to confirm needle placement before the chymopapain injection. The chymopapain must be refrigerated up to the time of mixing with distilled water that has been at room temperature. The mixed solution must be used immediately and cannot be stored. The dosage is 4000 U or 2 ml per disk, injected over 3 to 4 minutes.

Postoperative Care

The patient is encouraged to be as active as pain permits. A stiff canvas corset, oral analgesics, and antiinflammatory drugs are prescribed. Many patients require a few days of in-hospital care and a few may require intramuscular narcotic analgesics.

SELECTIVE NERVE ROOT INJECTION

It is technically possible to inject all lumbar nerves and the first sacral nerve. This procedure is occasionally helpful to identify which particular spinal nerve is the cause of leg pain in patients who have no objective neurological deficit. It is especially useful in patients with vague symptoms and CT scan findings of borderline lateral stenosis at two or more levels. The L4, L5, and S1 nerves are the ones most commonly injected.

Information is obtained by irritating the nerve with the needle tip and contrast medium and then blocking the nerve with local anesthetic. The success in finding the target nerve is confirmed by a clear radiculogram and by a sensory or motor deficit that corresponds to the particular nerve. This requires repeated reexamination before and after each nerve block. The most reliable evidence is quadriceps weakness for L3, knee jerk loss for L4, weak toe extension for L5, and ankle jerk loss for S1. We have not been able to obtain reliable information concerning the nature of the particular pathological process from the dye outline or pattern.[19]

Before and after each root is injected, the patient is questioned and examined. In addition to sensory and motor tests, the range of spinal movement and straight leg raising is tested each time. This requires reprepping and redraping the skin before each nerve is injected. A great deal of patience and cooperation is required from the patient.

Technique

The procedure is carried out in the Radiology Department with two-plane image intensifier guidance under local anesthesia. Excessive preoperative sedation may reduce the patient's cooperation and invalidate the information. The patient is positioned prone with two folded sheets under the hips.

The needle placement is the same for all the lumbar nerves. The L5 nerve may require a technique similar to the "bent needle" technique described above. A 22-gauge needle is introduced 3 to 4 cm lateral to the midline, level with the spinous process. The needle is directed at 90° to the skin surface toward the base of the transverse process. When the needle is felt to strike the transverse process, the position is confirmed on AP and lateral views. The needle is retracted 1 cm and redirected caudad and medially. The needle tip is felt and seen to advance anterior to the transverse process and into the intervertebral foramen (Figs. 16-54, 16-55). The patient may experience radiating leg pain, and he is questioned about its character and distribution. Lateral and AP views should confirm that the needle tip is located immediately inferior to the pedicle. A 1 or 2 ml dose of 60% Conray is injected and the patient may experience pain again. AP films are taken and 2 to 3 ml of 1% lidocaine are injected. The leg pain disappears and the patient is stood up and examined (Fig. 16-56).

The S1 nerve requires a different approach through the S1 posterior foramen of the sacrum. The image intensifier and needle are directed 45° caudad to allow for the backward tilt of the sacrum. This view superimposes the posterior on the

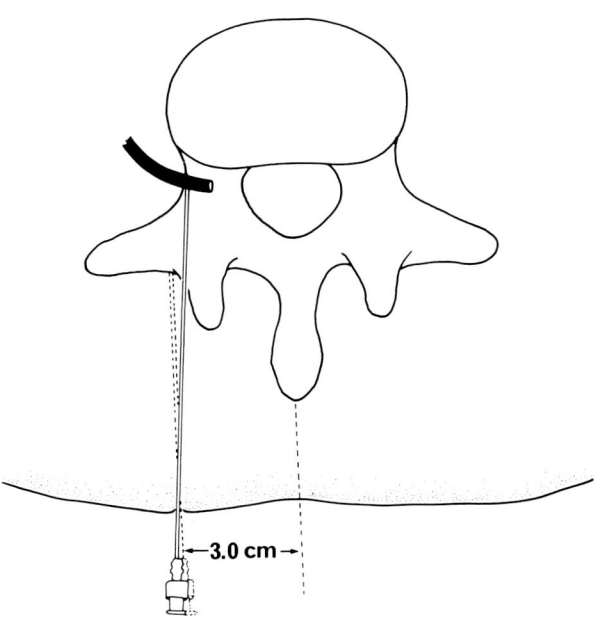

Fig. 16-54. Technique of selective lumbar spinal nerve block. (see text)

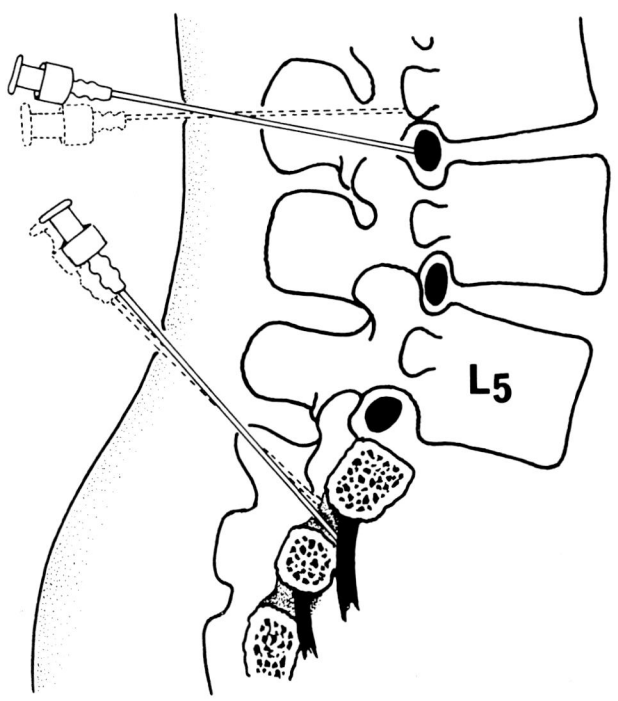

Fig. 16-55. Technique of selective third lumbar spinal nerve and first sacral nerve block. The sacrum has been cut away in a saggital plane through its anterior and posterior foramina.

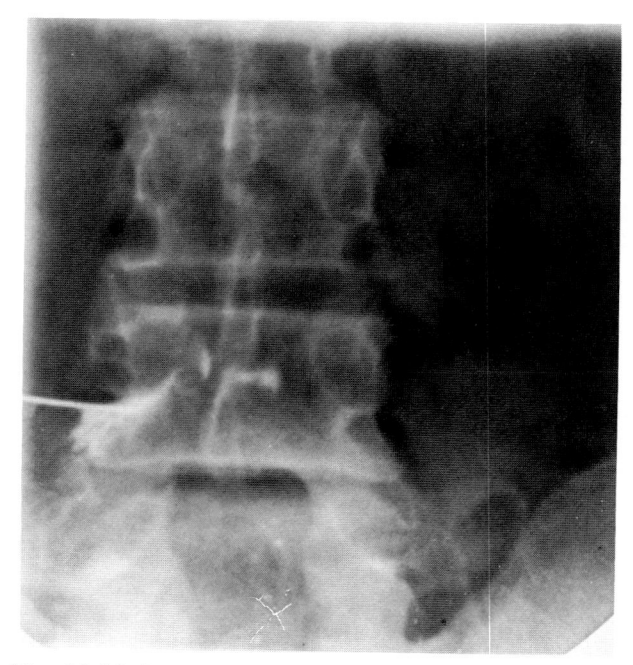

Fig. 16-56. L4 spinal nerve block. Needle placement and a radiculogram are shown.

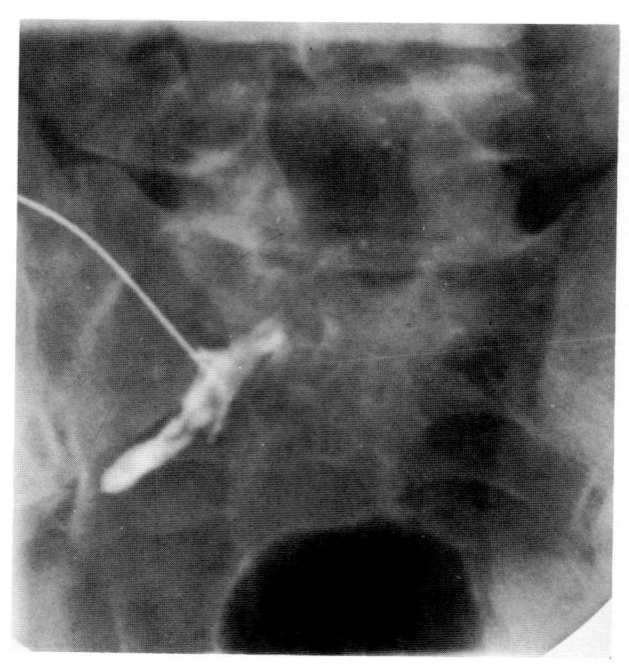

Fig. 16-57. S1 spinal nerve block. Needle placement and a radiculogram are shown. Patient had a previous L5 laminectomy.

anterior sacral foramina to produce a clearer image. The needle is introduced 2 to 2.5 cm lateral to the midline, level with the L5 spinous process. It is directed 45° caudad to contact the edge of the posterior sacral foramen. The needle is adjusted to enter the foramen, then advanced 2 cm so that its tip lies in the anterior foramen. X-ray confirmation is made and the contrast and local anesthetic are injected as described above (Figs. 16-55, 16-57).

No special postoperative care is necessary.

POSTERIOR JOINT INJECTION

Injecting the posterior joints is an easy procedure. The injection is placed around the joint capsule and sometimes probably into the joint cavity. At least two pairs and usually three pairs of joints are routinely injected, each with 12.5 mg prednisolone acetate (Meticortelone) and 5 ml of 0.25% bupivacaine (Marcaine).

The injection is carried out as an outpatient procedure in the Radiology Department under local anesthesia with fluoroscopy guidance. The patient is placed in the lateral position with folded sheets under the flank to straighten the spine. The skin entry points are infiltrated with a local anesthetic. A 4-inch 18-gauge needle is inserted level with the interspinous space 5 to 6 cm lateral to the midline. The needle is directed 60° to the skin towards the posterior joints until the needle tip encounters the bone of a facet. The needle tip position is confirmed with fluoroscopy. All the needles are positioned before the injection is made. If a needle has to be repositioned, its tip is retracted near to the skin before it is redirected and reinserted.

PIRIFORMIS INJECTION

The injection is placed in the belly of the piriformis muscle, just lateral to the edge of the sacrum and medial to the course of the sciatic nerve. Prednisolone acetate (Meticortelone) 25 to 50 mg and 0.25% plain bupivacaine 3 to 5 ml are injected

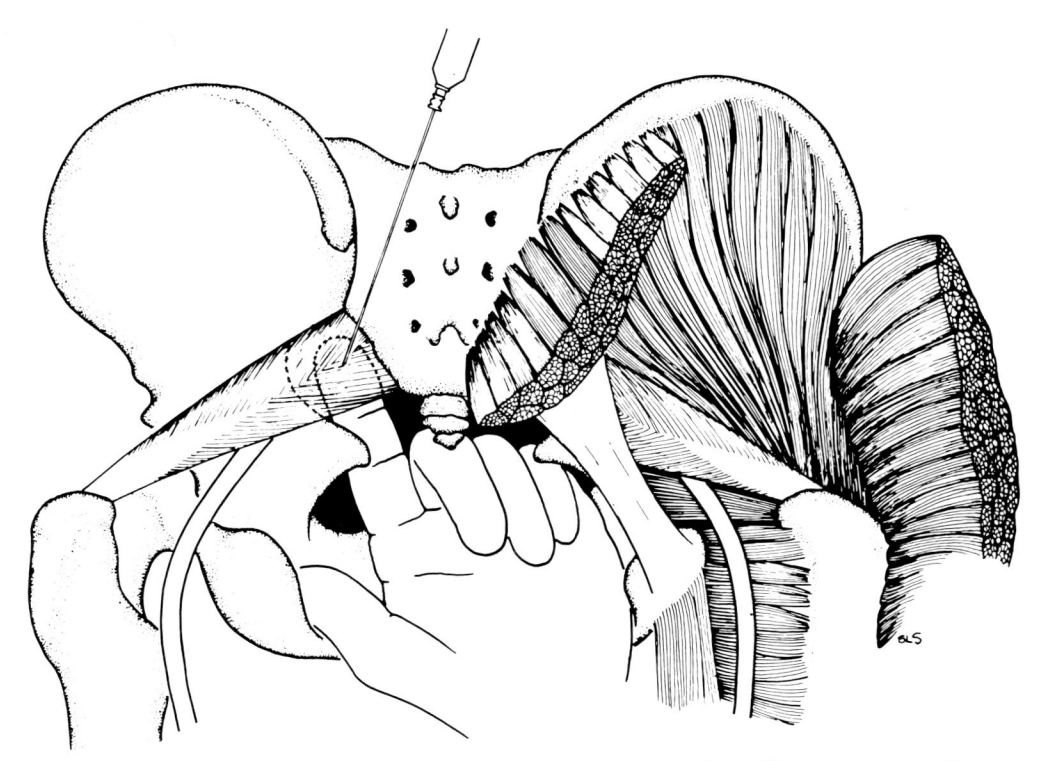

Fig. 16-58. Technique of piriformis injection. (After Wyant GM: Chronic pain syndromes and their treatment. III. The Piriformis Syndrome. Can Anaesth Soc J 20:305, 1979.)

under aseptic technique as an outpatient procedure.[20]

The patient is positioned on his side, with hips and knees flexed and the affected side uppermost. The skin is prepped and all drugs are drawn up in syringes before the next step. The physician then inserts the index finger of his (or her) nondominant hand into the rectum and palpates the lateral edge of the sacrum high in the sciatic notch. This will be the site of maximum tenderness. With the dominant hand, a 6-inch 20-gauge needle is directed perpendicular to the skin at a point on the buttock skin overlying the finger pulp in the rectum. The needle is advanced to stop 2 to 3 cm short of the finger pulp and the injection placed there. If the needle hub is repeatedly wiggled as it is advanced, the movement of the needle tip will be felt by the finger placed in the rectum, and in this way the physician can safely estimate the distance of the needle from the finger and avoid penetrating the rectal mucosa (Fig. 16-58).

REFERENCES

1. Yong-Hing K, Kirkaldy-Willis WH: Osteotomy of lumbar spinous process to increase surgical exposure. Clin Orthop 134: 218, 1978
2. MacNab I, Dall D: The blood supply of the lumbar spine and its application to the technique of intertransverse lumbar fusion. J Bone Joint Surg 53B: 628, 1971
3. Yong-Hing K, Reilly J, de Korompay V, Kirkaldy-Willis WH: Prevention of nerve root adhesions after laminectomy. Spine 5: 59, 1980
4. Rathke FW, Schlegel KF: Surgery of the Spine. Philadelphia, WB Saunders, 1979
5. Kirkaldy-Willis WH, Thomas G: Anterior approaches in the diagnosis and treatment of infections of the vertebral bodies. J Bone Joint Surg 47A: 87, 1965
6. Crock HV: Anterior lumbar interbody fusion: indications for its use and notes on surgical technique. Clin Orthop 165: 157, 1982
7. Goldner LJ, Wood KE, Urbaniak JR: Anterior lumbar discectomy and interbody fusion: indications

and technique, Current Techniques in Operative Neurosurgery. Edited by Schmidek HH, Sweet WH. New York, Grune and Stratten, 1977
8. Wiltse LL: The paraspinal sacrospinalis-splitting approach to the lumbar spine. Clin Orthop 91: 48, 1973
9. Hastings DE: A simple frame for operations on the lumbar spine. Can J Surg 12: 251, 1968
10. Kirkaldy-Willis WH, Wedge JH, Yong-Hing K, Tchang S, deKorompay V, Shannon R: Lumbar spinal nerve lateral entrapment. Clin Orthop 169: 171, 1982
11. Wiltse LL, Jackson DW: Treatment of spondylolisthesis and spondylolysis in children. Clin Orthop 117: 92, 1976
12. Cloward RB: The Cloward technique, Low Back Pain, 2nd Edition. Edited by Finneson BE. Philadelphia, JB Lippincott, 1980
13. Lin PM: A technical modification of Clowards posterior interbody fusion. Neurosurgery 1: 118, 1977
14. Cloward RB: Discography: technique, indications and evaluation of the normal and abnormal intervertebral disc. Am J Roent 68: 552, 1952
15. Simmons EH, Segil CM: An evaluation of discography in the localization of symptomatic levels in discogenic disease of the spine. Clin Orthop 108: 57, 1975
16. Wiley JJ, MacNab I, Wortzman G: Lumbar discography and its clinical applications. Can J Surg 11: 280, 1968
17. McCulloch JA, Waddel G: Lateral lumbar discography. Am J Rad, 51: 498, 1978
18. McCulloch JA: Chemonucleolysis: experience with 2000 cases. Clin Orthop 146: 128, 1980
19. Tajima T, Furukawa K, Kuramochi E: Selective lumbosacral radiculography and block. Spine 5: 68, 1980
20. Wyant GM: Chronic pain syndromes and their treatment, III. The piriformis syndrome. Canad Anaesth Soc J 26: 305, 1979

17 Psychological Treatment of Back Pain and Associated Problems

A. J. R. Cameron
L. F. Shepel
R. C. Bowen

Many psychological treatments for pain and disability have been developed recently.[1-7] Rather than attempting an exhaustive review, we shall present only basic information about psychological treatment approaches. Our goals are to describe very briefly the sorts of treatments psychologists or psychiatrists offer, and, as far as possible, to provide suggestions for management that can be implemented by physicians or surgeons.

Pain is a complex experience that incorporates sensory, behavioral, cognitive, and emotional elements. Therapeutic change in any of these domains may have a salutary effect. For heuristic purposes, we shall organize our chapter by considering in turn treatments designed to modify (1) sensory, (2) behavioral, (3) cognitive and (4) emotional aspects of pain and disability. In practice, of course, this compartmentalization is quite artificial, since any given treatment is likely to have a complex effect. For instance, patients who learn to reduce sensory discomfort may well report concomitant improvement in behavior, attitudes, and emotional state.

The most realistic goal of treatment often is to enable patients to cope more effectively with continuing discomfort and disability. It is frequently not possible to achieve the ideal outcome of complete, permanent relief. It is important to recognize this at the outset in order to avoid inflated expectations that may lead to disappointment and an unwarranted sense of failure. Learning to live more comfortably and normally is a good outcome, even if residual problems are present.

Many of the treatment techniques described below are educational in nature. The aim is to help patients find ways to help themselves. In general, this usually involves helping them learn how to avoid self-defeating patterns of thought and behavior, to respond more adaptively, and to create conditions conducive to their own well-being. Patients must become collaborative participants in the process if such treatments are to have any chance of success. A detailed discussion of strategies for establishing collaborative relationships with patients is available elsewhere.[4]

ALTERING PAIN SENSATIONS

Some interventions are designed to reduce physical discomfort. Relaxation training and transcutaneous electrical stimulation are the major treatments in this category.

Relaxation Training

Relaxation training appears to be effective in reducing a number of types of clinical pain.[5,8,9] The mechanism(s) of action is unclear. There are at least three possibilities, which are not mutually exclusive:

1. Muscle tension may cause or exacerbate pain; if so, relaxation of involved muscles should reduce pain.[10] However, no consistent relationship has been found between the amount of muscular relaxation achieved during training and the degree of subjective relief.[8,9]
2. Relaxation may result in a sense of serenity that increases the patient's sense of well-being.[11]
3. Relaxation training apparently induces changes in the sympathetic nervous system;[12] it is conceivable that unspecified alterations in the nervous system underlie the subjective sense of improvement.

Two methods of relaxation training, EMG biofeedback and progressive relaxation training, are used widely.

EMG Biofeedback. Attempts have been made to train people to relax muscles by providing them with ongoing information about EMG levels of target muscles.[8-10] Commercial equipment that transforms EMG readings into auditory or visual signals is available. The patient may, for instance, hear a clicking signal that increases in rate as EMG level rises and decreases as EMG level falls. The patient's task is to learn to relax with the assistance of this feedback.

This treatment has not been evaluated adequately with back problems. The limited available data suggest that while some back patients benefit considerably from this treatment[13,14] a substantial proportion do not.[11,15] Refinement in patient selection and treatment procedures could conceivably lead to more predictable results. However, at present the credibility of the approach is open to question since no consistent relationship has been found between EMG changes and subjective improvement.[8,9,11] Also, progressive relaxation training may be a more cost-efficient alternative to EMG feedback.[8,9]

Progressive Relaxation Training. Jacobson introduced progressive, or deep muscle, relaxation training.[16] A number of procedural variations have been developed.[17] All involve having the patient learn to relax major muscle groups throughout the body. Relaxation instructions[18] may be delivered by the therapist or by tape recording.

Progressive relaxation training appears to be used widely to treat patients with back pain. However, surprisingly little information exists about its effectiveness with this population.

A recent report describes results of treatment with 111 chronic low back patients.[19] The progressive relaxation training was supplemented with EMG biofeedback. The biofeedback was used "to help patients become more aware of excessive muscular activity in specific muscle groups, to concentrate on relaxing these muscle groups, and to increase motivation to practice general relaxation procedures." Patients learned to relax not only while reclining but also while sitting, standing, and walking. The average number of treatment sessions was 10.6. Biofeedback was faded gradually from the program, so that patients were relaxing without the equipment by the end of treatment.

Steps were taken to promote the use of relaxation skills in environments other than the immediate treatment situation. For instance, patients were asked to practice at least twice a day on their own using taped relaxation instructions. Also, they were given adhesive-backed dots to place in conspicuous places in their natural environment: these dots were to cue them to engage in a "mini-practice" technique, which involved relaxing while carrying on normal activities. Patients were encouraged to learn to relax first in situations where relaxation was relatively easy (e.g., while lying down), then to progress to relaxing under conditions that tended to increase pain (e.g., walking relatively long distances).

By the end of treatment, average pain ratings dropped 29%, 49.2% of patients decreased medication use, and 63.2% reported increased activity. EMG levels dropped with treatment, but patients with good outcomes did not have greater EMG reductions than those who responded poorly.

Comparison of good and poor responders revealed that the good responders had (1) fewer years of continuous pain, though they did not differ from poor responders in number of years since onset; (2) a lower incidence of multiple surgery; and (3) a lower incidence of disability payments. Good and poor responders did not differ in MMPI scores, incidence of psychiatric diagnoses, or anatomical plausibility of pain descriptions.[19]

Our clinical experience suggests that several

things can be done to enhance patients' involvement in relaxation training. First, if the original relaxation induction can be conducted under conditions that produce a marked result, this seems to increase the credibility of the procedure, thereby motivating the patient to both learn and use the skill. For instance, we have sometimes seen patients who reported that because of their pain they had had little sleep for several days, despite taking soporific medications; when a leisurely relaxation induction put them into a sound sleep, they were subsequently very impressed by and enthusiastic about the procedure. Second, asking patients to rate and record levels of subjective distress and serenity before and after relaxation may help to maintain a sense of progress even if residual discomfort remains. Third, patients wary of psychological formulations of their problems may be reassured by the introduction of supplementary EMG feedback: the equipment tangibly communicates the physical focus of the treatment.

Transcutaneous Electrical Stimulation

As the name suggests, transcutaneous electrical stimulation (TES) involves the application of electrical current using surface electrodes. Melzack found that among a group of patients with long-standing, intractable back pain, TES yielded an average pain decrease of 60%, although outcomes were variable and unpredictable.[20] Relief was sometimes short-lived, sometimes more enduring. Approximately 50% of patients seemed to experience continuing benefit 6 to 18 months after treatment ended. Greatest relief may be experienced by patients with minimal previous medical or surgical treatment.[21] Although TES seems to be used most commonly to treat chronic pain, a recent controlled study suggests that the technique may also be useful for helping to relieve postoperative pain among back patients.[22] TES seems to produce more pain relief than placebo.[20,23]

Clinical guidelines for TES therapy emphasize the need to explore different electrode placements with each patient. Melzack placed electrodes (1) over trigger zones (areas that trigger pain, identified through palpation) in the painful region; (2) over distant trigger zones (a map of trigger zones was used to search for these if no local zones were found); (3) over major peripheral nerves associated with the painful area; or (4) over acupuncture points. Melzack noted that there was considerable correspondence between trigger zones and acupuncture points designated for the same pain patterns and that these regions tended to lie over major sensory nerves. With the electrodes in place, voltage was increased gradually until the patient found it painful, then lowered slightly to a level that the patient thought would be tolerable for 20 minutes. Each treatment session lasted 20 minutes, with voltage adjusted up or down as necessary to maintain intense but tolerable stimulation. Most patients had one to three treatments per week; some had two sessions a day over 4 consecutive days. Some apparently had few treatments; others were treated over a period of weeks or months. Those who responded were allowed to borrow a stimulator for home use, with instructions to use it once daily for 20 minutes.

TES appears to be quite safe.[24] However, it has been recommended that the technique not be used with patients who have demand cardiac pacemakers or who are in the first trimester of pregnancy; also, electrodes should not be placed over the carotid sinus.[24]

The mechanism by which TES works is not understood, although there are a number of hypotheses.[20,25] For example, Melzack has speculated that the analgesic effect may result from the disruption of abnormal central neural activities related to chronic pain.[20] Evidence from animal experiments suggests that peripheral electrical stimulation may elicit enkephalins.[26]

REDUCING PAIN BEHAVIOR

An important treatment goal, in addition to pain relief, is to help the patient restablish or maintain a lifestyle that is as normal and satisfying as possible. Two general treatment strategies, not mutually exclusive, may be used to this end. The first, operant treatment, emphasizes the importance of creating an environment where "pain behaviors" are disregarded and "well behaviors" are actively encouraged. The second, adaptive response training, concentrates more on the patient than on the environment: it involves training the patient how to deal more effectively with personal difficulties.

Operant Treatment

Wilbert Fordyce and his colleagues developed a treatment program based on the principles of operant conditioning.[1,27] The basic premise of the program is that behaviors leading to positive consequences tend to persist or to increase in frequency, while behaviors that are followed by neutral consequences tend to decrease in frequency or even to disappear altogether. For instance, in a familiar application of these basic principles, it is often noted that if a child's temper tantrums pay off, they become more frequent; if ignored, they tend to become less frequent and usually stop entirely.

Formal operant treatment of pain patients is conducted on an inpatient basis over a period of weeks. Staff members are trained to ignore pain behaviors (e.g., complaints, wincing, groaning, limping); "well behaviors" (e.g., socializing, physical activity) are expected and systematically encouraged. Detailed records of ongoing progress are maintained for the benefit of patients and staff alike; Fordyce has published a detailed description of his program and procedures.[1]

The operant approach to detoxification is noteworthy. Medication is not provided on demand. This arrangement makes pain relief (a positive experience) contingent on pain complaints and may therefore serve to maintain or increase complaints. Instead, drugs are provided at fixed intervals. Medications are mixed with a flavored syrup in a "pain cocktail" that makes it possible to reduce active medication gradually without the patient's awareness (although the patient should know in advance what is planned and agree to the tapering).

Operant programs seem to result in improvement in difficult patients. For instance, Fordyce described results obtained with 36 patients who had had two to seven major operations for pain and who had had pain for 92.7 months on average. With treatment, average weekly "up-time" (i.e., time not reclining) increased from 59.2 hours to 88.9 hours; average daily walking distance doubled to more than a mile; use of analgesic medication dropped to approximately one-sixth of pretreatment levels. Patient follow-ups after discharge were encouraging, though incomplete. Results that are generally similar have been obtained in response to similar programs in other settings.

Although the cumulative results seem impressive, it is difficult to interpret the data with confidence.[6,28,29] For instance, all reports are based on uncontrolled outcome studies, with the exception of one very small scale controlled investigation.[30] Since operant programs have been used with other treatments (physiotherapy, vocational therapy, etc.), the absence of control groups makes it impossible to know how much of the apparent treatment effect is the result of the operant program itself.

There are drawbacks and limitations to operant treatment. It is costly, time consuming, and complex (despite its conceptual simplicity, all staff members in contact with the patient need to be cooperatively involved in the program). Although treatment seems to reduce pain behavior, patients still report considerable discomfort.[27] Finally, treatment gains may be reversed quickly if people interacting with the patient discontinue the systematic encouragement of normal behaviors.[30] Fordyce attempts to forestall such relapse by training members of the patient's family to respond selectively to normal behaviors.[1]

Even though it is not feasible to offer a formal operant program in many settings, it should be noted that the basic principles can be implemented in the context of other common treatments (Fordyce's book contains specific, practical suggestions). The general practice of systematically monitoring and encouraging gains in normal behavior, while carefully avoiding inadvertent encouragement of pain behaviors, appears prudent.

Adaptive Response Training

Patients sometimes appear to be engaging in self-defeating patterns of behavior that exacerbate their general malaise or deprive them of rewarding experiences. In such cases, treatment may focus on establishing more adaptive behavior patterns. In recent years, psychologists have become interested in the therapeutic value of training in basic adaptive skills (e.g., effective communication strategies, general problem-solving skills).[31] The potential role of adaptive response training can be illustrated in relation to two problems commonly experienced by back patients, namely, social inhibition and insomnia.

People who feel shy, insecure, sexually inadequate, etc. may discover that their pain enables them to avoid stressful situations in a socially acceptable way. If such patients can acquire the skill and confidence required to deal directly with stressful situations, they may benefit considerably. For example, a recent patient reported that she had difficulty refusing unreasonable requests. In the past, she had found herself yielding to pressures to take on commitments that she resented and worried about. She also had trouble resisting demands from her family, especially her aging parents who lived nearby. After she developed pain, however, she discovered that she was asked to do less and others were willing to help more. Her pain seemed to serve to fend off others and enlist their cooperation without her appearing to be "offensive" or "selfish." The treatment program included training in how to be directly assertive in ways that would be satisfactory both to her and to those with whom she interacted. The value of training pain patients to respond more effectively in social relationships has not been systematically evaluated. However, a follow-up of 81 patients treated in a rehabilitation program revealed that those who improved were more likely to have received assertive skill training than those who had not improved.[32]

Insomnia. Adaptive responding may also be used in the treatment of insomnia, a common complaint among patients with back pain. People who experience insomnia may exacerbate their sleep difficulties in a variety of ways. For instance, they may compensate for lost sleep by napping through the day or by oversleeping in the morning, so that they are not tired at bedtime. Sleep difficulties have been treated with some success by training poor sleepers how to establish routines, skills, and conditions conducive to a normal sleep pattern.[33-35] The following guidelines, for instance, have been recommended:[33]

1. Lie down to sleep only when sleepy.
2. Do not do anything (aside from sexual activity) in bed except sleep.
3. If you are not asleep within 15 minutes after getting into bed, get up and leave the bedroom.
4. If still unable to sleep, repeat Step 3 as often as necessary.
5. Set the alarm for the same time every morning and get up then, regardless of how much sleep time was achieved.
6. Avoid daytime naps.

It may also be prudent to avoid caffeine and alcohol before retiring.

Adaptive response training may serve to enhance the general quality of the person's life even if there is no clear evidence that the pain or associated problems are being aggravated by maladaptive behavior patterns. For instance, we have sometimes worked with patients who were interested in improving relationships or in personal productivity. Although no demonstrable decrease in pain or pain behavior occurred, some of these people reported that it was satisfying to have a positive focus and to see evidence of constructive change in their lives. They hurt as much as ever and had to continue restricting activities, but somehow, in the overall context of their lives, these things seemed to bother them less.

THE PATIENT'S THOUGHTS AS A FOCUS FOR TREATMENT

The way the patient thinks about problems may influence the way he or she feels and behaves. Our main objectives are to promote realistic thinking and a sense of personal control.

Encouraging Realistic Expectations and Attitudes

Patients' expectations and attitudes may affect treatment response, whether the treatment is physical or psychological.

Those who have unrealistically optimistic expectations about treatment may be disappointed with what would normally be regarded as a good outcome if there are lingering problems that they hadn't anticipated. Similarly, those who have serious reservations about treatment (e.g., those who are unusually apprehensive about surgery because they have known people whose operations seemed to worsen their problems) may overreact to residual difficulties if these are misinterpreted as evidence that the treatment really was ill-conceived. Patients with misgivings about proposed treatments may be reluctant to express them unless they are actively encouraged to discuss questions or concerns.

Realistic expectations can be promoted through careful pretreatment discussion of the probable outcome of successful treatment, with emphasis on any residual difficulties or limitations that are likely. Patients who are very apprehensive may gain confidence if they are encouraged to get a second opinion or given an opportunity to talk to patients sucessfully treated with the procedure.

Misinterpretations that lead patients to overestimate the severity of their problems also cause difficulties occasionally. A rather dramatic case illustrates this point. A man was admitted to a surgical ward for nonsurgical treatment. He was a source of concern because he was subdued, withdrawn, and appeared to be surprisingly incapacitated. During the course of a long interview he eventually said that he was distressed because he was receiving what he erroneously perceived to be mere palliative treatment rather than "corrective surgery." He had misconstrued all this as meaning that he was beyond surgical help ("I guess they can't operate or they'll paralyze me or something") and on a degenerative course. Unearthing and correcting such misunderstandings may have therapeutic value.

Patients who make sinister misinterpretations of their symptoms may sometimes benefit from structured opportunities to engage in experiences that invalidate their fears. For instance, an athletic middle-aged woman who had surgery discovered that her back subsequently bothered her when she was active. She saw this as evidence that she had a permanent disability that would make it impossible to engage in vigorous activity, so she gave up sports. She became reclusive and depressed, since much of the personal recognition and social contact she received came through participation in athletic competition. We encouraged her to attribute her activity-related discomfort provisionally to being out of shape and urged her to see if it could be relieved by systematically working back into good condition. She resumed athletic activities gradually, under supervision, and was soon fully active with minimal discomfort. The improvement had been maintained at a two year follow-up. Graduated resumption of normal activities with reassuring supervision appears to be a useful strategy for managing patients who are overly cautious and self-restricting.

Fostering a Sense of Control

Patients whose pain and disability cannot be eliminated may feel overwhelmed, helpless, and desperate. There is evidence that a sense of helplessness in the face of adversity may have wide-ranging debilitating effects.[36,37] People who believe that they can do nothing about their difficulties tend to give up. The less they do to help themselves, the worse the problems become, and the more overwhelmed and hopeless they feel. This can become a vicious cycle.

A major challenge of rehabilitation is to reverse or forestall this cycle, to promote a sense that patients can, indeed, take effective action on their own behalf. Much psychological research is currently being devoted to clarifying the processes involved in the development of self-efficacy.[38,39] Although a detailed discussion of this work is not possible here, it would appear that at a gross level of analysis two conditions must be met before patients can be expected to help themselves.

First, they must recognize that there is something constructive they can do. Pain and disability tend to be seen as medical problems requiring professional treatment. It may not be evident to patients that they themselves often have it within their power to reduce their own discomfort and to counteract secondary psychological or interpersonal difficulties. Any psychological (e.g., relaxation training) or other rehabilitative treatment (e.g., physiotherapy exercises) that explicitly equips them to help themselves has the potential to enhance their morale and sense of control. Making such treatments available, and presenting them with enthusiasm, may boost the patient's morale and lay the groundwork for self-help behavior.

Second, given that patients have the capacity to respond effectively, and recognize this, they must put this capacity to use by actually engaging in efforts to help themselves. Clear evidence of progress may be the best spur to continued effort and confidence.[38] A sense of progress may be engendered by setting realistic, attainable goals (e.g., walking progressively longer distances beginning with a distance well below potential and increasing slowly and steadily). Modest, specific, short-term goals (e.g., to walk a half mile this morning) are more likely to be useful in this process than more ambitious, vague, long-term goals (e.g., to be back to normal by the end of June).[40] Once initiated, continued progress may be encouraged by keeping records of daily accomplishments: patients who continue to experience diminished walking endurance, for instance, are less likely to become discouraged if they have authentic evidence that walking endurance has been increasing steadily. It may be advantageous to monitor positive (how much the patient was able to accomplish) rather than negative (level of discomfort or amount of continuing restriction) indexes of progress, since the latter may contribute to preoccupation with pain.

Stress inoculation training[4,41,42] refers to a treatment strategy specifically designed to establish and promote self-help capabilities and a sense of control. Patients go through an educational or conceptualization phase, during which they carefully examine their own experiences with pain. The data of their own experiences are then used to educate them, in a collaborative way, about the complex nature of pain. This is followed by a skills acquisition and rehearsal phase, which involves having patients learn and practice strategies for coping with the various aspects of the pain experience. Finally, there is an application phase during which the patient gains experience testing out the skills in pain-engendering situations under clinical supervision. More detailed descriptions of this approach are available elsewhere.[4,41] Laboratory studies[4,42] and an uncontrolled clinical trial with chronic headache patients[43] suggest that the treatment procedures hold promise.

TREATMENT OF NEGATIVE EMOTIONAL STATES

People who experience back pain are often depressed, anxious, or irritable. These dysphoric emotional states may warrant treatment, especially if they are pronounced. It is common to regard mistakes in diagnosing a physical lesion as a grave error but to view mistakes in diagnosing depression or anxiety as a trivial matter. The correct diagnosis and management of negative affect is an important issue, because the complaint of chronic pain is as likely to be a symptom of a psychiatric disorder as that of a physical problem.[3,44] Pharmacological treatment should be considered if the emotional problem appears to have a biological basis.

Depression

It is agreed that depression and pain are closely associated,[3,44,45] but there is no consensus about the proportion of pain patients who are clinically depressed and require treatment. The figures vary from a low of 10%[46] to a high of 100%.[45] At least one-half of psychiatric patients complain of pain and in approximately one-half of these the pain is a presenting complaint.[3] Most studies have found that the back is the most common or the second most common site of pain in patients with psychiatric problems.[3] It is unclear whether depression and chronic pain are manifestations of an underlying psychobiological disorder[47] or whether the depression is secondary to the pain problem. Chronic pain does lead to despondency and despair, but chronic pain patients may deny or minimize depression,[47] "Sure I'm depressed, Doc, you'd be too, if you had this pain as long as I have."[48] Antidepressant drugs are not likely to help unless evidence of the biological depressive syndrome is present.

Indicators of a biological depressive syndrome are

1. Changes in appetite and weight, sleep changes, a diurnal mood fluctuation, anergia and lassitude, and the inability to feel pleasure
2. A positive family history for depression or alcoholism[49]
3. A history of spontaneous remissions and exacer-

bations, since most chronic affective disorders run a cyclic course
4. A previous history of depression or of response to antidepressants or electroconvulsive therapy

Choice of Drug. More than ten antidepressants are now available and several more will be marketed in the near future; no single drug may be the best for all patients. Amitriptyline (SK Amitryptyline), one of the older drugs, has been the most widely used, and because it is available as a syrup, it is contained in the "pain cocktails" of many pain clinics. Its sedative side effects may be an advantage, but the effect on cardiac conduction and the prominent anticholinergic side effects are relative disadvantages.

Chloripramine (Anafranil) is a selective serotonin re-uptake inhibitor, and there are theoretical reasons for using this drug that relate to serotonin-mediated pain-inhibitory pathways. Theory has been supported by a few empirical studies.[51] A disadvantage is that chloripramine produces motor restlessness in a small proportion of patients. Alternative drugs are doxepin (Adapin, Sinequan) (quite sedative with less of a cardiac conduction effect) and desipramine (Norpramin, Pertofrane) (few anticholinergic side effects and less tendency to produce postural hypotension).

The dosage range and side effects are similar for all four of these drugs. Start with a daily divided dose of 30 to 75 mg and gradually increase this over 2 weeks to 150 mg a day. Older patients are more sensitive to side effects and usually reach therapeutic serum levels at doses of 75 to 100 mg a day. Some authors suggest that the therapeutic response is improved if a neuroleptic is used concurrently, and perphenalzine (Trilafon) 2 mg or fluphenazine (Moditen) 2 mg two or three times a day could be tried.[52,53] There is some theoretical support for the use of these drugs related to the effect of dopaminergic neurons on pain perception.[54] The risks of inducing tardive dyskinesia should be considered.

Some studies have reported very favorable results from treating chronic pain patients with antidepressants[44,50] and others disappointing results.[55] If improvement does not occur in 3 to 6 weeks, referral to a psychiatrist familiar with the management of chronic pain patients might be considered. Issues to pursue include the use of recent drugs, the determination of serum levels, tests for biological markers of depression,[56] and the use of lithium carbonate or monoamine oxidase inhibitors.[57]

Anxiety

Most studies have found that anxiety problems are almost as common in chronic pain patients as depression.[55] When the anxiety is generalized, training in relaxation techniques and adaptive response training are recommended. The benzodiazepines (diazepam, chlordiazepoxide, etc.) should be prescribed only for short periods of a few weeks, and are most useful when there is a situational cause for the anxiety (e.g., surgery). They do not help patients to learn how to cope, and they may be habituating.[58] They are also not generally indicated for patients with panic attacks.

Panic attacks are discrete episodes of severe anxiety that approach terror; they usually last for a few minutes but may last longer and are accompanied by many of the psychophysiologic symptoms of anxiety such as palpitations, chest pain, shortness of breath, and symptoms of hyperventilation. Some patients with panic attacks go on to develop multiple fears and restrictions in mobility and then use pain as the reason for their restriction to bed or home. These patients fear that too much effort or leaving a place of security will precipitate a panic attack. Relatively small doses of imipramine (Tofranil) (a tricyclic antidepressant, up to 75 mg a day) or phenelzine (Nardil), (a monoamine oxidase inhibitor, up to 45 mg a day) have a blocking effect against the occurrence of panic attacks.[59]

We do not intend to suggest that these drugs should be used in isolation. In fact, they may be more effective if used in conjunction with psychological techniques including those mentioned above. Even though negative affect such as depression and anxiety may be associated with the development of pain, changes in coping patterns, life style, and relationships (i.e., chronic pain behaviors) may become established in their own right. One should not assume that these problem behaviors will necessarily disappear just because the negative affect has been treated with psychotropic drugs.

Psychological Treatment of Depression and Anxiety

Psychological treatment of severe, chronic depression or anxiety is likely to require the services of staff with specific training. Since such treatment is not likely to be provided by surgeons or family physicians, it will not be described in detail here, except to say that treatment often is focused on establishing adaptive patterns of thought and behavior. Although the efficacy of psychological treatments for depression is still being evaluated, the early evidence suggests that psychological treatment can compare favorably with antidepressant medication.[60]

A PERSPECTIVE ON PSYCHOLOGICAL TREATMENT

The preliminary evidence that is available suggests that psychological and psychiatric treatments may be useful for managing patients with back pain. Although a scientific literature is developing, current clinical practice often goes beyond well established findings. It is to be hoped that, whenever possible, rehabilitative programs will be structured so that they permit reasonable evaluation of the treatments offered. A self-critical approach appears prudent if we are to be self-correcting (i.e., to ensure that management programs are revised on an ongoing basis to enhance their efficacy and economy).

ACKNOWLEDGMENT

We are grateful to C. Barr Taylor for his valuable comments on an earlier draft of this material.

REFERENCES

1. Fordyce WE: Behavioral Methods for Chronic Pain and Illness. St Louis, CV Mosby, 1976
2. Roy R, Tunks E, (Eds): Chronic Pain: Psychosocial Factors in Rehabilitation. Baltimore, Williams & Wilkins, 1982
3. Sternbach RA: Pain Patients: Traits and Treatment. New York, Academic Press, 1974
4. Turk, D, Meichenbaum D, Genest M: Pain and Behavioral Medicine. New York, Guilford Press, in press.
5. Turner JA, Chapman CR: Psychological interventions for chronic pain: a critical review 1. Relaxation training and biofeedback. Pain 12: 1, 1982
6. Turner JA, Chapman CR: Psychological interventions for chronic pain: a critical review 2. Operant conditioning, hypnosis, and cognitive-behavioral therapy. Pain 12; 23, 1982
7. Weisenberg M: Pain and pain control. Psychol bull 84: 1008, 1977
8. Jessup BA, Neufeld, WJ, Mersky H: Biofeedback therapy for headache and other pain: an evaluative review. Pain 7: 225, 1979
9. Turk DC, Meichenbaum DH, Berman WH: Application of biofeedback for the regulation of pain: a critical review. Psychol. Bull. 86: 1322, 1979
10. Budzynski TH, Stoyva JM, Adler CS: Feedback-induced muscle relaxation: application to tension headache. J Behav Ther Exp Psychiatr 1: 205, 1970
11. Hendler N, Derogatis L, Avella J, Long D: EMG biofeedback in patients with chronic pain. Dis Nerv Sys 38: 505, 1977
12. Hoffman JW, Benson H, Arns PA, et al: Reduced sympathetic nervous system responsivity associated with the relaxation response. Science 215: 190, 1982
13. Gentry WD, Bernal GAA: Chronic pain, Behavioral Approaches to Medical Treatment. Edited by Williams RB, Gentry WD. Cambridge, Mass, Ballinger, 1977
14. Nigel AJ, Fischer-Williams M: Treatment of low back strain with electromyographic biofeedback and relaxation training. Psychosomatics 21: 495, 1980
15. Peck CL, Kraft GH: Electromyographic biofeedback for pain related to muscle tension: a study of tension headache, back, and jaw pain. Arch Surg 112: 889, 1977
16. Jacobson E: Progressive Relaxation. Chicago, University of Chicago Press, 1938
17. Borkovec TD, Sides J: Critical procedural variables related to the physiological effects of progressive relaxation: a review. Behav Res Ther 17: 119, 1979
18. Ferguson JM, Marquis JN, Taylor CB: A script for deep muscle relaxation. Dis Nerv Syst 38: 703, 1977
19. Keefe FJ, Block AR, Williams RB, Surwit RS: Behavioral treatment of chronic low back pain: clinical outcome and individual differences in pain relief. Pain 11: 221, 1981
20. Melzack R: Prolonged relief of pain by brief, intense transcutaneous somatic stimulation. Pain 1: 357, 1975

21. Wolf SL, Gersh, MR, Rao VR: Examination of electrode placements and stimulating parameters in treating chronic pain with conventional transcutaneous electrical nerve stimulation (TENS). Pain 11: 37, 1981
22. Schuster GD, Infante MC: Pain relief after low back surgery: the efficacy of transcutaneous electrical nerve stimulation. Pain 8: 299, 1980
23. Thorsteinnson G, Stonnington HH, Stillwell GK, Elveback LR: The placebo effect of transcutaneous electrical stimulation. Pain 5: 31, 1978
24. Rosenberg M, Curtis L, Bourke DL: Transcutaneous electrical nerve stimulation for the relief of postoperative pain. Pain 5: 129, 1978
25. Callaghan M, Sternbach RA, Nyquist JK, Timmermans G: Changes in somatic sensitivity during transcutaneous electrical analgesia. Pain 5: 115, 1978
26. Woolf CJ, Barrett GD, Mitchell D, Myers RA: Naloxone-reversible peripheral electroanalgesia in intact and spinal rats. Eur J Pharmacol 45: 311, 1977
27. Fordyce W, Fowler R, Lehmann J, et al: Operant conditioning in the treatment of chronic clinical pain. Arch Phys Rehab 54: 399, 1973
28. Cameron R: Behavior and cognitive therapies. Chronic Pain: Psychosocial Factors in Rehabilitation. Edited by Roy R, Tunks E. Baltimore, Williams & Wilkins, 1982
29. Turk DC, Genest M: Regulation of pain: the application of cognitive and behavioral techniques for prevention and remediation. Cognitive-Behavioral Interventions: Theory, Research, and Procedures. Edited by Kendall PC, Hollon SD. New York, Academic Press, 1979
30. Cairns D, Pasino JA: Comparison of verbal reinforcement and feedback in operant treatment of disability due to low back pain. Behav Ther 8: 621, 1977
31. Goldfried M: Psychotherapy as coping skills training, Psychotherapy Process. Edited by Mahoney MJ. New York, Plenum, 1980
32. Morgan CD, Kremer E, Gaylor M: The behavioral medicine unit: a new facility. Compr Psychiatry 20: 79, 1979
33. Bootzin RR, Nicassio PM: Behavioral treatments for insomnia, Progress in Behavior Modification, Vol 6. Edited by Hersen M, Eisler RM, Miller PM. New York, Academic Press, 1978
34. Borkovec TD: Insomnia. Behavioral Approaches to Medical Treatment. Edited by Williams RB, Gentry WD, Cambridge, Mass, Ballinger, 1977
35. Thoresen CE, Coates TJ, Zarcone VP, Kirmil-Gray K, Rosekind MR: Treating the complaint of insomnia: a behavioral self-management approach, The Comprehensive Handbook of Behavioral Medicine, Vol 1. Edited by Ferguson JM, Taylor CB. New York, Spectrum, 1980
36. Lefcourt HM: Locus of Control: Current Trends in Theory and Research. New York, Erlbaum, 1976
37. Seligman MEP: Helplessness. San Francisco, Freeman, 1975
38. Bandura A: Self-efficacy: toward a unifying theory of behavior change. Psychol Rev 84: 191, 1977
39. Bandura A: Self-efficacy mechanism in human agency. Am Psychol 37: 122, 1982
40. Bandura A, Simon KM: The role of proximal intentions in self-regulation of refractory behavior. Cognitive Therapy Research 1: 177, 1977
41. Meichenbaum D, Cameron R: Stress-inoculation training: toward a general paradigm for training coping skills, Stress Prevention and Management. Edited by Meichenbaum D, Jaremko M. New York, Plenum, in press.
42. Meichenbaum D, Turk D: The cognitive behavioral management of anxiety, anger and pain. The Behavioral Management of Anxiety, Depression, and Pain. Edited by Davidson PO. New York, Brunner/Mazel, 1976
43. Bakal DA, Demjen S, Kaganov JA: Cognitive behavioral treatment of chronic headache. Headache 21: 81, 1981
44. Delaplaine R, Ifabumuyi OI, Merskey H, Zarfas J: Significance of pain in psychiatric hospital patients. Pain 4: 361, 1978
45. Ward NG, Bloom VL, Friedel RO: The effectiveness of tricyclic antidepressants in the treatment of coexisting pain and depression. Pain 7: 331, 1979
46. Pilowsky I, Chapman CR, Bonica JJ: Pain, depression, and illness behavior in a pain clinic population. Pain 4: 183, 1977
47. Blumer D, Heilbronn M: Chronic pain as a variant of depressive disease: The pain prone disorder. J Nerv Ment Dis 170: 381, 1982
48. Sternbach RA, Wolf SR, Murphy RW, Akeson WH: Aspects of chronic low back pain. Psychosomatics 14: 52, 1973
49. Schaffer CB, Donlon PT, Bittle RM: Chronic pain and depression: a clinical and family history survey. Am J Psychiatry 137: 118, 1980
50. Johansson F, Von Knorring L: A double-blind controlled study of a serotonin update inhibitor (Zimelidine) versus placebo in chronic pain patients. Pain 7: 69, 1979
51. Carasso RL, Yehuda S: Chloripramine and amitriptyline in the treatment of severe pain. Int J Neurosci 9: 191, 1979

52. Clarke IMC: Amitriptyline and perphenazine (Triptafen DA) in chronic pain. Anaesthesia 36: 210, 1981
53. Merskey H, Hester RA: The treatment of chronic pain with psychotropic drugs. Postgrad Med J 48: 594, 1972
54. Murphy MF, Davis KL: Biological perspectives in chronic pain, depression, and organic mental disorders. Psychiatr Clin North Am 4: 223, 1981
55. Large RG: The psychiatrist and the chronic pain patient: 172 anecdotes. Pain 9: 253, 1980
56. Blumer D, Zorick F, Heilbronn M, Roth T: Biological markers for depression in chronic pain. J Nerv Ment Dis 170: 425, 1982
57. Bielski RJ, Friedel RO: Depressic sub-types defined by response to pharmacotherapy in affective disorders. Psychiatr Clin North Am 2: 483, 1979
58. Schuckit MA: Current therapeutic options in the management of typical anxiety. J Clin Psychiatry 42: 15, 1981
59. Strain JJ, Liebowitz MR, Klein DF: Anxiety and pain attacks in the medically ill. Psychiatr Clin North Am 4: 333, 1981
60. Rush AJ, Beck AT, Kovacs M, Hollon SD: Comparative efficacy of cognitive therapy versus pharmacology in outpatient depressives. Cognitive Ther Res 1: 17, 1977

18 Neuroaugmentive Surgery

C. V. Burton

Pain is nature's way of informing the brain that something is amiss in a body part. Acute injury produces high intensity sharp pain that is well localized and elicits reflex withdrawal from the insult. A study of the brain's representation of body parts (the "homunculus") reveals that the cortical area for the low back is miniscule when compared with that for mouth, fingers, toes and special senses. This should not be surprising when we consider that during early life the storage banks of our brain "computer" are being programmed by a high volume of sensory information from the latter but not from the former. It is only in later decades of life that sensory information in the guise of pain is likely to be directed to the brain. Thus it is not difficult to understand that this input is deciphered as diffuse and nonspecific in light of the very small area of representation.

Following acute injury a phase occurs in which sharp, localizing pain is replaced by dull, aching discomfort (agony), which is nature's way of reminding us not to use or further injure the afflicted body part. We now appreciate that pain can be potentiated by many means, and the end perception represents an interplay of organic and functional entities. Pain is basically a protective system, but when constant and severe, it is a liability and can be destructive and incapacitating.

Pain-relieving analgesics and narcotics serve effectively to manage acute pain. They are, however, because of their endorphin-suppressing effect, a disaster for the chronic pain patient in whom they potentiate (rather than alleviate) the pain problem.

In the search for means of relieving incapacitating pain the medical profession turned to electrical stimulation over 2,000 years ago, as documented by the Roman writer Scribonius Largus.[1] Painful extremities (usually from gouty arthritis) were placed in buckets of water along with an electric eel (torpedo fish). The inevitable electrical "jolt" produced a state of immediate pain relief. It also often produced pain relief lasting for many hours. We know now that this phenomenon resulted from the release of endogenous opiates from the brain in response to the electrical stimulation.

In recent centuries scientists and physicians have tried mightily to harness electricity for pain relief. Benjamin Franklin was a famous student of this. Figures 18-1 and 18-2 show a battery-operated transcutaneous electrical nerve stimulator (TENS) manufactured in Paris by Gaiffe and described by Beard and Rockwell in 1871.[2] It is basicly similar to modern TENS devices with the exception that its maximum output was only about 3 milliamperes (modern devices output over 90 mamp with similar resistive loads). The "electreat," which has been manufactured in the United States since 1918 represents the first of recent TENS units (Fig. 18-3). The advent of solid

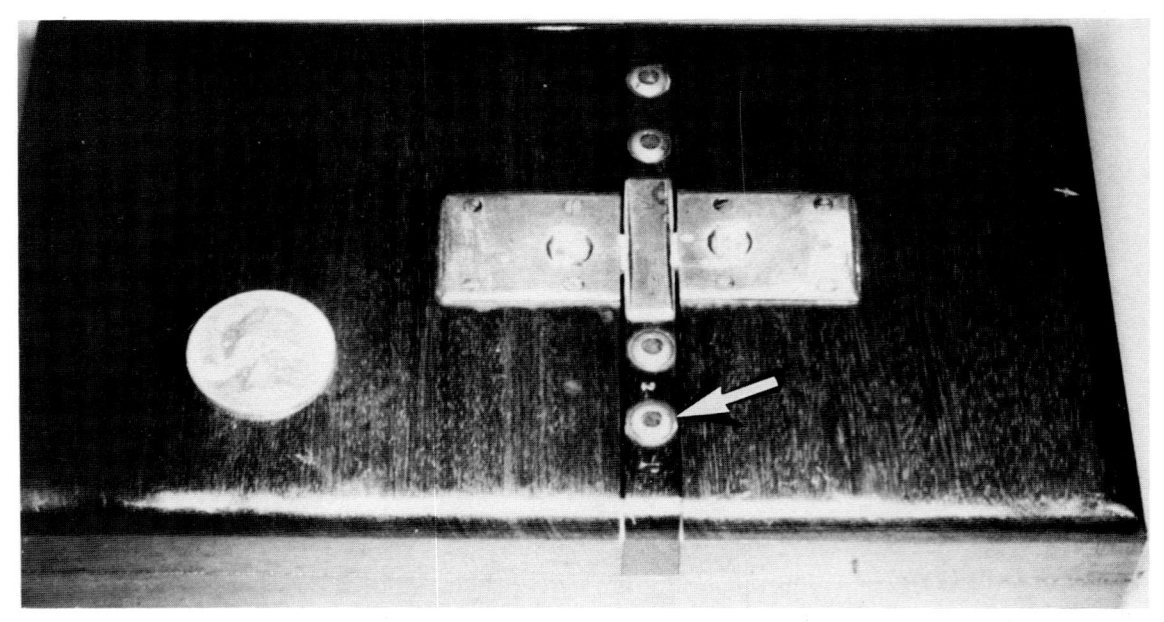

Fig. 18-1. A battery-operated TENS device manufactured in Paris by Gaiffe prior to 1871. Size is compared with a U.S. quarter. The arrow points to one of the lead wire "plug-ins."

state electronics after World War II and the development of the cardiac pacemaker allowed a modern refocusing of medical interest on electrical stimulation as a means of potentiating (augmenting) function of the intact nervous system. Present TENS units are solid state and designed to be used with a high level of safety.

Following the publication, in 1965, of the "Gate Theory of Pain" by Melzak and Wall[3] it was thought by many that the neuromechanism of electronic pain relief was evident. The discovery of endogenous opiate systems passing between brain and spinal cord has served both to enlighten and to confuse understanding of this complex subject.[4]

Modern TENS devices continue to have application as a reasonable means of producing pain relief when the pain is mild and is well localized to a single area. Although efficacy for acute use (60–80%) is higher than for chronic use (35–60%) the device has the advantage of enhancing (rather than depressing) endogenous opiates and is inherently safe. Basic efficacy, precautions, and practical limitations of TENS have been reviewed by Burton[5] who notes that the most common complication has been skin reaction to electrodes.[6]

In addition to pain relief TENS systems are now being used to potentiate bone healing[7] and for the electronic stimulation of muscle groups.[8] Muscle stimulation by this means has been used during surgery to avoid thrombophlebitis and to reduce risk of postsurgical pulmonary embolus.

IMPLANTED NEUROAUGMENTIVE DEVICES

In 1967 neurosurgeon C. Norman Shealy developed the first implanted electronic device intended to relieve pain.[9] Initial tests of his dorsal cord neurostimulator (DCN) were successful in relieving pain from metastatic carcinoma, and when these DCN units entered the commercial market in 1970[10] there was a high level of initial enthusiasm. Unfortunately, the lack of knowledge regarding patient selection and techniques of surgery combined with initially high device malfunction rates led to a subsequent period of disenchantment during which time device design, surgical techniques, and indications for use were improved.

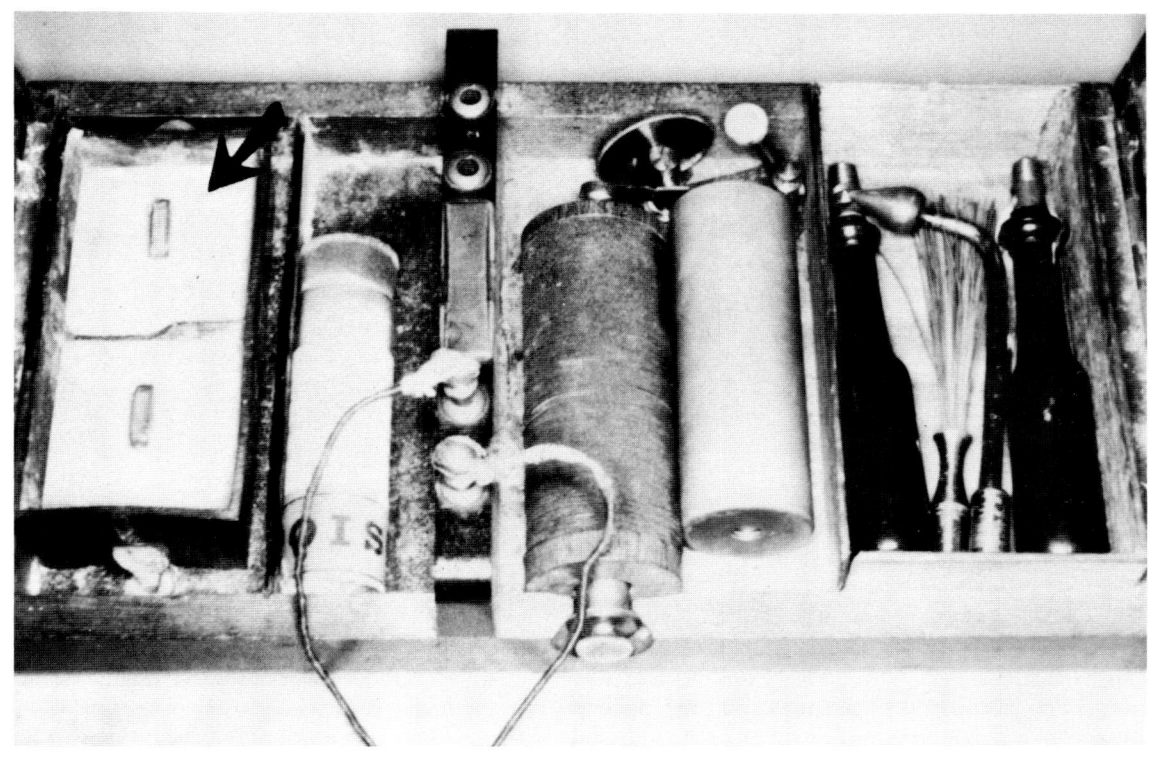

Fig. 18-2. The TENS components basically resemble modern units. The arrow points to a lead-walled battery containing mercury sulfate. The battery is removable and the contact points in the case are similar to those in modern flashlights. At the right is a vial of mercury sulfate and next to it a cylindrical inductorium. The last compartment contains contact probes and a wire brush with wooden handles. With a higher electrical output this TENS unit would have been clinically effective.

A major problem from the beginning was the difficulty in determining which patient with chronic pain was a potential candidate for a neuroaugmentive implant.[11] Although neural tissue-destructive procedures were still being used to treat some acute pain problems in the early 1970s (e.g. rhizotomy, cordotomy, tractotomy, thalamotomy) it became evident that these procedures had very little role in managing chronic pain because they produced deafferentation pain states. These problems, of which anesthesia dolorosa is an example, were often more disabling than the original chronic pain problem. It also became evident that the DCN was not capable of relieving *all* pain. Patients using these devices were able to appreciate sharp and localized pain (neo-spinal–thalamic) normally with the device activated, but were relieved of the dull and aching pain (paleo–spinal–thalamic). It was also found that patients on narcotic medications often felt the electrical parasthesias but obtained no pain relief and that pain relief could sometimes be enhanced by using nutritional supplements and tricyclic anti-depressant medications that potentiated endorphin release and action. A significant disadvantage was the inability to determine by testing prior to implantation of the DCN if a patient would benefit from its use. TENS devices were tried for such screening but proved unreliable.

In 1973, Hoppenstein[12] first reported on the use of percutaneously inserted epidural neurostimulating electrodes (PENS) that could be implanted on a temporary basis under local anesthesia to allow the patient to determine the degree of pain relief. Through rapid development and improvement, PENS systems have become the most extensively used neuroaugmentive devices for pain relief. Although the usual period of testing for an

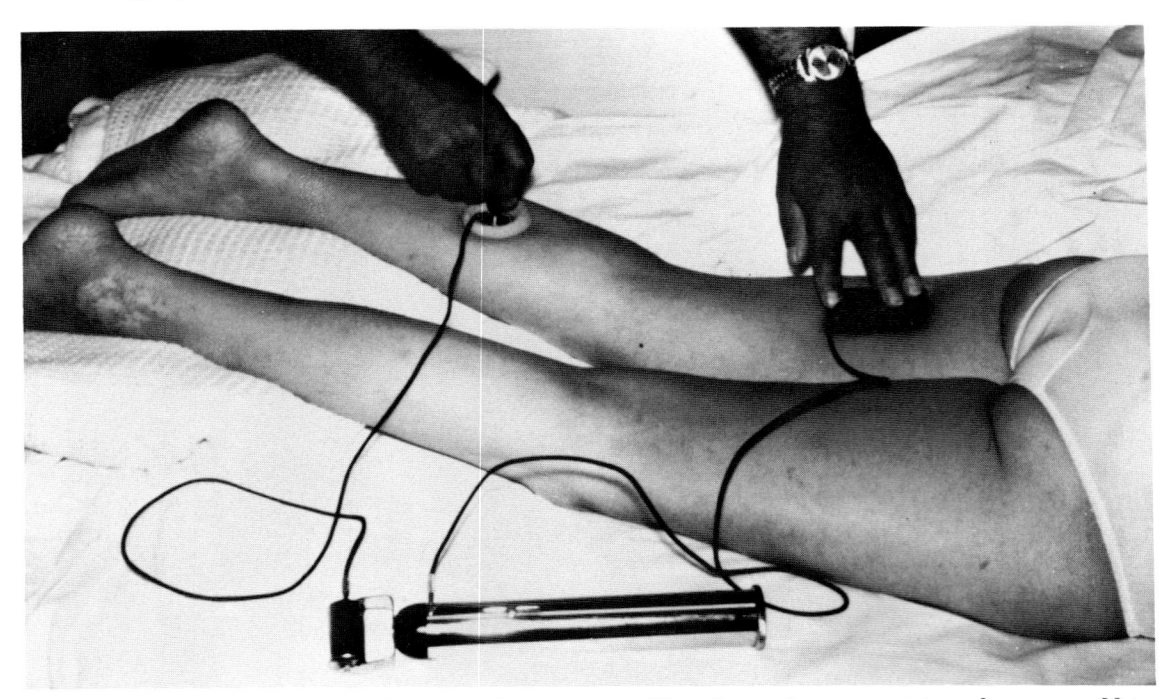

Fig. 18-3. The "electreat" TENS unit is shown in use. The electrodes are moistened sponges. Note the roller at the end of the unit used for electrical "massage." It is estimated that over 300,000 of these devices have been sold since 1918. Although crude, they are capable of producing pain relief where TENS is of value.

ambulatory patient is 2 to 5 days, in debilitated patients it is possible to maintain the epidural electrodes with their percutaneous extensions for many months. Normally, after the testing period the epidural electrodes are internalized and can serve as a definitive electronic pain relief device. Today many PENS systems have been functional for more than 5 years. If after internalization a malfunction occurs (approximately 30% of cases) the clinical efficacy information is utilized to place a directly implanted dorsal cord neurostimulator system optimally with the electrode placed either epidurally or within a dural pocket (endodural). DCN systems are the most stable, effective, and long-lasting when used in conjunction with PENS systems for screening. DCN development has been well documented in a number of publications.[13]

Although spinal neurostimulators are the most frequently used neuroaugmentive devices to relieve low back and/or leg pain, there are occasional patients whose pain is so severe and widespread throughout the body that deep brain neurostimulators (DBS) are necessary. In these cases the stimulating electrode is usually located in the periventricular gray matter (limbic system) or in a thalamic sensory nucleus. DBS systems are the most effective in relieving pain but also carry the highest risk.[14] They are, however, potentially capable of relieving some elements of sharp, well localized pain. The DBS appears to function more by endogenous opiate release than by "gating," which seems to be more characteristic of spinal stimulators.

Peripheral nerve stimulation (PNS) devices have been used for pain relief in some patients over the past decade but have been significantly limited in use because of the common complication of muscle spasm accompanying pain relief. A very important advantage of spinal stimulation over PNS has been the consistent observation that the former is capable of not only relieving pain but also increasing peripheral blood flow into impaired extremities.[15,16] This phenomenon is particularly noticeable in patients with causalgia of an extremity because of both the neurologic and vascular bundle injuries. Existing tissue anoxia and chronic ulceration usually disappear within 1 to 2 weeks following initiation of stimulation. The author has seen a number of cases where patients with peripheral arteriosclerotic vascular disease have been referred for treatment of a post-amputation pain syndrome (usually due to neuroma). Following the initiation of spinal cord stimulation for pain relief, blood flow in the impaired contralateral extremity has dramatically improved. The improvement in blood flow appears to reflect a direct modification of autonomic function at the spinal level and promises to be an important area for future investigation.

PATIENT SELECTION

As previously noted, patients with constant dull and aching pain (often referred to as "agony") tend to obtain the best results from neuroaugmentive devices. This type of pain is typical of a number of clinical entities involving nerve injury. Causalgia is an example of this. The term was coined by neurologist Weir Mitchell during the U.S. Civil War. He observed and described the "burning and searing" agony produced by incomplete lesions of peripheral mixed nerves. The author believes that causalgia is caused by atypically patterned sensory information (resulting from partial injury to the conducting system) reaching the brain and being interpreted in an adverse manner. This entity is often dramatically alleviated by electrical nerve stimulation that modifies the pattern of information being sent to the brain.

One of the most difficult therapeutic problems known, and unfortunately a problem affecting approximately 25% of patients who have undergone lumbar spine surgery in the past, is the "failed back surgery syndrome" (FBSS). This is a complex entity reflecting organic and functional disease as well as learned pain behavior and socioeconomic incentives which tend to enhance incapacitation. From the work of Burton et al.[17] many of the primary organic causes of FBSS have been identified in large populations of patients who were referred for rehabilitation. While the majority of patients (57–58%) were found to have lateral spinal stenosis (potentially treatable by surgical decompression), 6 to 16% had adhesive arachnoiditis and 6 to 8% epidural fibrosis as the primary pathologic process* responsible for chronic pain. The last two are pathologic entities which are usually not improved by surgical treatment, and the associated pain reflects the chronic nerve impairment resulting from swelling and irritation. These particular problems are the most difficult therapeutic challenges. It is this group of patients who are, following alleviation of functional and chemical dependency and abuse problems by special programs, primary candidates for implanted neuroaugmentive pain relief devices. The lateral spinal stenosis patients may also have permanent nerve injury and may require neuroaugmentive devices as a secondary procedure. Statistics at our institute indicate that over the past 5 years approximately 11% of FBSS patients being referred for rehabilitation have had a neuroaugmentive device implanted as part of the comprehensive rehabilitative process.

A comprehensive 9-year summary of the application and efficacy of neurostimulation at our institution has recently been published by Ray et al.[18]

TECHNIQUE

As previously noted, PENS systems have the advantage of being relatively easy to implant and test. Their disadvantage is their instability in the spinal canal. Approximately 30% need to be replaced by a surgically placed DCN because of malfunction.

In Figure 18-4 a monopolar electrode has been passed under local anesthesia through a guide needle into the epidural space. This should be carried out under bi-plane fluoroscopic control. For back and leg pain control one or more electrodes are passed to approximately the thoracic 8-level and multi-parameter (multiple locations and variable) testing is performed. Most optimal results are obtained at the thoracic 9–10 levels. Figure 18-5

---

* It was not possible to document intraneural fibrosis clinically.

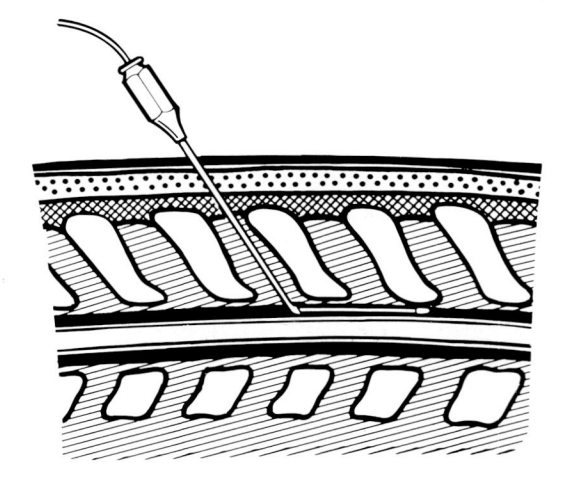

Figure 18-4. Under local anesthesia an epidural guide needle is passed to the epidural space. The flexible PENS electrode is passed to the appropriate level, usually in the midline. Skew of position to either side usually produces an appreciation of stimulation only on that side. (Courtesy of Cordis Corp.)

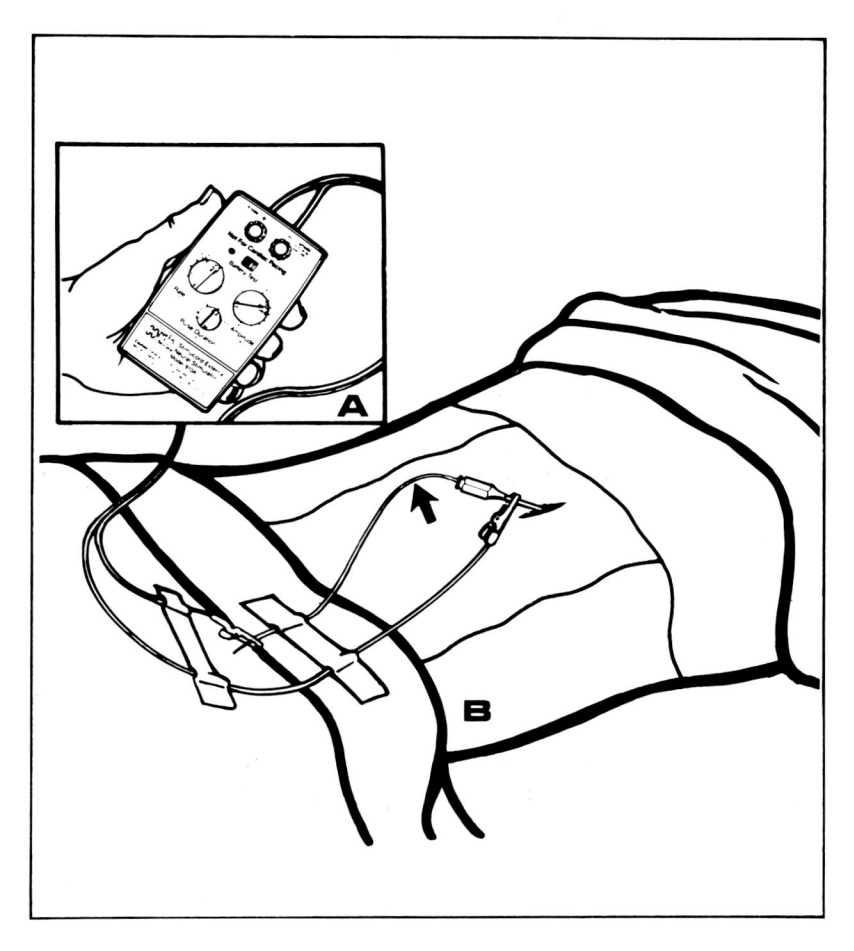

Fig. 18-5. A solid-state battery operated pulse generator is used for initial testing. Amplitude, frequency, and pulse width of waveform are usually varied as part of multi-parameter testing at different spinal levels and locations (Insert A). In Insert B a flexible PENS electrode (arrow) has been passed through the guide needle. In this case, monopolar testing is in progress using the guide needle as "ground." (TENS skin electrodes may also be used for this purpose). If initial testing is successful, the guide needle is removed leaving the epidural electrode(s) in place. Extension leads are connected to the end of the electrode and placed under the skin so that the ends of the extension pass through the skin and can be connected to a pulse generator for ambulatory testing. (Courtesy of Cordis Corporation.)

Neuroaugmentive Surgery 247

ized (Fig. 18-6). Recent advances in technology have also provided the option of having a totally implanted system (Figs. 18-7, 18-8) whose battery life is estimated at 5 years. The stimulation parameters of the total implant can be changed by an external programmer and the patient turns the system on and off by bringing a magnet close to the skin.

Because of continuing improvements in materials and designs, the efficacy of neuroaugmentive devices has progressively improved. In 1977, Ray reviewed the approximate number of patients in whom neurostimulators had been used and estimated degrees of improvement (Table 18-1).[19] The figures given are still basically correct, al-

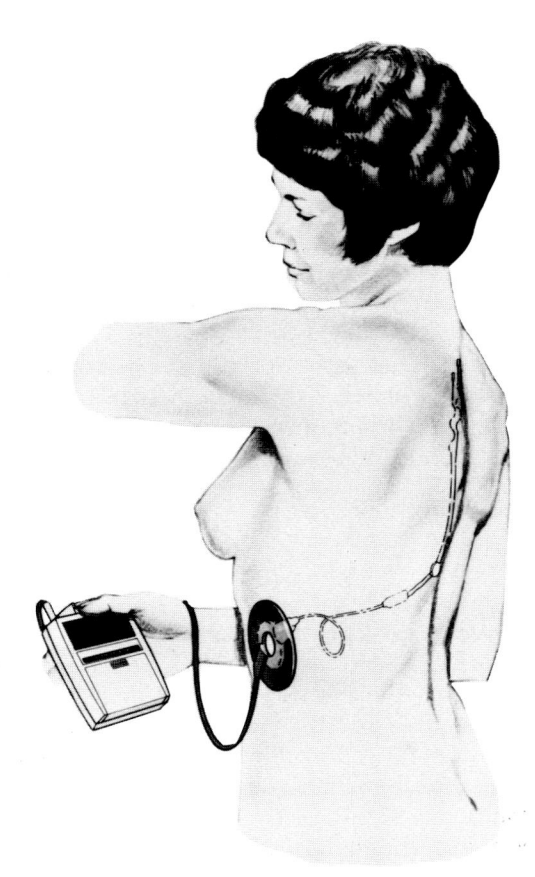

Fig. 18-6. In this illustration the twin epidural electrodes (bipolar) have been connected to a subcutaneous radio-frequency receiver. The battery-operated pulse generator is external and patient controlled. The silicone antenna is placed over the skin and the signal is pulsed through the skin, received, demodulated, and passed to the epidural electrodes. In actual use the tips of the electrodes are separated by at least one vertebral level. (Courtesy of Medtronic, Inc.)

shows a single electrode (monopolar) being tested with the guide needle serving as "ground." A solid-state pulse generator provides the electrical stimulation. Should initial testing provide pain relief, the epidural electrodes can be connected to extension leads that run under the skin and exit laterally where they can be connected to a pulse generator operated by the patient. At our institute, twin leads (bipolar) are usually preferred to a single lead (monopolar). Successful ambulatory testing indicates that the system can be internal-

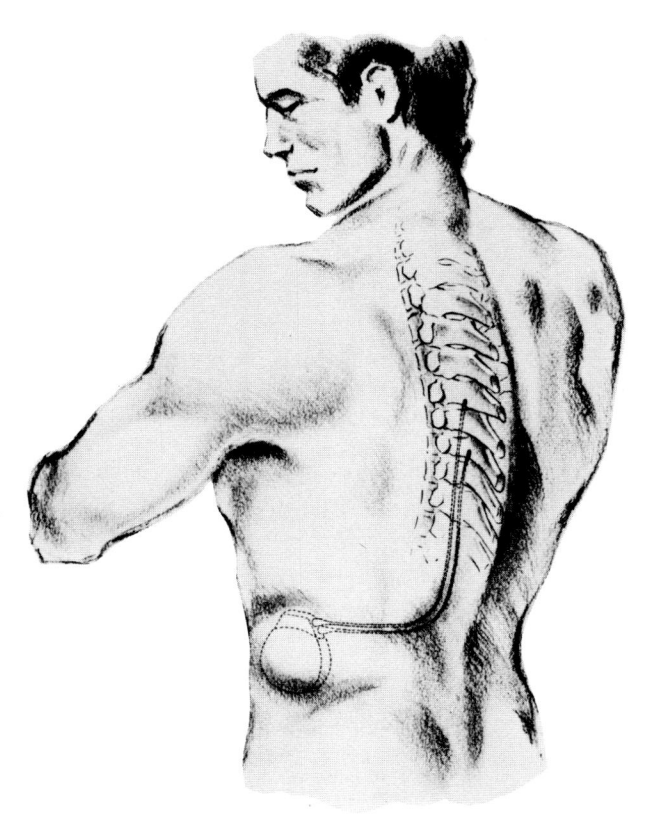

Fig. 18-7. A more recent option is a totally implanted system that can be programmed from an external device and turned on and off by an external magnet. With small size and high output the total implant is becoming increasing popular. In this case the system is bipolar. After 5 years the chest incision must be opened and the batteries replaced. (Courtesy of Cordis Corporation)

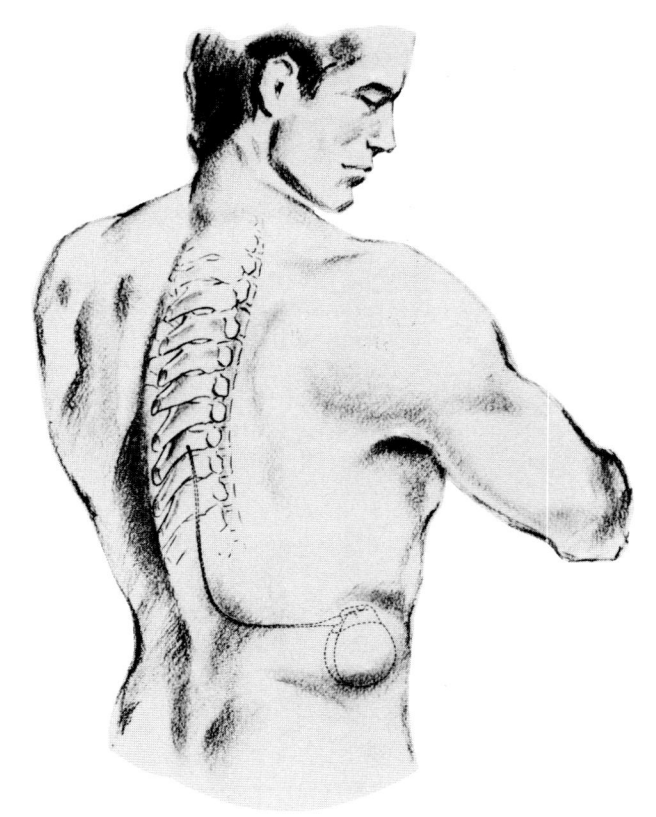

Fig. 18-8. A monopolar system is represented here. The pulse generator itself serves as the opposite pole of the circuit. This basic system is a forerunner of the future "smart" implant systems. (Courtesy of Cordis Corporation.)

though with better screening the long-term significant improvement with TENS can be increased to approximately 45% and the present figure for PENS is probably 50 to 60%.

All of the neuroaugmentive devices in present use are controlled by the patient and turned on and off according to need. Intermittent, rather than continuous, use during the day is recommended to optimize the endorphin effect. Basic research is now underway to develop a "smart" generation of neuroaugmentive devices functioning on a biofeedback basis, in which the output is governed by circulating levels of endogenous opiate or monitored neurophysiologic responses.

SUMMARY

As currently used to treat chronic pain, neuroaugmentive devices represent a modern means of potentiating function of the intact nervous system. Limitations in their effectiveness require careful patient selection. Success of use depends also on the training and experience of the surgeon, and results are significantly higher when these devices are used in conjunction with comprehensive facilities and programs with adequate medical and technical support personnel.

Table 1. Neuromodulation: Use and Estimated Improvement

Pain Control Device	Estimated Number Worldwide	Short-Term %	Long-Term %
Transcutaneous electrical nerve stimulator (TENS)	100,000	80	35
Percutaneous epidural neurostimulator (PENS), acute and chronic	1,200	80	†
Dorsal cord neurostimulator (DCN)	7,500	80	35
Peripheral nerve neurostimulator (PNS)	500	80	50
Depth brain neurostimulator (DBS)	100	90	70

* Significant improvement = 50% or more (moderate to marked) improvement in pretreatment pain. Criteria are variable and depend on patient population, clinical pain problem, selection criteria, device used, and method of use. Long-term improvement averages over 2 years in patients who continue to use the device.

† Thought to be about 50–60%.

ACKNOWLEDGMENTS

The author would like to take this opportunity especially to express to Dr. Charles D. Ray, friend and colleague over many years, Director of the Neuroaugmentive Surgery section of the Institute for Low Back Care, our appreciation for the many contributions made to the field of neurostimulation. Dr. Ray has been an innovative pioneer in this area and much of the present state of the art reflects his contributions.

Appreciation for support and consideration is also directed to Drs. Alex Lifson and Harvey Aaron, Mr. Kevin Gracie, and the staff of the Institute for Low Back Care, and to Medtronic, Inc. and the Cordis Corporation for use of illustrations and quality products for our patients.

REFERENCES

1. Scribonius L: De compositione medicamentorum liber. Translated in Kellaway P: The part played by electric fish in early history of bioelectricity and electrotherapy. Bull Hist Med 20: 112, 1946
2. Beard GM, Rockwell AD: A Practical Treatise on the Medical and Surgical Uses of Electricity. New York, William Wood, 1871
3. Melzak R, Wall PD: Pain mechanisms: a new theory. Science 150: 971, 1965
4. Burton CV, Ray DC: Neurostimulation, Cancer: Principles and Practice of Oncology. Edited by DeVita V, Hellman S, Rosenberg SA. Philadelphia-Toronto, JB Lippincott, 1982
5. Burton CV: Transcutaneous electrical nerve stimulation to relieve pain. Postgrad Med 59: 105, 1976
6. Burton CV, Maurer DD: Pain suppression by transcutaneous electronic stimulation. JEEE Trans Biomed Engin BME-21: 81, 1974
7. Bassett CAL, Pawluk RJ, Pilla AA: Acceleration of fracture repair by electromagnetic fields: a surgically non-invasive method. Ann NY Acad Sci 238: 242, 1974
8. Burton CV, Maurer DD: Solvent-activated current passing tape electrode for transcutaneous electrical stimulation of the peripheral nervous system. JEEE Trans Biomed Eng BME-33: 346, 1976
9. Shealy CN, Mortimer JT, Reswick JB: Electrical inhibition of pain by stimulation of the dorsal columns: preliminary clinical report. Anesth Analg (Cleve) 46: 489, 1967
10. Shealy CN, Mortimer JT, Hagfors NR: Dorsal column electroanaglesia. J Neurosurg 32: 560, 1970
11. Ray, CD (ed): Electrical stimulation of the human nervous system for the control of pain. Minneapolis Pain Seminar. Surg Neurol 4: 61, 1973
12. Hoppenstein R: Percutaneous implantation of chronic spinal cord electrodes for control of intractable pain. Preliminary report. Surg Neurol 4: 171, 1973
13. Burton CV, Ray CD, Nashold BS: Symposium on the safety and clinical efficacy of implanted neuroaugmentive devices. Neurosurg 1: 185, 1977
14. Ray CD, Burton CV: Deep brain stimulation for severe, chronic pain. Acta Neurochir [Suppl] 30: 289, 1980
15. Cook A, Oygar A, Baggenstros P, et al: Vascular disease of extremities: electric stimulation of spinal cord and posterior roots. NY State J Med 76: 366, 1976
16. Dooley DD, Kasprak M: Modification of blood flow to extremities by electrical stimulation of the nervous system. South Med J 69: 1309, 1976
17. Burton CV, Kirkaldy-Willis WH, Yong-Hing K, Heithoff KB: Causes of failure of surgery on the lumbar spine. Clin Orthop 157: 191, 1981
18. Ray CD, Burton CV, Lifson A: Neurostimulation as used in a large clinical practice. Appl Neurophysiol 45: 160, 1982
19. Ray CD: New electrical stimulation methods for therapy and rehabilitation. Orthop Rev 6: 29, 1977

19 Back Pain and Work

W. H. Kirkaldy-Willis

SOCIOLOGICAL FACTORS

The psychological factors that affect people with low back pain have been considered at some length in chapter 6 (Psychological Assessment). Sociological factors are also very important both within and outside the work environment. The role of the patient in the home and the help and support he or she gets from the family affect very considerably his or her attitude to the present disability, the speed of recovery, and the necessary adjustment to any residual disability. An unhappy home environment can and often does delay the patient's recovery. Similarly, the personality characteristics of the patient and the way in which he or she interacts or fails to interact with friends, neighbors, other people in community activities such as clubs and associations for games, and with members of a church community play a very important role. Part of the task of the physician and the psychologist is to give the patient advice about these matters and to encourage an active role in all these situations. All the factors mentioned above can interact significantly with the efforts of the employer and of compensation boards to get the patient back to work.

Our Environment

Our environment is the atmosphere in which we live and work and play. In this modern age we live in an environment that is full of stress and noise and bustle. To be bigger is equated with being better. Fortunately, some among us are rebels and seek a life that is not full of stress, that is quiet, and that proceeds at a slower tempo regardless of financial gain. Many men and women work for a firm, a business, or an industry in which profit is the main concern of management. For many the workplace represents an environment where they are not consulted; they do not enjoy their work; and subconsciously they are ready for any excuse not to work. North American industry could well take a look at the new approach now common in Japan, in which management considers the well-being of their employees, tries to make work interesting for them, consults them, and plans to make them feel that their place of work is one to which they belong.

The Work Atmosphere

For many the environment at work operates in such a way as almost to set the stage for the first attack of low back pain before it ever takes place. In a sense, the man or woman caught up in such an environment almost hopes to be afflicted by something like low back pain as a means of escape.

It operates also in another way. The patient laid up by a first attack of low back pain often has little incentive to recover and return to the impersonal, boring grind. Pain, fear, lack of understanding, and uncertainty make matters worse. The author recently stood in the wings and observed a young man with a moderately severe episode of posterior joint dysfunction. Before the attack he worked as a plasterer for a company that demanded a full day's work or nothing. Simple measures of treatment dealt with the pain but not with the sense of despondency he felt. After some weeks it suddenly occurred to him that he could work for himself and start by doing half a day of work each day. Almost immediately he ceased to have any problem with his back and the worry and anxiety left him. What appeared to be a very difficult matter for the physician suddenly ceased to be a problem at all for physician or patient.

Delay in Obtaining Adequate Treatment

Fortunately most patients with an episode of low back pain (dysfunction) recover quickly on rest, aspirin, and reassurance. One figure given is 17 to 21 days, depending on the measures employed. A small percentage of patients do not respond to simple measures in what is considered a reasonable period of time. These plague both the physician and their employers. Symptoms and signs are often minimal and the radiograph is considered normal. It is in fact very difficult to say what adequate treatment is for such patients. Some years ago the author himself had a minor episode of low back pain. After a week of rest at home, he was able to return to work as a physician. Certain activities—getting in and out of the car, sitting in a boat, attempts at gardening—were painful for many weeks. He was aware that he would not have been able to work as a carpenter, plasterer or laborer for 3 months.

One result of an apparently unavoidable delay in seeking expert help in such cases is a back that is stiff and painful in a patient who is fearful and apprehensive.

In some patients the pain becomes "fixed" and a point is reached at which no form of treatment is effective in returning the patient to work.

The Return to Work

Returning to work depends on the attitudes of both the patient and the employer. The patient must want to go back to work. This is much less of a problem for people who are self-employed and who thus can gradually increase the amount of work done in a day until they are back to normal. The incentive is greatest in someone like a farmer: it is often impossible to prevent him from engaging in activities that are not wise at the stage reached in his recovery, but it is better to let him run some risk—riding his tractor or lifting bales of hay—than to have him champing at the bit. Work has a therapeutic value. During all work, and especially that involving physical exertion, muscles contract, joints move, and the mechanoreceptors are stimulated and tend to close the gate to pain impulses (see chapter 4).

The attitude of the employer is also vitally important. Fortunate the patient who has an employer considerate of his well-being. A phone call from the doctor helps. The employer should be asked if he can arrange things so that the patient does a half day's work for 2 or 3 weeks and so gradually reconditions himself for the job. Activities that produce pain should be avoided. The principles learned during the Spine Education Program in regard to standing, sitting, lifting, and resting to relax after a few hours of work should be practiced. Under these conditions return to work is much more rapid. Recently, the author saw two patients in one afternoon. Both were recovering from minor episodes of posterior joint dysfunction. Both were apprehensive about their return to work. They were told that at this stage in their recovery return to work was an important part of treatment. The writer then phoned both employers, explained the situation, and arranged for a gradual return to work under the employer's supervision.

Many employers and supervisors say that they are unable or unwilling to make special concessions that would enable the employee to return to work until he or she is completely fit for the job. Inevitably this means that time off work is prolonged for weeks or months. Days spent at home without employment are bad for the patient mentally and physically, compound the problem, and sometimes result in the patient never returning to work.

Some large business concerns, such as the Vauxhall Company in the United Kingdom and the Volvo Company in Sweden, encourage consultation between the physician and the steward on the shop floor. A program of work is planned that is within the patient's capability and it is gradually increased till he is back to a full day of normal work. This is ideal. We need a quiet but persistent publicity campaign to make this enlightened approach common practice in industry. A Saskatchewan firm, recently stimulated by one of its employees who had undergone treatment for a disk herniation, asked for help in setting up a day's program of instruction in Spine Education for supervisors and workers in the factory.

Insurance Companies and Compensation Boards

These should be, and often are, concerned not only with financial assistance while the patient is unable to work but also with making it as easy as possible for him to return to work. Often there is a lack of understanding and a lack of liaison between the physician and the officer of the company or board. Both can be at fault. Part of the difficulty is that each looks at the problem from a different point of view. The result can be many additional weeks away from work.

Compensation Board officers do try to help the patient back to work. In talking to employers they often encounter the difficulties referred to above. Perhaps more thought and more effort should be directed to this aspect of their work.

In some patients the spinal disorder, though not grave, makes it impossible for a laborer or heavy worker ever to return to the job he did before his injury. Here it is of vital importance to find lighter work for the patient or to retrain him for other work that is within his capacity. In the writer's opinion, companies and boards are sometimes slow to make such essential arrangements. On other occasions their officials encounter the very real problem of decreasing opportunities for employment in a shrinking economy.

There is value in making a final decision regarding the degree of permanent disability as quickly as possible. It may not be possible for the physician to produce the necessary information for some weeks or months. At this stage further official delay often takes place. It can be tough but is often effective to make a definite decision, compensate the patient, and leave him on his own to sink or swim. The chances are greater that the patient will swim.

PREVENTION OF LOW BACK PAIN

Introduction

The writer has to admit to a sense of shame that he wrestled for years with the etiology, diagnosis, and treatment of low back pain before he realized that to prevent low back pain was much more important than to treat it. Two factors have to be considered: (1) communicating the necessary knowledge of the causes and management of this condition to individuals, the community, and those responsible for industrial plants and factories; and (2) practising basic spine mechanics by individuals in the community and in industrial environments.

The Spine Education Program

This program has been described in some detail as it applies to the management of low back pain in chapter 12. It is designed not only to relieve an existing episode of pain but also in practice to prevent future attacks of pain. The knowledge gained of the normal back and the way it functions, of the abnormal back and the ways in which pain results, of exercises that maintain the back in a healthy condition, and of basic spine mechanics that reduce the risk to the back during daily activities is the most effective way of preventing back pain for the individuals who have attended the sessions of such a program. There is of course room and need for many more such programs in every country.

Publications on Back Care for the Lay Public

A number of books are now available. The individual who reads and carefully studies one of these should understand the problem much better and be able to put what he has read into practice. Undoubtedly to attend a well planned Spine Education Program is of greater value than reading the best of books but the Program is so far only available for a limited percentage of any population.

Spine Education Program for School Children and the Lay Public

Programs for children in school, adapted from that described above, would certainly be most useful. Some such programs are already run for adults in institutions such as the Y. M. C. A. We need to develop and increase the number of such programs. At the present stage quality (a well-run program) is probably more important than quantity (starting a large number of poorly run programs).

Television Programs

Television authorities are beginning to appreciate the value of educational broadcasts for both school children and adults. The writer knows of two such programs now being planned in Canada. A great deal of thought and hard work is being put into these. Any such program needs to be as short and as simple as possible, based on the Spine Education Program described above.

Spine Education in Industry

The Spine Education Center in Dallas, Texas has already started to arrange educational sessions in factories in that area. This is an example that many of us should follow. As mentioned above the Vauxhall and Volvo factories have been doing this for a number of years. Management, i.e., shop stewards and employers, need to know as individuals the things that are taught in the Spine Education Program and the knowledge that is available needs to be put into practice in the factory. Each task should be planned so that it can be done with minimum risk to the back. Poorly designed plants that place the worker's back at risk should be replaced. To do this requires much tact on the part of advisors from outside. Clearly management must want to make changes. In the long run the company will benefit not only from a decrease in absenteeism due to back pain but also from a happier, more contented group of workers. Industrial psychologists have been working as advisors in factories for at least 50 years, but the problem of low back pain has not yet received adequate attention. It should be no more difficult to persuade management that our present problem needs attention than it has been in the past to convince them of the importance of temperature, light, space, and noise in affecting the health and the output of their employees.

A Combined Approach for the Future

The author approaches this section with some initial hesitancy. All too often the "combined approach" results in a great deal of energy and time expended by many experts with little final achievement. It has been stated frequently, and with good reason, that, when a group of specialists, let us say in a hospital, wishes to make no change, the best way to be certain of maintaining the status quo is to appoint a committee. This should not and must not apply as we study together what now needs to be done for the further prevention of low back pain. We need to be aware of the dangers.

It seems likely that the teams should consist of communications experts; sociologists; psychologists; including industrial psychologists; and physicians, surgeons, and allied therapists concerned with and interested in this field.

The immediate need is for further research into every aspect of the problem of prevention. A great deal of research has been done over past years into the basic science and clinical aspects of low back pain. Much time and energy—some say too much—has been expended on devising new and more effective surgical procedures. Research into prevention demands a new slant and a new approach. We do not yet know what form this will assume.

Research in this field will lead to practical applications. Indeed it will intermingle with the latter. Much of this research will have to be undertaken in the environment in which individual persons or the group of people live, work, and play.

CONCLUSION

In this book a number of different aspects of the management of low back pain have been considered and a large number of facts have been described. They all lead to this conclusion—what are we going to do from now on to prevent the lesions that we have tried to understand and to treat?

Index

Page numbers followed by *f* denote figures; page numbers followed by *t* denote tables.

Abdominal muscles in control of buckling, 13
Aching in legs, 49
Activity diary, 72f
Adaptive response training, 232–233
Adhesion
  intra-articular, 25
  postoperative, 200–201, 202f
Aging and degeneration, 19
Amitriptyline, 236
Aneurysm, abdominal aortic, 130–131, 132f
Annular substance loss, 20
Annulus fibrosus
  circumferential tear in, 29, 30f
  compression loading and, 15–16
Anxiety, 236
Arthrokinetic reflex, 48
Articular cartilage degeneration, 25
Articular process, superior and inferior, 18
Attitudes, realistic, 233–234
Axial rotation, torsional failure due to, 19

Back Easer Footstool, 172, 173f
Bed, getting in and out of, 169–170

Behavioral data in pain assessment, 71, 72f
Bending forward, 170–171
Biofeedback, EMG, 230
Biomechanics of lumbar spine, 9–21
Bleeding, surgical, 200
Body mechanics, 167–170
Bowstring test, 101
Braces and supports, 185–190
Braggard test, 101
Brushing teeth, 168
Buckling of lumbar spine, 13, 14f
Burning pain, 49

Capsule laxity, 25
Car, getting into, 170
Carcinoma, metastatic
  colon, 135f
  renal, 135f
Chair back brace, 188f, 190
Chemonucleolysis, 153, 223–224
Chloripramine, 236
Chronic psychosomatic pain syndrome, 45
Circumferential tear in annulus fibrosus, 29, 30f
Cold in low back pathophysiology, 24
Compensation boards, 253

Compression
  axial, disk in, 15–16
  as mechanism of injury, 24
  results of, 20
Conservative treatment, 147–148
Control, sense of, for patient, 234–235
Coughing, 171
Creep deformation, 20
Crock's sausage, 207, 209f
CT scan, 111, 116f–125f
  in needle biopsy, 136f
  of osteoid osteoma, 138f
Cushion for back, 171–172, 173f

Decompression
  central canal, 211–212, 211f–212f
  lateral canal, 212–214, 213f
  in spondylolisthesis, 215, 215f
Deep brain neurostimulators, 244
Defensiveness of patient, 64–65
Deformation, 13
Degeneration of spine
  aging and, 19
  three phases of, 75–89, 76f
Degenerative disk disease, 92, 97
Denervation of posterior joints, 151

255

Index

Depression
  in pain patients, 70
  treatment of, 235–236
Diabetic neuropathy, 129–130
Diagnosis, 54t, 109–127, 110t
Diagnostic labels, 63
Differential diagnosis, 129–143
Disk
  axial compression loading and, 15–16
  changes in, facet joint interaction in, 29–37, 33f–35f, 97
  degenerative disease of, 92, 97
  herniation of. See Herniation of disk.
  loss of height of, sequelae of, 31–32, 35f
  motion at, 16, 17f
  pathologic changes in, 29, 29f–32f
  resorption of, 29, 32f, 98f
  spectrum of pathological changes in, 4f
  surgical removal of, 201f
Diskectomy, 209–211, 210f
Diskography, 222–223, 223f–224f
Diskotomy, 153–155, 154f
Do's and don'ts, 170–171
Dorsal cord neurostimulator, 242–243
Double knee-to-chest or low-back stretch, 166
Driving, 170
Dysfunctional phase, 75–80
  mechanisms of, 75–76, 76f
  posterior facet syndrome and, 91–92
  radiographic changes in, 76–80, 77f–79f, 79t
  specific lesions of, 92t
  symptoms and signs of, 76, 79t
  treatment in, 148–151, 149t

Education program, spine, 147–148, 161–174, 253–254
Elasticon garment, 164f, 185–189, 186f–187f
Electreat unit, 241, 244f
Electromyelography, 111, 117
EMG biofeedback, 230
Emotional states, negative, 235–237
Endplate compression forces, 15
Evoked potential, spinal, 117
Exercise program, 165–167, 172
Expectations, realistic, 233–234
Extraperitoneal approach, anterior, 203–204, 204f–205f

F-wave technique, 117
Facet joints
  center of motion for, 19
  changes in, disk interaction in, 29–37, 33f–35f, 97
  CT scan of, 116f–117f
  denervation of, 151
  injection of, 110, 149, 226
  innervation of, 150f
  nerves of, 150f
  progressive degenerative changes in, 25, 25f–28f
  shear and torsion at, 18
  spectrum of pathological changes in, 4f
  strain, 162
  subluxation of, in lateral nerve entrapment, 33, 35f, 38f
Family interview in pain assessment, 71
Fears of patients, 70
Feet, supports for, 172, 173f
Fibrosis
  CT scan of, 119f
  in multi-operated back, 159f
  periarticular, 25

Fixed-deformity of spine. See Stabilization phase.
Fluorosis, 39
Fluphenazine, 236
Foramen, intervertebral, reduction in size of, 32, 35f
Fusion
  anterior interbody, 221–222, 221f–222f
  CT scan in, 123f–125f
  posterior lumbar interbody, 216–221, 217f–220f
  posterolateral, 215–216, 216f
  spinal, role of, 152
  surgical, 215–222

Gate control theory of pain, 46, 47f, 162–163
Gravity lumbar reduction, 191–197
  applications of, 193
  contraindications to, 196–197
  efficacy of, 194–196, 195f–196f
  for in-patients, 193–194, 194f
  for out-patients, 194, 194f–195f
  technique in, 193–196, 194f–196f

H-reflex technique, 117
Hamstring stretch, 166–167
Hastings frame, modified, 206, 209f
Heat in low back pathophysiology, 24
Herniation of disk, 93–96, 95f
  CT scan in, 118f–119f
  gravity lumbar reduction of, 193
  manipulation in, 177–180, 179f–180f
  myelography in, 110, 112f
  pain drawing in, 56, 59f
  pathogenesis of, 29, 34f
  positions of, 210f

posterior facet syndrome and, 92
    treatment of, 152–155, 154f
Hip extensor muscle, 10, 10f
Hydraulic system of vertebral body, 15
Hypertension, venous, 39, 41

Infection
    in low back pain, 137–140, 140f–141f
    of posterior joints, 110
    wound, 201
Injection, 111
    facet, 110, 226
        in posterior facet syndrome, 149
    nerve root, 224–226, 225f–226f
    piriformis, 226–227, 227f
    in sacroiliac syndrome, 150
    technique for, 224–226, 225f–226f
Insomnia, 233
Instability of spine. See Unstable phase.
Insurance companies, 253
Intensive therapy, 172–174
Internal oblique muscle, 12
Intervertebral joint
    biomechanics of, 15
    early changes in, 23–24
    instantaneous center of motion for, 19
    phases of degeneration in, 24–25, 25f
    stable and unstable injuries to, 18–19, 18f
Intrathecal tumor, 131f

Knee-to-chest, double, 166

L4–5 joint, 24
L5–S1 joint, 24
L5 nerve. See Lateral spinal nerve entrapment.

L5 vertebrae, high vs low, 78f, 79
Lasegue test, 101
Lateral spinal nerve entrapment, 31–33, 34f–40f, 98–101, 98f–100f. See also Stenosis, lateral.
    combined factors in, 39
    fixed deformity with, 33, 38f–39f
    instability with, 31–33, 36f–37f
    in isthmic spondylolisthesis, 158f
    levels of, 155, 155f
    two nerve, 122f
Legs, aching in, 49
Leg raise, sidelying, 166
Lesion, site and nature of, 91–107
Lifting, 169
    balance between muscle and ligament in, 12–13, 12f
    hip extensor muscle in, 10, 10f
Ligament
    muscle and, in lifting, 12–13, 13f
    of spinal mechanism, 10–12, 11f
Light cast jacket spica, 189f, 190
Low-back stretch, 166
Low back syndromes, distinguishing features of, 102t
Lumbar spine
    biomechanics of, 9–21
    buckling of, 13, 14f
    injury to, 162, 163f
    normal, 161–162, 162f
    stability of, 13–15, 14f
    transverse section of, 35f
Lumbodorsal fascia in spinal mechanism, 12
Lumbosacral corset, 188f, 189–190
Lying, 171

McGill Pain Questionnaire, 66, 67f
Manipulation, 175–183
    on abnormal joint, 177–181, 179f–180f
    indications for, 181
    on normal joint, 176–177, 177f–178f
    in posterior facet syndrome, 148–149
    results of, 181, 182t
    in sacroiliac syndrome, 150
    what is it? 175–176
    zones and barriers of, 176, 176f
Mechanism of injury, 24
Mechanoreceptors, effect of manipulation on, 181
Medication overuse, 70
Meningioma, 131f
Metacarpo-phalangeal joint cracking, 176–177, 178f
Metastasis causing low back pain, 133, 135f–136f
Midline approach, posterior, 206–209, 209f
Minnesota Multiphasic Personality Inventory, 65–66
Misconceptions of patients, 70
Moment
    balance of, 12f
    in weight lifting, 10, 10f
Mood of pain patients, 70–71
Mountain and sag, knee to elbow, 166
Multifidus muscle, 24
Multi-operated back, 158–159, 159f
Muscle
    ligament and, in lifting, 12–13, 13f
    in low back pain, 24
Myelography, 110, 112f–115f
    of intrathecal tumor, 131f
Myeloma, multiple, 131, 133f–134f

Natural history of spinal degeneration, 3–8
Needle biopsy, 136f
Negative emotional states, 235–237
Nerves, posterior joint, 150f
Nerve block. See Injection.
Nerve irritation, 164f
Nerve root
  selective injection of, 224–226, 225f–226f
  surgical damage to, 119, 200f
Neural arch forces, 18, 18f
Neurilemmomata, 129
Neuroaugmentive surgery, 241–249
  implanted, 242–245
  patient selection in, 245
  technique in, 245–248, 246f–248f, 248t
Neurofibromata, 129, 130f
Neurogenic back pain, 129–130, 130f–131f
Nucleus pulposus
  herniation of. See Hernation of disk.
  radial tear in, 29, 31f
Nonscientific approach to low back pain, 53

Obesity, 165
Occupational therapy, 173
Operant treatment of pain, 232
Osteoblastoma, 138f
Osteoid osteoma, 133, 137f–138f
Osteomyelitis, vertebral, 137–140, 140f–141f
Osteopenia, diffuse, 131, 133f, 134f
Osteophyte
  on facet joint, CT scan of, 116f
  lateral nerve entrapment and, 33, 38f, 98, 99f
  subperiosteal, 25
Osteoporosis, 137, 139f

Pain, 162–165, 162t, 165t
  altering sensations of, 229–231
  attempting to cope with, 71
  benefits from, 69
  central modulation of, 47–48
  in dysfunctional stage, 76
  expression of, 68
  gate control theory of, 46, 47f
  of mechanical and psychological origin, pain drawing in, 56, 60f
  patient description of, 48–49
  patient thoughts and, 233–235
  perception of, 45–49
  peripheral modulation of, 46–47
  personality of patient and, 54–55
  physical vs psychological, 45
  psychological
    entirely, 61, 62f
    mechanical and, 56, 60f
  radicular, 48, 101
  reducing behavior of, 231–233
  referred, 48, 101
  types of, 49
Pain clinic, 174
Pain drawing, 56, 56t, 57f–61f, 62
Panic attacks, 236
Paraspinal muscles in spinal mechanism, 10
Pars interarticularis defect, 105f
Pathogenesis of spinal degeneration, 4, 4f
Pathophysiology
  of early joint changes, 23–24
  of lumbar spine dysfunction, 23–24
  role of muscle in, 24
Patient
  defensiveness of, 64–65
  fears and misconceptions of, 70
  thoughts in pain control, 233–235
Patient-physician rapport, 55–56
Pelvic tilting, 165
Pelvis, anterior-posterior diameter of, 10
Percutaneous epidural neurostimulation (PENS), 243–244
Peripheral nerve stimulation, 244–245
Peripheral vascular disease, 131
Perphenalzine, 236
Pheasant test, 99, 100f, 102
Physician-patient rapport, 55–56
Piriformis injection, 226–227, 227f
Piriformis syndrome, 96–97, 151
Posterior facet syndrome, 91–92
Posterior joint syndrome
  manipulation in, 177, 182t
  pain drawing in, 56, 57f
  treatment of, 148–149
Posterior joint. See Facet joint.
Posterior joint syndrome. See Posterior facet syndrome.
Posterolateral approach, 204–206, 206f–208f
Posture, good vs poor, 164f
Prevention of low back pain, 253–254
Psychogenic back pain, 131
Psychological assessment, 63–73, 126
  behavioral data in, 71, 72f
  indications for, 63–64
  interview in, 66–71
  purpose of, 63
  referral for, 64–65
  tests and questionnaires in, 65–66

Psychological treatment, 229–239
Psychotherapy, 173–174
Punched-out lesions, 131, 133f–134f
Push more than pull, 168

Quadratus lumborum syndrome, 97
  manipulation in, 177
  treatment of, 150–151

Radial tear in nucleus pulposus, 29, 31f
Radioisotope bone scan, 133, 137f
Reaching, 168
Recurrence of back pain, 171
Reexploration, 214, 214f
Referral for psychological assessment, 64–65
Relaxation position, 161, 161f
Relaxation training, 229–231
Retrospondylolisthesis
  in isthmic spondylolisthesis, 106f
  in lateral stenosis, 98f
  manipulation in, 180
  in unstable phase, 80, 83f–84f
Rhythm in intensive therapy, 172
Rotational strain as mechanism of injury, 24

Sacroiliac joint
  structure and function of, 92
  tests for fixation of, 94f
Sacroiliac syndrome, 92–93, 94f
  manipulation in, 177, 182t
  pain drawing in, 56, 58f
  treatment of, 149–150
Sacrospinalis muscle in weight lifting, 10
Schmorl's node, 96
Scientific approach to low back pain, 53

Scoliosis, generalized spondylosis with, 103
Severe injury results, 20–21
Shearing forces, 16–19, 18f
Sit-ups, modified, 165
Sitting, 167–168, 170, 171
Shock absorption by vertebral body, 15
Sleeping positions, 169
Sneezing, 171
Sociological factors in back pain, 251–253
Spica, light cast jacket, 189f, 190
Spinal degeneration
  natural history of, 3–8
  three phases of, 24–25, 25f
  throughout life, 5f
Spinal evoked potential, 117
Spinal mechanism, 9–13
  hip extensor muscle in, 10, 10f
  ligamentous system in, 10–12, 11f
  lumbodorsal fascia in, 12
  muscle vs ligament in lifting, 12–13, 13f
  trunk musculature in, 10
Spine-Bac, 171
Spine education program, 147–148, 161–174, 253–254
Spondylitis, ankylosing, 140, 142f
Spondylogenic back pain, 131–140, 133f–142f
Spondylolisthesis
  degenerative, 41f, 104, 104f
    manipulation in, 180
    treatment of, 156–157, 157f
    unstable phase and, 80, 82f
  isthmic, 41f, 104–106, 105f–106f
    manipulation in, 180
    treatment of, 157–158, 158f
  surgical treatment of, 214–215, 215t, 215f
Spondylolysis, 19

Spondylosis, 103f
Stability of lumbar spine, 13–15, 14f
Stabilization phase, 25, 85–86, 86t, 86f–88f
  lateral nerve entrapment in, 33, 38f–39f, 98
  mechanisms of, 85, 86f
  radiographic changes in, 86, 86t, 87f–88f
  signs and symptoms of, 85, 86t
  specific lesions of, 92t
  treatment in, 152, 152t
Standing, 167
Stenosis
  central, 33, 37, 38f–40f, 101–103, 103t, 103f
    CT scan in, 120f–121f
    decompression in, 211–212, 211f–212f
    manipulation in, 180, 182t
    myelography in, 110, 112f–115f
    treatment of, 155–156, 155f–156f
  developmental, 33, 37, 39f
  enhancing factors and direct factors in, 43f
  lateral, 38f, 98–101, 98f–100f. See also Lateral spinal nerve entrapment.
    CT scan in, 120f–121f
    decompression in, 212–214, 213f
    dynamic, CT scan in, 122f
    manipulation in, 180, 182t
    treatment of, 155–156, 155f
  multilevel, 33, 38f
  post-fusion, 39, 40f, 158
  post-traumatic, 40f
Strains, treatment of, 164f, 165, 165t
Stress
  at intervertebral joint, 15
  in low back pathophysiology, 24
Stress inoculation training, 235

Subluxation of joint surfaces, 25
Supports and braces, 185–190
Supports for feet, 172, 173f
Supraspinous-interspinous ligament system attachment, 11
Surgical techniques, 199–228
   anterior extraperitoneal approach, 203–204, 204f–205f
   anterior transperitoneal approach, 201–202, 203f
   approaches in, 201–209, 202f
   complications of, 199–201, 200f–202f
   posterior midline approach, 206–209, 209f
   posterolateral approach, 204–206, 206f–208f
Swimming exercises, 167
Symptoms, pathological changes vs, 4–6, 5f
Synovial fold, 25
Synovial joint, shear forces and, 18
Synovitis, 25
Synthesis of diagnostic tests and clinical examination, 126

TENS, 231, 241–242, 242f–244f
Tension in low back pathophysiology, 24
Tests for diagnosis, 110t
Therapy, intensive, 172–174
Three-joint complex
   biomechanics of, 19
   mechanism of injury at, 24
Torque, generation of, 13
Torsion, 16–19, 18f
Torsional failure, 19
Torsional injury, 20
Transcutaneous electrical stimulation (TENS), 231
   historical, 241–242, 242f–244f
Transperitoneal approach, anterior, 201–202, 203f
Treatment
   comprehensive outline of, 147–160, 148t
   in different stages of pathogenesis, 6, 7f
   expected results from, 6, 7f
Trunk musculature in spinal mechanism, 10

Unstable phase, 80–85, 81t, 81f–85f
   due to facet degeneration and disk disruption, 34f
   lateral nerve entrapment in, 31–33, 36f–37f, 98
   manipulation in, 181, 182t
   mechanisms of, 80, 81f
   posterior facet syndrome and, 92
   radiographic changes in, 80–81, 81t, 82f–85f
   signs and symptoms of, 80, 81t
   specific lesions of, 92t
   treatment of, 151–152, 151f

Vasculogenic back pain, 130–131, 132f
Vertebral body
   compression strength of, 15
   hydraulic system of, 15
Viscerogenic back pain, 129

Weight shift and diagonal (vacuuming), 168
Work and back pain, 251–254